The Health Care of Homeless Persons

Our Funders

This manual is a testament to the generous benefaction of:

Blue Cross Blue Shield of Massachusetts Foundation

Created in 2001, the mission of the Blue Cross Blue Shield of Massachusetts Foundation is to expand access to health care in Massachusetts through grantmaking and policy initiatives.

The Pfizer Foundation

An independent charitable foundation established by Pfizer, Inc., the Pfizer Foundation is committed to promoting access to quality health care and programs that are committed to advancing this mission.

The US Department of Housing & Urban Development

Support for the Manual is provided by the US Department of Housing and Urban Development through a grant from the Health Resources and Services Administration to the National Health Care for the Homeless Council.

The Yawkey II Foundation

This Foundation was founded by Jean R. Yawkey and has a long history of supporting community health centers and medical research programs.

The Health Care of Homeless Persons: A Manual of Communicable Diseases and Common Problems in Shelters and on the Streets is an original publication of The Boston Health Care for the Homeless Program.

For further information, contact The Boston Health Care for the Homeless Program, 729 Massachusetts Avenue, Boston, MA 02118 or visit us at www.bhchp.org

Project Editor: James J. O'Connell, MD
Assistant Editors: Stacy E. Swain, MPH, and Christine Loeber Daniels
Copy Editing by Joslyn Strupp Allen, MSW
Photo Research by Joslyn Strupp Allen, MSW
Design and Production Coordination by Patricia Mullaly, MFA, Circle Graphics

Printed by Guthrie Nixon Smith Printers, Boston, MA
Distributed by The National Health Care for the Homeless Council

ISBN 0-9711650-8-4

Library of Congress Control Number 2004103317
The Health Care of Homeless Persons: A Manual of Communicable Diseases and Common Problems in Shelters and on the Streets / edited by James J. O'Connell

The *Health Care* of Homeless Persons

A Manual of Communicable Diseases *&* Common Problems in Shelters *&* on the Streets

James J. O'Connell, MD, Editor

with
Stacy E. Swain, MPH
Christine Loeber Daniels
Joslyn Strupp Allen, MSW

The Boston Health Care for the Homeless Program
with The National Health Care for the Homeless Council

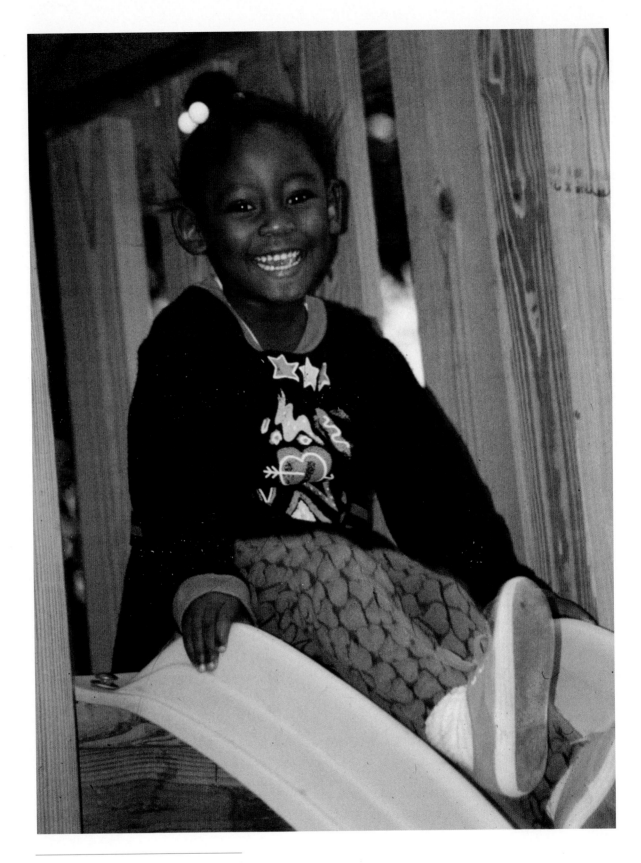

A child in the playground of a motel for homeless families.

Table of Contents

Part One: Communicable Diseases & Selected Infections

Alphabetical List of Chapters

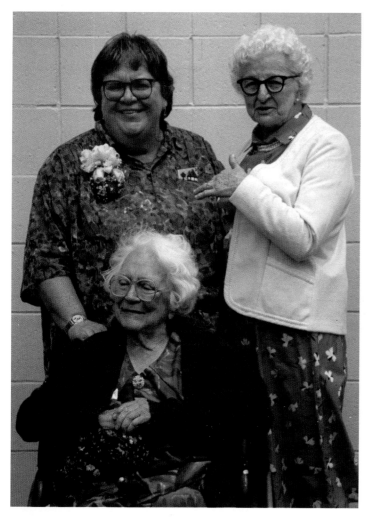

Dedication to
Barbara M. McInnis, RN

Dedication Ceremony, Barbara McInnis House, 1993. Barbara (left) beams with her family upon fulfilling her longtime dream of a safe place for sick homeless persons to heal.
Photo by James O'Connell MD

Boston mourns the loss of a beloved and irreplaceable treasure. Barbara McInnis, RN, died late last summer from complications of minor surgery to repair a leg fractured when she was hit by an inebriated driver. We have been struggling to find our equilibrium ever since.

Barbara is the only true saint I ever met: funny, loving, brilliant, frumpy, gentle, irascible, wise, humble, stubborn, unpredictable, and always (as we used to marvel while watching Miami Vice every Friday night after clinic) dynamically present to the Cosmic Unfolding. She was always herself, whether talking with dignitaries such as Mother Theresa, comforting those suffering under a bridge or down a dark alley, or regaling us with stories at Doyle's Pub. Long the soul of Boston's inner city, Barbara was known and trusted by every homeless person and had earned the respect of the local and national health care community.

Several years ago while visiting friends in England, I stumbled upon Theodore Zeldin's book, *An Intimate History of Humanity*. Unbeknownst to me, the author had made a journey to America to seek examples of men and women who had changed the world around them. I was stunned that he had discovered Barbara in the inner city of Boston, and I could only marvel at the words she used to deflect his praise: "I make no plans. I have no dream of a different society. I never think about that. I'm busy surviving, like the guests. I am intuitive…we are overwhelmed." She worked quietly and exhaustively, helping those most in need, never seeking office or honor or position.

Our lives have been enriched and transformed by her presence. Barbara has been mentor, muse, friend, and conscience since the day our program began almost two decades ago. Emblazoned in my memory is the first night I arrived at Pine Street Inn in the summer of 1985, when a group of nurses offered a stern welcome and then read me the riot

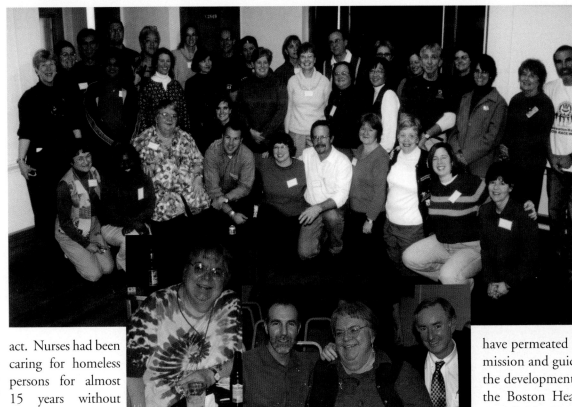

act. Nurses had been caring for homeless persons for almost 15 years without help of hospitals or doctors, and with time and patience I might learn the art necessary to match my newly acquired clinical skills. I was dumbfounded, but watched and learned as Barbara's apprentice. It was perhaps the best thing that ever happened to me.

Barbara drilled us on the basics incessantly and relentlessly. The core of the healing art is the personal relationship. Doctors need to leave the traditional clinics and venture out to join the nurses in places familiar to persons living in shelters and on the streets. Seek every opportunity to share food or coffee, be present in the lives of others, and listen to their stories. Offer care and relieve suffering, but never judge. We are not in the business of changing people, she would chide us, but rather in gently offering hope and options. From our very beginning, Barbara's wisdom and compassion have permeated the mission and guided the development of the Boston Health Care for the Homeless Program. I was never as proud as the day we opened the Barbara McInnis House in 1993, our 92-bed medical respite that fulfilled Barbara's dream of a refuge for homeless persons suffering from medical illnesses and injuries.

The death of Barbara McInnis is still too fresh to comprehend. She lived life in abundance and called out the very best in each one of us. We have been blessed by her presence and enjoined by her to embrace the care of those forgotten and ignored. Maybe her skepticism that society will never change is correct, but our lives have been forever transformed by her generosity and her mercy. Peace to you, Barbara.

- JJO'C   Boston, June 2004

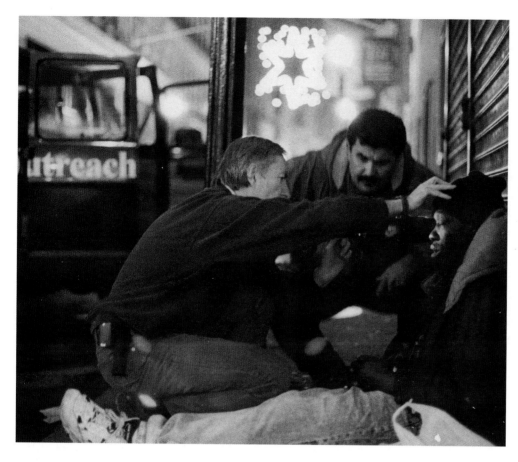

Acknowledgements

W̲e are deeply grateful to our many friends and colleagues whose vision, support, and encouragement made the second edition of this manual possible. So much has changed since we first gathered in the Boston Foundation in the fall of 1988 to dream about creating a health care manual for clinicians and other staff serving homeless persons in shelters and on the streets.

The impetus for this second edition came from two very special people in our lives: Jean Hochron of the Office of Minority and Special Populations of the Bureau of Primary Health Care in the Health Resources and Services Administration, and John Lozier, Executive Director of the National Health Care for the Homeless Council. Jean has been our guardian angel, shepherding the growth of the Bureau's Health Care for the Homeless Program to over 160 projects that are now located in every state as well as Puerto Rico. John has been the soul and the muse of health care for the homeless projects throughout the country, and a tireless advocate for the basic rights of all persons to decent housing and affordable health care. Jean and John, working with the Health Care for the Homeless Clinicians' Network, articulated the need for a new and expanded manual for the growing number of providers and workers in shelters and encouraged

us to pursue this goal. They have been steadfast in their support, guiding us throughout the two years it has taken to complete this effort.

A very special thanks to Patricia Mullaly of Circle Graphics. Captured and conscripted at the very first meeting at the Boston Foundation with Sister Margaret Leonard of Project Hope in the autumn of 1988, Pat crafted our first edition from unimaginably humble and scattered beginnings. We did everything on our little Macintosh 512, ferried the floppy disks to her office in Hull, and then she worked her magic. When we were asked to do this new version, we immediately sought refuge in Pat's new digs in Hingham. Surrounded by large scanners, massive monitors, and breathtaking posters, she bravely embraced us. And we've put her through the ringer once again. Despite innumerable changes and insufferable delays, Pat always smiles wryly and encourages us to persist. Without Pat, this manual

Street Medicine on Pine Street Inn's Outreach Van. Photo by Rick Friedman

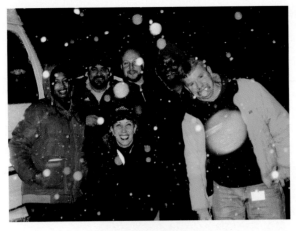

The Pine Street Inn Outreach Van staff travel under bridges and down back alleys every night from 9PM until 5AM, offering soup, sandwiches, clothing, and transportation to Boston's "rough sleepers" who avoid the shelters and live on Boston's streets. The BHCHP Street Team joins these dedicated workers three nights each week.
Photo by Sharon Morrison RN

would never have been possible.

The photographs in this book have been the gifts of many generous people throughout the years. We have kept many pictures from the first edition and added many new ones. Hearty and hale thanks to Dr. Irwin Freedberg of New York University School of Medicine, Dr. Howard Koh of Harvard School of Public Health, Dr. Nicholas Fiumara and Dr. Jon Fuller, SJ, of Boston University School of Medicine, Melissa Shook, Rick Friedman, David Comb, Stan Grossfeld, Stephen Savoia, Michael Hintlian, and Webb Chappell. Carmen Cleary NP, Deborah Langston MD, Norma Laurenzi, Jessie McCary MD, Sharon Morrison RN, Robert T. Souther, and Carol Waldmann MD.

We have been blessed with many partners throughout our city and state. The hospital community has welcomed us, and we continue to hold our clinics at Boston Medical Center, Massachusetts General Hospital, and the Lemuel Shattuck Hospital. Likewise we have been welcomed into the family of community health centers. Jim Hunt, the Executive Director of the Massachusetts League of Community Health Centers, invited us into the primary care association many years ago after visiting our sites and following us through our clinics. Along with the health center directors, he has stood resolutely by our sides in creating partnerships to improve the health of homeless persons throughout the state.

Boston's Mayor Thomas Menino, Elaine Ullian, President and CEO of Boston Medical Center, and John Auerbach, Executive Director of the Boston Public Health Commission, have been sources of constant support while assuring the integration of BHCHP into the fabric of the city's health care system. Dr. Anita Barry, Director of the Communicable Disease Control of the Boston Public Health Commission, embraced our original embryonic efforts in 1988 and has continued to guide and support us through these years. She once again has been a true mastermind behind this manual.

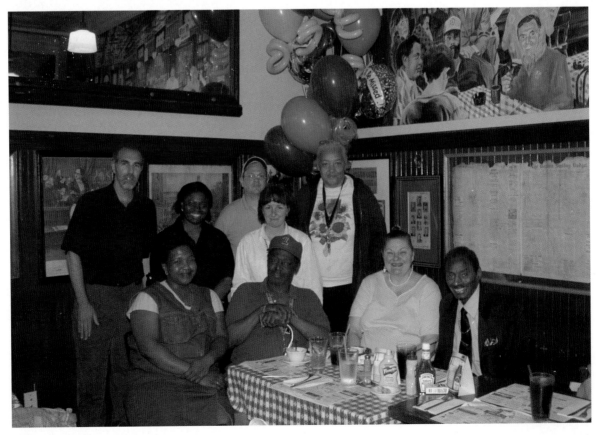

BHCHP's Consumer Advisory Board convenes under the mural of famous Boston politicians at Doyle's Restaurant and Pub.
Photo by James O'Connell MD

Eliza Greenberg and Jim Greene of the Emergency Shelter Commission of the City of Boston have been our constant friends.

We also thank the many agencies of the Commonwealth of Massachusetts who have worked so diligently to create better services for homeless persons, including the Departments of Transitional Assistance, Public Health, Mental Health, Medical Assistance, and Corrections.

Philip Mangano, Mary Ellen Hoombs, Leslie Sarofen, David Foster, MD, and Joseph Finn, JD from the Massachusetts Housing and Shelter Alliance have been stalwart in their support of BHCHP and tireless in advocating for the abolition of homelessness. Mr. Mangano is now in Washington serving as the Director of the Interagency Council on Homelessness.

Very special thanks to the evanescent David Bozzi of the Center for Educational Technology at Harvard Medical School. David, always friendly and immensely patient, is the computer genius extraordinaire who helped us scan and edit the slides and photographs that bring such warmth and light to this manual.

We thank all of our friends and colleagues working in the over 70 shelters and soup kitchens where BHCHP is privileged to conduct our clinics. They inspire us each day and constantly call out the best in each of us.

Robert Taube, our longsuffering Executive Director, has been a resolute champion of this effort, a devoted friend and colleague, and true unsung hero. His wisdom and serenity (except during home games at Fenway Park) have guided BHCHP through these years of tumult and change in health care delivery.

Greg Wagoner, MD, our Medical Director, and Barry Bock, RN, our Director of Clinical Operations, have been fully engaged and overwhelmingly supportive throughout these efforts. BHCHP has now grown to include over 250 staff members, creative and energetic professionals who have been willing to devote their days and evenings and nights to caring for the health needs of homeless families and individuals. The talent of these doctors, nurse practitioners, physician assistants, dentists, nurses, social workers, outreach workers, and administrative staff is truly staggering, and the success of BHCHP through the years is a testament to their excellence, teamwork and perseverance. We cannot thank them enough, and can only wish that the readers of this book could share in the fun and competence

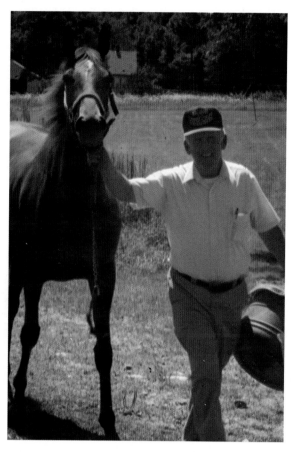

Jim Green, founder with Shirley Edwards of the Eighth Pole, walks his horse at Suffolk Downs Racetrack in Boston. Greene and Edwards enticed BHCHP to begin clinics at the racetrack for the backstretch workers. Photo by James O'Connell MD

that abound at our meetings and infuse this work with joy.

I am proud and humbled to offer a very special thanks to Ellen Dailey and the Consumer Advisory Board of BHCHP. This group of dedicated and diverse individuals receive their health care from our doctors, nurses, and clinicians. They meet once each month to tackle the myriad issues facing health care for the homeless programs everywhere. The CAB vetted all of our ideas for this manual and has conducted focus groups with families, persons with HIV, the street folks, the racetrack workers, and many other groups to understand the needs of homeless individuals and families. Two members of the CAB are members of the BHCHP Board of Directors, Marilyn Jones and Ellen Dailey. Ellen has been a fierce advocate who has traversed the country helping to launch the National Consumer Advisory Board for the HCH Program. Ellen has also been courageous enough over the past several years to share her remarkable story with the incoming class at Harvard Medical School during orientation week.

The success of BHCHP is a direct reflection of the creativity and utter commitment of our Board of Directors, led by Chair Sarah Anderson, Co-Chair Ellen Dailey, Len Simons, Peter Meade, Stephen

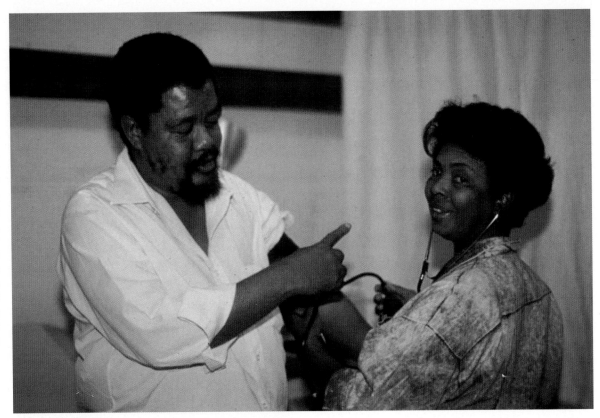

Betty Snead, our original respite aide in the Shattuck Shelter, checks a blood pressure at McInnis House. Betty, beloved by our guests and cherished by her colleagues for her humor, irreverence, and care, died in 1997. Our women's respite care program at McInnis House is known as the Betty Snead Wing.
Photo by David Comb

Tringale, Louis Riley MD, Bruce Bullen, Deborah O'Hara-Rusckowski RN, Barbara Blakeney RN, and Marilyn Jones. I shudder to think of the untold hours they have volunteered to guide us through these two tumultuous decades in health care.

I owe a personal debt of thanks to Stacy Swain, Christine Daniels, and Joslyn Strupp Allen. Stacy was our conscience and our guide, calming stormy waters and bridging deep chasms throughout this journey. Stacy was the steady hand at the helm of our research department for five years who kept my life from careening out of control. In December 2003 she assumed the role of Director of Family Services for BHCHP. Christine Daniels has divided her time working with our nascent Development Team at BHCHP and serving as the conductor of this effort. Her enthusiasm has been extraordinary and her organizational skills stunning. Joslyn Strupp Allen joined us in the fall of 2003 and has been a breath of fresh air, not to mention a dynamo whose contributions to this manual have been simply superb.

With deep sadness and longing, I want to remember four of our BHCHP colleagues who have died since the publication of the original Manual: Betty Snead, Dr. Thomas Bennett, Ann Allison, and Patricia Allison. They imbued us with a lasting enthusiasm and we hope that this manual will be a tribute to their memory and the remarkable legacy they left for us.

Finally and most importantly, we offer humble thanks to the heroic individuals and families whose strength and character have proven indomitable in the struggle against the ravages of poverty while deprived of the basic right to housing. The clear lesson of two decades of caring for homeless persons is straightforward: housing is health care. If safe and affordable housing and access to quality health care were available for all, most of the communicable diseases and medical conditions described in this manual would be rare and easily managed. ◼

- JJO'C   Boston, June 2004

Foreward

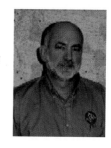

John Lozier

This important manual responds to disturbing realities. Each year millions of our neighbors lose their homes, and many seek refuge in crowded emergency shelters or on the streets. There they are exposed to deadly communicable diseases such as tuberculosis, hepatitis and influenza, and to other grave health threats such as infestations or frostbite. Their personal health deteriorates, and the threat of epidemic spread of communicable disease always lurks.

The health care system is ill-equipped to deal with the challenge of homelessness. The vast majority of homeless people – like 46 million other Americans – do not have health insurance, hampering their use of 'mainstream' health care providers. Primary care clinics for indigent people generally operate beyond their capacity, are not well-located to serve people staying in shelters, and are not prepared to deal with the complex conditions often presented by homeless people. The public health system, which made great strides in the 20th century by eliminating unhealthy living conditions, seems ill-equipped to contend with the teeming shelters that are a throwback to the 19th century.

Since 1985, intrepid health care workers have been developing interventions intended to improve the health of homeless people. Beginning with a 19 city demonstration effort funded by private foundations, and continuing now with federal funding to 161 grantees throughout the country, the Health Care for the Homeless (HCH) Program has worked diligently to assure that homeless people have access to primary care, substance abuse treatment, mental health and dental services, case management and supportive services. These local projects, which now reach about 550,000 homeless people per year, emphasize outreach and have established an important presence in numerous emergency shelters.

The original version of this manual was produced by the Boston Health Care for the Homeless Program in response to needs its workers observed in shelters. Because the danger of contagion is so great in shelter settings, it is crucial that shelter staff and guests be able to recognize communicable diseases, know when to seek medical assistance, and understand disease transmission and infection control. This edition has been expanded to help clinicians, shelter providers and homeless people cope with a somewhat broader range of health problems frequently associated with homelessness, including non-communicable medical conditions such as frostbite and hypothermia. It also contains a new exposition of the successful approaches to management of chronic diseases developed through the Health Disparities Collaboratives in which numerous HCH projects are participating.

By preparing this manual and making it available nationally, our visionary colleagues in Boston continue their long tradition of protecting displaced individuals and the public from potentially lethal health problems that can flourish in congregate living settings. With them, we hope and work for a day when the miseries of mass homelessness will be unknown and the right to health care will be realized for everyone.

John N. Lozier, MSSW
Executive Director
National Health Care for the Homeless Council
Nashville, Tennessee

The National Health Care for the Homeless Council is a membership organization consisting of HCH projects, the HCH Clinicians' Network, and the National Consumer Advisory Board. Additional resources are available at www.nhchc.org.

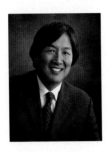

Foreward

Howard Koh

The health care of homeless persons requires an integration of medicine and public health. One person living in a shelter or on the streets who contracts influenza or tuberculosis requires expert medical care. Just as important is a well coordinated public health plan to prevent and control further illness and suffering among this very vulnerable and impoverished population.

The Commonwealth of Massachusetts established the country's first state board of health in 1869, and our state has long been an innovative leader in addressing the major public health epidemics of the past century, including measles, polio, rheumatic fever, syphilis, and tuberculosis. Our Department of Public Health understands the need for working closely with academic teaching hospitals, universities and medical schools, community health centers, and the myriad non-profit organizations that are dedicated to the direct care of our poorest neighbors.

In the bitterly cold winter of 1998-1999, more than a dozen homeless persons died tragically on the streets of Boston and Cambridge. We viewed this tragedy as a public health crisis and convened a monthly working group comprised of officials from city and state agencies, shelters and human service providers, the police and emergency medical services, street outreach workers, medical and mental health teams, substance abuse experts, advocates and homeless persons, and many others. This remarkable group worked collaboratively to identify those at greatest risk for death on the streets and to design appropriate services. In the four years since that time, we have seen a marked decline in the number of deaths due to hypothermia on the streets of Boston. This is a testament to the commitment of literally hundreds of dedicated persons working together to overcome the immense obstacles to health faced by those who are struggling to survive on our streets and in our shelters.

This second edition of the Manual continues to underscore the critical importance of providing health care to those living in crowded shelters and offers very practical approaches to controlling and treating the major communicable and other diseases that are seen all too commonly among homeless individuals and families. I am proud to share in this innovative endeavor.

Howard Koh, MD, MPH
Commissioner of Public Health
Commonwealth of Massachusetts, 1997-2003
Associate Dean for Public Health Practice and Professor of Health Policy and Management
Harvard School of Public Health

Contributing Authors

Toni Abraham, RN, CS, ANP, has been a nurse practitioner with BHCHP since 1996 and is currently the Associate Medical Director responsible for representing the NP/PA interests at the management level. A suburban mother of three grown children, she is a nurse from the 1960s, who lived through the Beatnik Era and neither smoked nor inhaled. Her vanishing spare time is spent reading, exercising, and visiting her children.

Daniel P. Alford, MD, MPH, is an Assistant Professor of Medicine and a member of the Clinical Addiction Research and Education Unit of the Section of General Medicine at Boston University Medical Center. He is the Medical Director of the Frontage Road Methadone Clinic and an expert in pain management and the management of opioid dependency. He trained in Internal Medicine at Boston Medical Center and served as Chief Medical Resident. Dan enjoys photography, gardening, and playing with his dog, Nellie. If his wife Barbara is reading this, he also enjoys going to museums and the theater.

Robin K. Avery, MD, is a staff physician and specialist in transplant infectious diseases in the Department of Infectious Disease at the Cleveland Clinic Foundation in Cleveland, Ohio. Robin was a full-time physician for BHCHP in 1988-89, helping to set up programs for homeless persons living with HIV. The interns and residents at Boston City Hospital honored her with an award for the best attending physician. A Schweitzer Fellow who spent several months in Gabon, Central Africa, during medical school, Robin has been a volunteer physician at Care Alliance (formerly known as Cleveland Health Care for the Homeless) since 1996.

Johnye Ballenger, MD, FAAP, is an Instructor in Pediatrics at Harvard Medical School and a pediatrician in general practice. Her interests include

ADHD and international and domestic adoptions. She completed her residency in Pediatrics and a fellowship in Ambulatory Pediatrics at Boston City Hospital, before joining the department of General Pediatrics at Children's Hospital in Boston. She was the clinical director for Project Better Health, a multidisciplinary, mobile, medical outreach program that joined BHCHP in serving families placed in motels from 1989-1991. Johnye was featured in Sara Lawrence-Lightfoot's book *Respect* and has been dabbling in learning languages. Quilting and gardening are much beloved but rarely enjoyed in her busy life.

M. Anita Barry, MD, MPH, is Director of Communicable Disease Control for the Boston Public Health Department. She has been a leader in public health prevention and treatment programs for homeless individuals and families throughout the city and state. Anita completed a residency in Internal Medicine and a fellowship in Infectious Diseases at Boston City Hospital. She is an Assistant Professor of Medicine and Public Health at Boston University. In addition to being a wife and mother, Anita also serves as a volunteer home visitor for Yankee Golden Retriever Rescue, a non-profit organization placing abused, abandoned, and other Golden Retrievers in need.

Joel Bass, MD, completed his residency in Pediatrics at Children's Hospital in Boston and is currently Chair of Pediatrics at Newton-Wellesley Hospital and Associate Clinical Professor of Pediatrics at Harvard Medical School. He has provided care for family shelters in the Framingham and Newton areas and is the principal author of "Pediatric Problems in a Suburban Shelter of Homeless Families."

John Bernardo, MD, erstwhile mechanic at Toyota of Weymouth and former Volkswagen afficionado, also doubles as a pulmonologist and Professor of Medicine at Boston University Medical Center. He serves as the Tuberculosis Control Officer for the Commonwealth of Massachusetts and a Research Professor of Biochemistry at Boston University School of Medicine. John has been a national leader in tuberculosis prevention and control in homeless shelters and has conducted a TB Clinic at Pine Street Inn once each week since 1984.

Monica Bharel, MD, is the Medical Director of BHCHP's Barbara McInnis House. She trained in Internal Medicine at Boston University Medical Center and served as Chief Medical Resident. She left for the University of California in San Francisco, and it took us five years to finally lure her back to Boston. Monica is a Clinical Instructor at MGH and an Assistant Clinical Professor at Boston University Medical Center. She is an amateur photographer and avid world traveler. Her best views in the world (so far) are from the peak of Mount Kilimanjaro.

Patricia MacWilliams Bowe, RN, MS, is the nurse manager of BHCHP's clinic at Pine Street Inn, New England's largest shelter for homeless adults. Trish began volunteering at Pine Street Inn while a student at Boston College and worked in the Nurses' Clinic there after completing her RN at New England Baptist Hospital. She has been with BHCHP since 1994, and she pioneered our clinics at two local thoroughbred racetracks that provide care to the backstretch workers who live and work in the barns and stables. Not surprisingly, she is a Sagittarius who loves animals (cats, monkeys, and horses) and loves to travel.

David Buchanan, MD, completed his training in Internal Medicine at the University of California, San Francisco. During residency, he performed medical outreach by bicycle to homeless people in Golden Gate Park. Though he continues to bike to work everyday, David is currently the Head of the Section of Social Medicine at John Stroger Hospital of Cook County (formerly Cook County Hospital). He serves as the Medical Director for two shelter-based clinics in Chicago and is currently supported by a Soros Advocacy Fellowship to pursue policy work on access to respite care for homeless individuals. David recently started learning to surf.

Michelle Canning, RN, BSN, has been a public health nurse with the Boston Public Health Commission since 1999. Within the Communicable Disease Control Bureau, Michelle has participated in surveillance activities to identify occurrence of biologic events, education programs for health care providers as well as the general public, participated in vaccination programs, and supervised nurses for the Bioterrorism program as well as the Immunization program.

Claire J. Carlo, MD, is a staff physician with BHCHP. She is a mainstay of our HIV Team and has pioneered the development of our racetrack clinics at Suffolk Downs and Rockingham Park. Fluent in Spanish, Claire cares for the backstretch workers, many from Central and South America, who live in the barns and stables hidden behind the pageantry of the racetrack. Claire delivers primary care to homeless patients, including those who are HIV positive. She is the mother of three children ages 6, 9, and 10, who keep her busy when she is at home. In her free time, she enjoys walking, sewing, and decorating her Victorian house.

Carmen Cleary, NP, completed her nursing doctorate at Rush University College of Nursing. She is a certified family nurse practitioner and faculty member at Rush College of Nursing. She is a clinical instructor for Rush nursing students and provides on site clinical care for residents of a 350 bed shelter in Chicago.

Andrew Ellingson, BS, is an epidemiologist at the Cambridge Public Health Department (CPHD) working towards the completion of a Masters in Public Health at Boston University. At the CPHD he is responsible for monitoring reportable infectious diseases within the city and working with the public health nurses to assess and mitigate risks from these diseases within the city. He also collaborates with local emergency room physicians and the Boston Public Health Commission to monitor for possible bioterrorism and naturally occurring disease outbreaks in the region. Andrew was a Peace Corps volunteer in Nepal, where he developed his interest in public health and infectious diseases after noting the devastating effects of a cholera epidemic.

Louise J. Eutropius, RN, BSN, CIC, has been an infection control practitioner at the University of Utah Hospitals and Clinics (UUH&C) since 1987. Louise is responsible for a wide variety of prevention and control activities, including communicable disease surveillance and reporting. She serves as the UUH&C infection control liaison to the state and local health departments. Additionally, Louise has lectured extensively on topics related to infection control, blood-borne pathogens, and tuberculosis. An avid outdoors person, she enjoys skate skiing, backcountry skiing, road and mountain biking, hiking, and backpacking. Louise has accompanied a friend on several stretches of a continental divide trail quest and last summer went down the Colorado River - an experience of a lifetime!

Lori Fantry, MD, MPH, finished her residency in Internal Medicine at the University of Massachusetts Medical School in 1988 and was the Medical Director for the Homeless Outreach and Advocacy Project (HOAP) in Worcester until the summer of 1990. She is now an Assistant Professor in the Department of Internal Medicine at the University of Maryland Medical School. Lori is also the Medical Director at the Evelyn Jordan Center at the Institute of Human Virology.

Kathleen Fitch, MSN, APRN,BC, FNP, has been a nurse practitioner with BHCHP since 2001. She grew up in Yakima, Washington, the most recent location of the Mad Cow disease scare. She loves knitting and knits anything from baby booties to 13-foot scarves. Traveling and planning trips helps her get through the long New England winters. Most recently she has been to India, Italy, and Thailand.

Robert Gamble, FNP, has been a nurse practitioner with BHCHP since 1999. He spent the first 3 years of his tenure working in our respite program at McInnis and Snead Houses and is now a key member of our Family Team. Robbie and the team work in two community health center clinics and venture out to provide direct primary and episodic care to homeless children and adults living in shelters and motels scattered throughout the greater metropolitan Boston area. Robbie has also done health care and human rights work in El Salvador and Peru. In his free time he enjoys writing poetry.

Laura M. Gillis, MS, RN, is currently the Health Care for the Homeless (HCH) Collaborative's Coordinator for the Health Care for the Homeless Clinician's Network, a national network of over 700 clinicians that Laura helped to found. She served as Chair of the Clinician's Network from 1996-1997. Laura provides technical assistance to HCH programs nationally that participate in the Health Disparities Collaboratives of the Bureau of Primary Health Care. Laura's expertise in the care of homeless persons is rooted in her 10-year

experience with the Baltimore HCH. Laura holds a master's degree in Community Health Nursing and Health Policy from the University of Maryland at Baltimore. When she is not "cutting the rug" dancing, Laura is either enjoying a foreign film or devouring female detective fiction.

Lawrence E. Gottlieb, MPA, MSW, has worked with community hospitals and health centers for more than 15 years in New Jersey and in Worcester, MA, where he currently serves as vice president of Community HealthLink. Larry is responsible for the administration of a 60-bed inpatient medical detoxification program, as well as the Homeless Outreach and Advocacy Project (HOAP). Before moving into a career of health care administration, Larry had the opportunity to travel extensively throughout Europe for two seasons while playing professional basketball for the city team of Ramat-Gan, Israel.

Maya Mundkur Greer, MSN, APRN,BC, worked as a Family Nurse Practitioner with BHCHP from 1988 until 1990. Since that time she has continued to work with disenfranchised populations, caring for individuals with HIV/AIDS at the Fenway Community Health Center, homeless adolescents and young adults at the Sidney Borum Jr. Health Center, and most recently at the Martha Eliot Health Center, where she coordinated the Ryan White HIV Primary Care program. Maya received her MSN at Yale University and completed a fellowship in adolescent medicine at Harvard Medical School. Over the past several years, she has used her time to travel the world, work as a publicist for a jazz band, and become a wife and mother.

Pedro Jose Greer, MD, is a physician, hepatologist, professor, MacArthur Fellow, author, father, and husband, better known as "Joe". His concern for those without access to health care fueled his passion to create various free clinics for persons who are homeless, undocumented, migrant, and poor in Miami. He did his undergraduate studies at the University of Florida, medical studies at La Universidad Catolica Madre and Maestra, and all his postdoctoral medical training at the University of Miami, where he was Chief Medical Resident. Joe is married to Janus, with two children, Alana and Joey, as well as a cat and a dog. They live in Coral Gables, Florida. Joe is the author of *Waking up in America*, an autobiographical account of his early years, recounting stories from under the bridges in

Miami to the White House. HBO is now making a movie of the book, starring Andy Garcia.

Susan Gregoire, RN, MSN, APRN,BC, was a nurse practitioner at BHCHP's McInnis House from 2001-2003 and is now one of four providers at a suburban internal medicine practice. In her time away from work, she can usually be found in the White Mountains, attempting to summit New Hampshire's 48 highest peaks. She has only 9 left to reach her goal.

Janet Groth, MS, CFNP, the irrepressible co-editor of our original manual, was a Family Nurse Practitioner and Public Health Consultant for BHCHP from 1988 to 1994. After a brief sojourn in family practice, she now works in rehabilitation and long term care, which she finds similar to caring for homeless people: multisystem disease, poor social supports, and institutionalized settings. Her night job is the much harder one and includes homework, laundry, groceries, and the talk-talk-talk that families need to keep balanced. She enjoys knitting and needlepoint and admits that she occasionally plays the piano and rarely skis. She swims a lot because no one can page her under water, and she enjoys her husband's cooking, as that's one of his major contributions to the family.

Adi Gundlapalli, MD, PhD, is board certified in internal medicine and infectious diseases and currently the Medical Director of the Wasatch Homeless Health Care in Salt Lake City, Utah, as well as an adjunct Assistant Professor of Medicine at the University of Utah School of Medicine. His research interests include infection control, the epidemiology of upper respiratory infections, public health surveillance, and health care for homeless populations. His work has been presented at national and international meetings, and he has been invited to lecture nationally on topics relating to infectious diseases and public health. Adi completed an internal medicine residency at the University of Connecticut before moving to Utah, where he completed a fellowship in infectious diseases and hospital epidemiology at the University of Utah School of Medicine.

Julia E. Gunn, RN, MPH, has been working with the Boston Public Health Commission in the Communicable Disease Control Program for over 10 years, assuming the position of Associate Director in 2003. During this time, Julia has contributed to dozens of publications and presentations enhancing our understanding of tuberculosis, HIV infection, food-borne illness, and other communicable illnesses, particularly among disadvantaged populations.

Carole Hohl, MHS, PA-C, has been a physician assistant with BHCHP since 1997. In addition to maintaining an active clinical practice, Carole served the program as Associate Medical Director for two years until becoming Director of the HIV Program. Carole's outstanding clinical skills and compassionate care earned her a Local Hero Award in 2002 from the National Health Care for the Homeless Council's Clinicians Network. Carole enjoys the symmetry of being the wife of one, mother of three, and grandmother of one.

Emily Hurstack, BSN, MS, NP, has been a nurse practitioner with BHCHP since 1994, providing primary care at two of our busiest clinics, Boston Medical Center and Saint Francis House, a soup kitchen located in downtown Boston. Over the years Emily has also acquired vast experience as an educator, teaching in public schools, hospitals, and schools of nursing. When not out in the community sharing her skills, Emily can be found hiking, kayaking, or reading quietly to her grandchildren.

Noreen A. Hynes, MD, MPH, completed her residency in Internal Medicine and a fellowship in Infectious Diseases at Massachusetts General Hospital and spent 2 years in the Epidemic Intelligence Service at CDC. She has spent over 25 years in government service, serving from 1997 until 2000 on an assignment from the CDC to the Baltimore City Health Department as the Director of Clinical and Preventive STD Services. In addition to her current duties as a government scientist, she serves on the faculty of Johns Hopkins University Schools of Medicine and Public Health. Noreen provides patient care, teaches a graduate level course on STD prevention and control, and authors and edits STD and genitourinary tract infection modules on the Johns Hopkins antibiotic web site.

Kathly M. Jean-Gilles, MSN, RN, RRT-NPS, FNP, has been a nurse practitioner at BHCHP's Barbara McInnis House since 2001. While caring for the comprehensive needs of her patients, Kathly emphasizes health promotion and disease prevention, including appropriate screening and preventive services. Kathly is also a registered respiratory therapist, with a specialty in neonatal and pediatric patients, and has worked in most of Boston's Level III NICUs. Kathly is a member of Sigma Theta Tau and hopes to enter a PhD program in the near future.

Stefan G. Kertesz, MD, MSc, is a homeless health care physician and health services researcher who enjoys Afro-pop music, long conversations, and the Daily Show with John Stewart. He is a Schweitzer Fellow, whose clinical work includes two periods of service in Sub-Saharan Africa and seven memorable years with the Health Care for the Homeless Programs in Boston, Massachusetts, and Birmingham, Alabama.

Stacy Kirkpatrick, MSN, ANP, RN, is a nurse practitioner who joined BHCHP after training at the Institute of Health Professions at Massachusetts General Hospital. She has worked at our Boston Medical Center clinic as well as at several local shelters and soup kitchens. Stacy has been the mainstay of our Diabetes Collaborative Team. Stacy can sing "Texas Our Texas" (the official song of the Lone Star State), believes that manual transmissions still rule, and loves to go hear live music (even on a school night).

Bruce D. Levy, MD, FACP, is a member of the Pulmonary and Critical Care Medicine Department at Brigham and Women's Hospital and Harvard Medical School. While a resident, he organized a volunteer clinic at the New England Shelter for Homeless Veterans, and he continues to care for homeless patients at that clinic. Bruce enjoys growing asparagus, berries, and sunflowers in his own urban Boston garden. Growing up in St. Louis, his first scientific endeavor was the collection of fireflies for luciferase isolation for Sigma Chemical Company.

Alison May, MD, has been a staff physician at BHCHP since 1994. She is a graduate of Harvard Medical School and completed a residency in Internal Medicine at Brigham and Women's Hospital in Boston. Alison has long been dedicated to the care of underserved populations and is another of our Schweitzer Fellows, having worked at the Albert Schweitzer Hospital in Gabon, Central Africa, during medical school. Alison currently maintains an active practice at BHCHP's clinic at Boston Medical Center and at Saint Francis House and cares for patients in a local detoxification unit as well as a methadone maintenance clinic.

Jessie McCary, MD, completed her residency in Internal Medicine at Boston Medical Center and served as Chief Medical Resident. She is an Instructor in Medicine at Boston University School of Medicine and serves as an attending physician on the medical service for several months each year. Jessie is a staff physician with BHCHP, caring for patients at Saint Francis House as well as Long Island Shelter and Father Bill's Place. She has been a champion of the Health Disparities Collaborative and has assumed a leadership role in improving the care of homeless persons with diabetes.

Margaret McNamara, NP, has been a nurse practitioner with BHCHP since 1989. She did graduate training at Boston College and Simmons College and holds both adult and family nurse practitioner certifications. Maggie has been a stalwart at our clinic at Saint Francis House and has spent many years working with homeless women who live on the streets and suffer from mental illness.

Sarah McSweeney-Ryan, MD, participated in the Boston Combined Residency Program at Boston Medical Center and Children's Hospital. During her residency, Sarah had the opportunity to spend clinical time each week at several homeless shelters in the Boston area. Sarah now lives in Portland, Maine, with her husband Ben, where she practices general pediatrics.

James J. O'Connell, MD, was a founding physician of BHCHP in 1985. He is a graduate of Harvard Medical School and completed his residency in Internal Medicine at Massachusetts General Hospital in 1985. He is President of BHCHP and has maintained a busy clinical practice with a focus on the care of those who avoid shelters and sleep on the streets. He admits that he is too tired to write another word.

Deborah Pavan-Langston, MD, FACS, is a Senior Surgeon, Director of Clinical Virology, and Attending Physician on the Cornea and Anterior Segment Unit of Massachusetts Eye and Ear Infirmary. She is Associate Professor of Ophthalmology at Harvard Medical School. Deborah trained in Internal Medicine at Columbia's Presbyterian Hospital in New York before completing her ophthalmic residency and fellowships at Harvard Medical School and the Massachusetts Eye and Ear Infirmary. She is the first woman to receive the international Castroviejo Medal and Europe's Van Alphen Award. Her bibliography includes over 220 publications and 10 books. Remarkably, Deborah still finds plenty of time to travel around the world photographing unusual and often magnificent places. Her work has been exhibited in several states and published in national magazines.

Denise A. Petrella, RN, CS, ANP, is a TV drama junkie. Some of her favorites include NYPD Blue, ER, and General Hospital. No one ever dreamed that Denny would end up in the medical field. She danced ballet for 22 years and everyone thought she would choose that as her career. In her high school year book, she was predicted to be the first dancing nurse on General Hospital. Denny has been a nurse practitioner with BHCHP since 1994. She has worked at McInnis House and was the first NP on our Street Team, caring for homeless persons living under bridges, in back alleys, and on the city's streets. She still insists that she is absolutely in love with her job at BHCHP.

Maria Pitaro, MD, was a staff physician with BHCHP for several years after completing her residency in Internal Medicine at Boston City Hospital, where she was President of the House Officer's Union. During her time with BHCHP, Maria was a leader in issues concerning the health of homeless women and was the program's representative on a task force to assure universal health insurance in Massachusetts. After leaving the program in 1991, Maria went on to work in both academic medicine and private practice. Maria is currently the Associate Medical Director of the Union Health Center in New York City, a multi-specialty ambulatory health care center providing care to active and retired members of the UNITE union and their families. Maria's numerous interests include cooking and gardening.

Phillip E. Pulaski, MD, has been a staff physician with BHCHP since 1994. He is the Medical Director of our clinic at Boston Medical Center and works at several shelter sites, including Saint Francis House and the racetrack clinic. Phil has been a leader and teacher in the care of homeless persons

with HIV/AIDS, and he has worked in the HIV specialty clinic at Boston Medical Center since 1994. Phil is one of our four Schweitzer Fellows who spent time in Gabon, West Africa. Before medical school, he worked for several years in Bolivia with his wife, Betty Ann. They now have three wonderful girls and live just outside of Boston.

Joseph Rampulla, MS, APRN,BC, is a nurse practitioner with BHCHP who has worked at our Massachusetts General Hospital Clinic since 1990. He has been caring for indigent populations for over 25 years and has a subspecialty in addictions. Joe enjoys bass fishing and gardening.

Richard F. Regan, PA-C, is a physician assistant and computer expert extraordinaire at BHCHP's Barbara McInnis House. A graduate of Mercy College of Detroit's Physician Assistant Program, Dick is a former high school teacher of social justice and social responsibility. He lived and worked for four years in the Andes Mountains of Peru doing pastoral work and village improvement projects, and his presentation to our program about his experiences during the Shining Path uprising was riveting and unforgettable.

Marisa Rogers, MD, MPH, is a clinical educator in Internal Medicine at the University of Pennsylvania. A graduate of Emory University School of Medicine, Marisa was a participant in a medical brigade to Honduras. She enjoys reading, music, and travel.

Jill S. Roncarati, PA-C, has been a physician assistant on BHCHP's Street Team since 2001 and spends most of her days and evenings combing the city and caring for homeless persons who are too frightened to go to the shelters. She began working with homeless persons in 1996 as a TB outreach worker and educator with Barbara McInnis at Pine Street Inn, and she remains the only person ever to understand and organize Barbara's legendary "filing" system. Jill still would rather be rowing or cycling, aspiring to complete a transcontinental ride.

Megan Sandel, MD, is a pediatrician at Boston Medical Center who has worked with the BHCHP Family Team since 1999. Her pediatric and adolescent practice focuses on the care of homeless and formerly homeless families, many of whom she met in the shelters and motels and continues to follow after they are permanently housed. She lives with her "boys" (husband John, son Conor, and another baby boy on the way) in the Boston suburbs. Her fervent desire is for the Red Sox to finally expunge the curse of the Bambino.

Ben Siegel, MD, has been the Pediatric Consultant for BHCHP since clinical services began in 1985. His vision and enthusiasm have been primarily responsible for the development of BHCHP's Family Team. Ben completed his residency in Pediatrics at Boston City Hospital and Montefiore Hospital in New York. He is an Associate Professor of Pediatrics at Boston University Medical Center. He has been nationally prominent in the evolution of pediatric residency training programs and the care of underserved populations.

Michael S. Singer, MD, PhD, is an ophthalmology resident at the Massachusetts Eye and Ear Infirmary in Boston. He also serves as Tutor-in-Residence at Eliot House at Harvard College, an interesting challenge for a graduate of Yale College. Upon finishing Yale University's MD/PhD program, he completed an internship in Internal Medicine at the Brigham and Women's Hospital in Boston. Michael has extensive international health experience, is proficient in eight languages, and has traveled extensively. His long list of accomplishments includes a photographic exhibit of portraits of children in developing countries and a pending patent on the "method and apparatus for predicting structure of transmembrane proteins."

Suzanne Strickland, MPH, is the Associate Director for the Office of Public Health Preparedness at the Boston Public Health Commission and formerly worked with Dr. Anita Barry as the Prevention Coordinator in the Communicable Disease Control Division. She has extensive experience in public health policy, as well as in education and training on a broad spectrum of public health topics. She is now enveloped in issues related to bioterrorism and preparedness planning. An escapee from the great State of Arkansas, Suzanne is the owner of a rescued greyhound ("the goofiest dog in the world") and a fan of bad English comedies.

Nancy Sullivan, MS, RN, FNP-C, is a nurse practitioner who served as BHCHP's Associate Director of Clinical Operations and Director of Nursing before becoming the Assistant Director of Health Services for Boston Public Schools. Nancy enjoys walking, aerobics, swing dancing, and reading.

Melinda Thomas, PA-C, completed her training as a physician assistant at Allegheny University in Philadelphia, where she became interested in the health care issues facing homeless persons. Melinda organized and coordinated the student and physician volunteers at a homeless shelter for women and children. Melinda has been with BHCHP since 1998, initially working at our Betty Snead House, a 18-bed medical respite unit for homeless women. She is currently on our Family Team, caring for homeless families in shelters and in motels.

Pat Petrosky Tormey, RN, MPH, is the Communicable Disease Program Manager and Public Health Nursing Supervisor for the Boston Public Health Commission. Pat has worked in the public health field for more than thirty years. She loves the ocean, biking, and hiking. She is hopelessly devoted to a great dog named Boyce.

Virginia A. Triant, MD, MPH, is a second year resident in Internal Medicine at Brigham and Women's Hospital in Boston. Virginia hopes to combine clinical practice and public health, focusing on the topic of health care access. Recent clinical activities have led her to a South African community clinic, the New Haven public school system, a homeless veterans shelter, and an Indian Health Service site in Montana. Virginia enjoys hiking and exploring national parks.

T. Scott Troppy, MPH, is an epidemiologist for the Boston Public Health Commission. A one year "visit" to Boston in 1990 from his native Texas has eclipsed more than a decade, although he still misses good Mexican food and the great city of Austin. His favorite vacation destination is Maui, Hawaii, where he enjoys scuba diving and lying on the beach.

Gregory A. Wagoner, MD, MBA, has been BHCHP's Medical Director since 2002. He has extensive experience in private practice, hospital practice, and has served as the Medical Director of several HMOs. Sprung from a long-line of farmers, Greg still treasures the therapy of working the soil. In addition, he enjoys traveling and playing tennis competitively.

Carol A. Waldmann, MD, has been a staff physician at BHCHP since 1995. After medical school at Case Western Reserve University, Carol completed her residency in Internal Medicine at Boston City Hospital. Prior to joining BHCHP, she served as the Field Medical Director with the International Medical Corps in Sudan. She maintains a hectic clinical schedule, caring for homeless patients in several shelter settings, our HIV clinic, and our clinics at Boston Medical Center and Massachusetts General Hospital. When not working or rowing on the Charles, Carol enjoys photography and writing poetry, for which she has received several awards and prizes.

Keith Williams, MD, MS, was a BHCHP staff physician from 1998 until 2003. He is now a Fellow in the new Master Educator Track of the General Internal Medicine Fellowship Program at Boston University Medical Center. He is a sailing instructor and a private pilot. Keith brews the best beer in the city, enjoys taekwondo, and has been known to cut a few rugs doing the lindy hop and swing dancing.

Jennifer Gordon Wright, DVM, MPH, DACVPM, is a veterinarian with a special interest in zoonotic diseases and their prevention. While completing her MPH, Jennifer worked part-time at CDC, part-time in veterinary practice, and was pregnant with her first child! She is currently an Epidemic Intelligence Service (EIS) officer and ready to respond at a moment's notice to investigate outbreaks of infectious disease. When not spending time with her child, she enjoys walking her dog, working in the yard, decorating her house, and designing the elusive home of her dreams. Had she not chosen veterinary medicine for her career, she probably would have become an interior designer.

Emily Zielinski-Gutiérrez, DrPH, is a behavioral scientist with the CDC Division of Vector-Borne Infectious Diseases. Emily holds doctoral and masters degrees in public health from the Tulane School of Public Health and Tropical Medicine in New Orleans, Louisiana. She concentrated her studies in medical anthropology, health communication, epidemiology, and tropical medicine, as well as Friday night zydeco. Prior to working with the CDC, she was a research assistant for Tulane's Department of International Health and Development, conducting research in Peru, Bolivia, Tanzania, and Nigeria; was a Fulbright Fellow with a Pan American Health Organization collaborating institution in Guatemala evaluating dengue prevention; and worked for the Louisiana Office of Public Health in HIV and prenatal care.

Gennine Zinner, RNC, ANP, has been a nurse practitioner with BHCHP since 1996 and has extensive experience working in our respite programs at Barbara McInnis House and the former Betty Snead House for women. Gennine is a graduate of the University of California at San Francisco, with a specialty in Mental Health. ▪

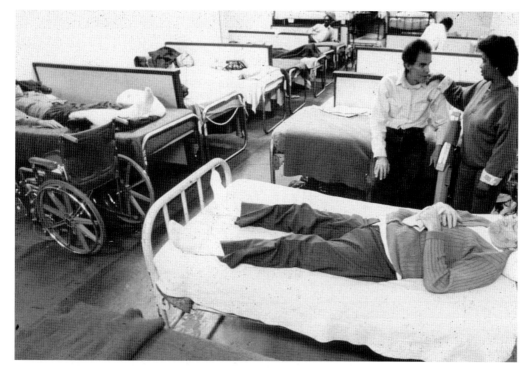

The Boston Health Care for the Homeless Program

T he chapters for the first edition of this shelter and street manual were written in 1990, which now seems an eternity ago. AZT was the only available medication for AIDS, with resistance and failure commonplace. The pills had to be taken every four hours around the clock, an overwhelming challenge for anyone living in a shelter or on the streets. Hepatitis C was still a mystery and usually called "non-A, non-B hepatitis". No vaccines were commercially available for chickenpox. Bioterrorism and "weaponized" bacteria and viruses were the fancy of science fiction novels. Outbreaks of mad cow disease and SARS were almost unimaginable.

The Medical Respite Unit at the Lemuel Shattuck Shelter, 1985-1992. Betty Snead, respite aide, shown with two patients recovering from heart failure and cellulitis at BHCHP's original 25-bed respite program, which began in September 1985 and was moved and expanded to 92 beds at BHCHP's Barbara McInnis House in 1993. Photo by David Comb

The Special Needs of Homeless Persons: Medicine Meets Public Health

Poverty remains a powerful social determinant of poor health, and persons struggling to survive without stable housing are particularly vulnerable.

Homelessness magnifies poor health, causes an array of medical illnesses and injuries, exposes those huddled in crowded shelters to communicable diseases such as tuberculosis and influenza, places individuals at risk for trauma and exposure to the elements, complicates the management of chronic illnesses such as diabetes and asthma, makes health care harder to access, leads to premature mortality, and presents vexing obstacles that exasperate health care providers and confound delivery systems.

Caring for homeless persons requires a deliberate blurring of the traditional boundaries between institutions and among health care disciplines and professions. While physicians, nurse practitioners, and physician assistants can diagnose and treat according to *Harrison's Principles of Internal Medicine*, a homeless person with a lower extremity ulcer and cellulitis needs access to antibiotics and a place to keep the leg elevated, an impossibility while living in shelters or on the streets. Thus the clinician's treatment plan is only as effective as the social worker who obtains the medications, the nurses who perform the twice daily dressing changes, and the shelter supervisor who permits the person to remain in the lobby during the day.

The Bureau of Primary Health Care of the US Public Health Service recognized the need to take health care directly to the shelters and the streets in order to overcome such barriers and now funds over 160 health care for the homeless programs across the nation, including every state as well

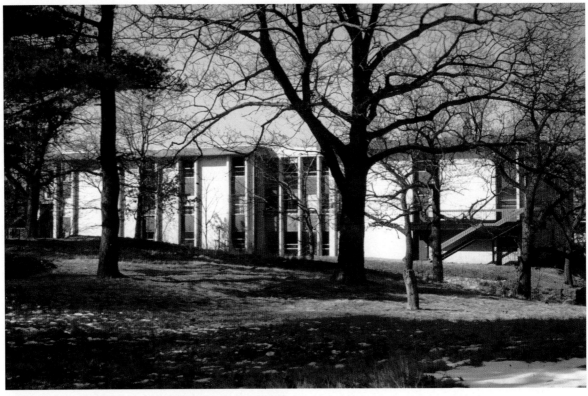

The Barbara McInnis House. This former nursing home was purchased by BHCHP in 1992 and is now a 92-bed respite care program that serves homeless persons in Boston and throughout the Commonwealth. Photo by James O'Connell MD

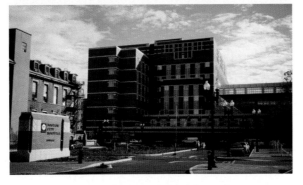

The New Boston City Hospital. This building opened in 1995 and replaced the cherished but antiquated inpatient wards. BHCHP continues to have a bustling daily clinic at the hospital, which is now called Boston Medical Center. Photo by James O'Connell MD

as Puerto Rico. Over 500,000 homeless persons receive care each year from these dedicated teams of intrepid clinicians and workers. In addition to these programs, literally hundreds of health professionals and workers continue to volunteer throughout the country in a heroic effort to serve our neighbors who are without homes.

This second edition of the manual is designed to be practical and readable to those working in shelters and on the streets, and each chapter has been written by clinicians familiar with the extraordinary challenges of providing health care in those settings.

The Boston Health Care for the Homeless Program (BHCHP)

BHCHP was one of 19 projects funded nationwide by the Robert Wood Johnson Foundation and the Pew Charitable Trust from 1985-1988. The Commonwealth of Massachusetts provided

matching funds. The mission has remained simple and direct: to provide or assure access to the highest quality health care for homeless individuals and families in Boston. The project was conceived by a broad-based coalition as a catalyst within the mainstream, working to integrate medical care in shelters and on the streets with the care provided by Boston's renowned academic teaching hospitals and neighborhood health centers. The coalition also charged the fledgling project to develop and implement a medical respite program to care for homeless persons too ill or injured to withstand the rigors of survival on the streets but not sick enough to require acute care hospitalization.

The BHCHP service delivery model utilizes three hospital-based clinics (Boston Medical Center, Massachusetts General Hospital, and the Lemuel Shattuck Hospital). Multidisciplinary teams, comprised of doctors, nurse practitioners, physician assistants, nurses, social workers, and outreach workers, venture out to provide direct care services at over 70 outreach and community sites throughout metropolitan Boston. These sites include adult and family shelters, soup kitchens and day centers, shelters for victims of domestic violence, motels and hotels, detoxification units and transitional programs. One team provides care for the backstretch workers who live in the barns of two local thoroughbred racetracks, while another team joins the day and night outreach workers who

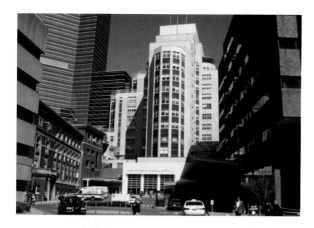

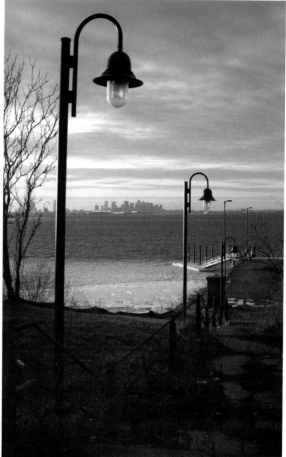

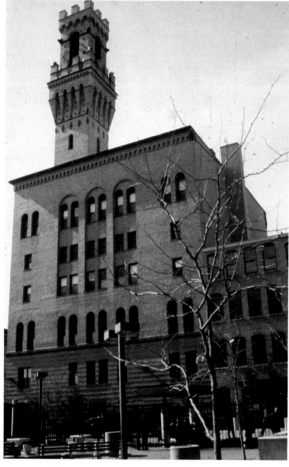

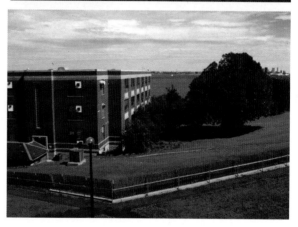

care for those sleeping rough under bridges, in back alleys, and on Boston's streets. Respite care, a word adopted by the homeless advocacy communities in Boston and Washington, DC, has come to mean acute, subacute, pre- and post-surgical, recuperative, rehabilitative, palliative and end-of-life care for homeless persons who would otherwise require costly acute care hospitalization. Respite care has emerged as a critical component in the continuum of services necessary for providing quality health care for homeless populations. BHCHP's original respite program (the first of its kind) began in September of 1985 with 25 beds nestled in a corner of the Shattuck Shelter, an arrangement which soon proved less than ideal given the increased acuity of illness as hospital lengths of stay rapidly decreased. In 1993 BHCHP opened the Barbara McInnis House, a free-standing 92-bed respite care facility. Now over 35 cities across the USA and Canada are developing respite programs, including those participating in a 10-city respite care demonstration program funded by the Bureau of Primary Health Care.

Comprehensive oral health care is provided in a state-of-the-art dental clinic at the South End Community Health Center as well as at two dental suites at the McInnis House. Mental health and psychiatric services are fully integrated into the primary care sites throughout the service delivery model. The Family Team works directly with several community health centers as well as the pediatric and family medicine clinics at Boston Medical Center to assure continuity and accessibility of care for families living in shelters and distant motels.

Coordination of care has been vastly improved since the implementation of an electronic medical record in 1996. All clinicians at any of the three hospital and 70 outreach sites enter data directly into each patient's chart, which is easily accessible over local area networks or traditional phone lines.

BHCHP serves more than 8000 unduplicated homeless persons each year. Our original staff of eight has now grown to over 250 individuals, including 12 MDs, 3 dentists, 19 NP/PAs, and over 30 RNs. ⊞

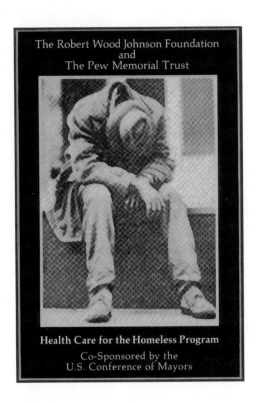

The Health Care for the Homeless Program, 1985-1988. The cover of the original RFP for this landmark 19-city grant of the Robert Wood Johnson Foundation and the Pew Memorial Trust.

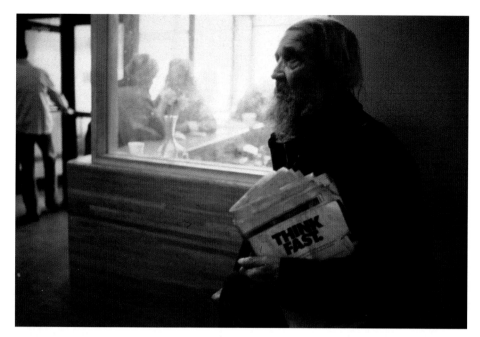

Introduction to the Manual

We have attempted to make this book easy to navigate and read. Most chapters are designed to be informative for clinicians and readable for shelter staff. This second edition of the manual acknowledges the profound effects that homelessness has on health; in addition to common communicable diseases, we have added several other illnesses and conditions confronted frequently by clinicians working on the streets and in the shelters. Esoteric "zebras" have been left for the more complete medical textbooks.

The manual is divided into seven parts. Part One contains discussions of 28 communicable diseases and 3 infections (cellulitis, pneumonia, and sinusitis) seen frequently among homeless populations. Each chapter has been written by clinicians experienced in the prevention and control of these infections and infestations in shelter settings. An attempt has been made to inform health care clinicians while also making these chapters readable to a more general audience, especially the staff and workers in shelters who are also exposed to these diseases. Each chapter briefly discusses the prevalence, transmission, diagnosis, treatment, and prevention of a particular communicable disease. A brief summary of the salient points concludes each chapter, followed by a few selected references for those who wish more in-depth knowledge.

A new feature of this edition is a list of the major medications in each chapter. Many clinicians bemoan the confusion caused by the interchangeable use of the generic and brand names of various medications, particularly with HIV medications,

antibiotics, and antihypertensive medicines. A list appears at the end of each chapter that includes the generic name of each medicine, the most common brand name products, and the relative cost. We have adopted the scale of $ to $$$$$ as utilized in the Tarascon 2004 Pocket Pharmacopoeia, in which:

$ = $25
$$ = $25-$49
$$$ = $50-$99
$$$$ = $100-$199
$$$$$ = $200 or more.

The relative costs were included in response to requests by clinicians concerned about judicious and cost-effective prescribing practices, particularly with poor and uninsured populations. Two caveats must be underscored with these medication lists: (1) the most common brand-name products are listed in alphabetical order, and the authors do not in any way endorse the use of any specific brand-name medications in this manual; (2) the relative costs are based on average wholesale costs for a month of maintenance therapy, such as diabetes and hypertension medications, or a course of short term treatment, such as antibiotics. These should be seen as rough guidelines only, as the cost of each medication can vary from state to state and from time to time, and can be dramatically influenced by the buying strategies of health plans, Medicaid and Medicare.

Part Two is new to this edition. Survival on the streets exposes homeless persons to the extremes of weather and the elements. This section discusses accidental hypothermia and frostbite, as well as hyperthermia and heat stroke.

The lobby of Pine Street Inn.
Photo by Melissa Shook

Part Three is another new addition to this manual and attempts to respond to an array of bewildering future and present challenges in shelter and street medicine. The emerging menace of bioterrorism is highlighted, as well as the perplexing array of nosocomial infections that can be spread easily in shelters. Recommendations on the proper use of antibiotics are offered in a chapter, while the two final chapters are designed to help clinicians manage chronic pain and recognize the subtle and debilitating consequences of traumatic brain injury.

Part Four addresses the management of chronic illnesses in a population without housing or a safe place to heal and store medications. The Chronic Care Model, developed through the Health Disparities Collaboratives of the Bureau of Primary Health Care, has some exciting new approaches to the organization and delivery of care for illnesses such as diabetes and depression. Several health care for the homeless projects have participated in this endeavor.

Part Five details the immunization schedules for children and adults, as well as some of the illnesses rendered rare by widespread vaccination programs, such as polio, diphtheria, mumps, rubella, and tetanus. Other resurgent or persistent vaccine-preventable infections, such as measles, pertussis, *Haemophilus influenzae* type b, and hepatitis B, are included with the common communicable diseases in Part One.

Food management in shelters and soup kitchens is the topic of Part Six, which includes practical suggestions for the proper handling, storage, and preparation of food in those settings. Periodic outbreaks of hepatitis A, including a recent one here in Boston, continue to make us aware of the critical importance of this topic.

Fact sheets for shelter guests are compiled in Part Seven. Now in Spanish as well as English, these simple instructions for families and individuals are intended to be photocopied and given to shelter guests during outbreaks of communicable diseases. These were very popular in our first edition, and we hope you will find them useful once again.

Our recommendations and suggestions are obviously not dogma. Most of our approaches are based on practical experience over these past two decades and have worked well in the shelters. We fully acknowledge that other approaches abound, many of which are perhaps better. We also understand that shelters differ in size, layout, staffing, rules for entry, and a host of other variables that are generally out of the control of health care clinicians. Our hope remains that this book, as the previous edition over a decade ago, will generate an open discussion among the growing number of clinicians in this field and will lead us all to more effective strategies for preventing and managing these illnesses and conditions in shelters and on the streets.

The pace of medicine has accelerated dramatically, and new treatments and approaches will inevitably supercede many of our current recommendations. We urge you to maintain a dialogue with your local health departments, hospitals, and community health centers in order to keep abreast of the most current methods of prevention, control, and treatment of communicable diseases in your cities and neighborhoods.

- JJO'C   Boston, June 2004

Part One

Communicable Diseases & Selected Infections

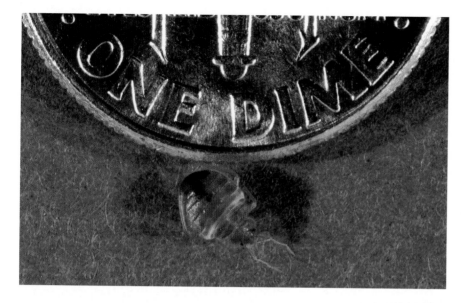

Bed Bugs

David Buchanan, MD
Carmen Cleary, NP

Cimex lectularis and *hemipterus*, or bed bugs, have plagued humankind since the beginning of recorded history. Although they have continued to affect people in developing countries throughout the modern era, bedbug infestations in the USA were relatively rare until recently. The resurgence is believed to have been caused by the use of less toxic pesticides, pesticide resistance, and the increase in international travel from countries where bed bugs are endemic. Bed bugs cannot fly and are transferred from place to place in luggage, bedding, and used furniture. Bed bugs feed primarily on human blood, but they can affect other mammals and birds.

Diagnosis

The diagnosis of bed bug bites is suggested by the history and physical exam and is confirmed by characteristic findings in the living space or by a positive identification of the offending bug. Patients typically present with multiple pruritic bites that are usually noticed when arising in the morning. The bites appear over areas which are not covered by clothing during sleep and generally spare the intertrigenous regions and areas under tight clothing that are commonly affected by scabies. Skin manifestations of the bites present in a variety of ways depending on the degree of immunological response.

The bites can present as:
*   pruritic wheals (like mosquito bites);
*   papules;
*   groups of small vesicles with surrounding erythema and induration;
*   bullous lesions which may resemble erythema multiforme;
*   asthma exacerbations, anaphylaxis, or other systemic responses.

Lesions often have a central punctum and are arranged in a linear fashion in groups of 3 (often called "breakfast, lunch, and dinner").

When bed bugs are suspected, the patient's living space should be inspected. Bed bugs feed on humans but live near the buttons and seams of mattresses, behind loose wallpaper or baseboards, and near electrical plates and cracks in walls. Over time, the areas where the bugs live become stained with human blood and bedbug feces. The stains appear oily with a reddish brown or black color and give off a distinctive sweet odor.

Definitive confirmation of the infestation can be made by capturing and positively identifying the bugs. This can be difficult because the bugs feed during the pre-dawn hours. The biting can occasionally interrupt sleep, but most commonly the bites are first noted in the morning after the bugs have returned to their hidden living spaces. We recommend giving patients a specimen container and asking them to capture the bugs that they notice near their sleeping area. Adult bedbugs can live for over a year without feeding and therefore can be easily saved for the clinician to examine

Cimex lectularis, the common bed bug, is brownish-red and approximately 5 mm in length. After a meal of human blood, the bed bug can swell to a length of over 7 mm. Photo by Carmen Cleary NP

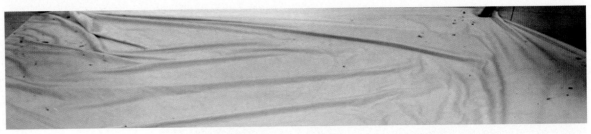

later. *Cimex lectularis*, the common bedbug, is light brown as a nymph and turns brownish red as it matures to adulthood. Before feeding, *Cimex lectularis* is approximately 5 mm in length and swells to over 7 mm after feeding. *Cimex hemipterus*, the tropical bedbug, is occasionally found in Florida and is distinguished by a longer pointed body.

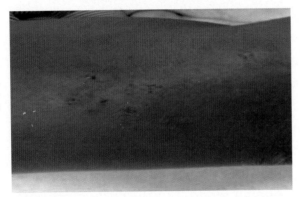

Treatment

The bites resolve spontaneously in 3-10 days without treatment. The pruritis or itchiness can be managed with antihistamines and topical steroids if symptoms are severe. Bed bugs feed multiple times during their life cycle and may be potential vectors for infectious diseases. Blood-borne viruses such as hepatitis B and HIV have been isolated in bed bugs who have fed on an infected host. However, this has not been proven scientifically; bed bugs have not been found to be vectors of disease in animal experiments, and the eradication of bed bugs has not been shown to reduce transmission rates of blood borne infections in heavily infested areas.

Control

The primary treatment for bed bug infestation is extermination. In addition to pesticide spraying, the bugs' living spaces should be eliminated by caulking cracks, removing peeling wallpaper, repairing loose floor boards, and cleaning or removing infested mattresses and upholstered furniture. Consultation with a professional pest control company is recommended.

Conclusion

Bed bugs are an increasingly common cause of pruritic rashes among homeless people in shelters. Diagnosis is suggested by finding bites on exposed areas upon awakening in the morning and by inspection of the affected bedding. Extermination of the bugs is necessary to prevent continued bites, but rashes from the bites resolve spontaneously. ▧

References

Jupp PG, Lyons SF. Experimental assessment of bedbugs (Cimex lectularius and Cimex hemipterus) and mosquitoes (Aedes aegypti formosus) as vectors of human immunodeficiency virus. *AIDS* 1987;1(3):171-174.

Krinsky WL. True Bugs (Hemiptera). In: Mullen G, Durden L, eds. *Medical and Veterinary Entomology*. Academic Press, Elsevier Science; 2002:80-84.

Robin J. PestWorld: Bedbugs Return Looking for Blood. National Pest Management Association; 2003. http://pestworld.org/news/article.sap?NewsID=1214

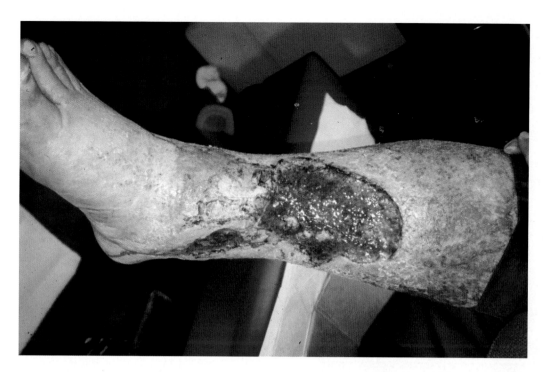

Cellulitis

Toni Abraham, ANP
Susan Gregoire, RN,
MSN, APRN,BC

Cellulitis is a rapidly spreading infection of the skin characterized by redness, pain, and swelling, and often accompanied by fever, malaise, chills, and headache. Abscess and tissue destruction are common complications when this infection is not treated with antibiotics.

Prevalence

A review of all patients seen by the Boston Health Care for the Homeless Program from January 1996 through August 2002 found that 7% developed cellulitis during that period. Of these patients, 45% were either hospitalized or admitted to BHCHP's Medical Respite Program at the Barbara McInnis House. Nine percent of this group left AMA (against medical advice) before completion of the course of prescribed antibiotics. Of those receiving treatment as outpatients in BHCHP's shelter and hospital clinics, 16% were lost to follow up.

No data could be found to quantify the incidence of cellulitis within the general population of the USA. Cellulitis accounted for 158 consultations per 10,000 persons in the United Kingdom in 1991. Additionally, skin and subcutaneous infections were responsible for 29,820 hospital admissions and a mean occupancy of 664 hospital beds each day.

Symptoms, Predisposing Factors, and Diagnosis

Cellulitis occurs anywhere on the skin. The most common clinical signs and symptoms include redness, generalized swelling, tenderness, and increased warmth. The differential diagnosis is broad: erysipelas, erythema serpens or erysipeloid (an infection seen in fisherman and meat handlers), deep venous thrombosis, and local skin irritation secondary to radiation treatment.

Cellulitis occurs when bacteria invade the skin, usually through an interruption in the epidermis such as a cut, abrasion, bite, needle injection, surgical incision, fungal infection, psoriasis, eczema, and many other things. The characteristics of the infection depend upon the specific location on the body and the nature of the invading pathogen(s). As the infection progresses, leukocytes infiltrate the area and debris is formed. Suppuration (formation of pus) and necrosis (localized tissue death), can follow when the infection is untreated. Occasionally an abscess is created that encapsulates the infection and theoretically safeguards the surrounding tissue. An abscess can rupture and form a furuncle, which communicates with the outside skin. Fistulas and chronic draining sinuses may also result from this infectious process.

Cellulitis can easily spread and disseminates along the paths of least resistance, especially veins, fascial planes, and the lymphatics. This spread along the lymphatics can cause a visible red streak that is known as lymphangitis. The regional lymph

Stasis Ulcer with Cellulitis.
This elderly man has venous stasis disease, marked swelling of both lower extremities, and a large stasis ulcer. He has been admitted to McInnis House with frequent episodes of cellulitis.
Photo by James O'Connell MD

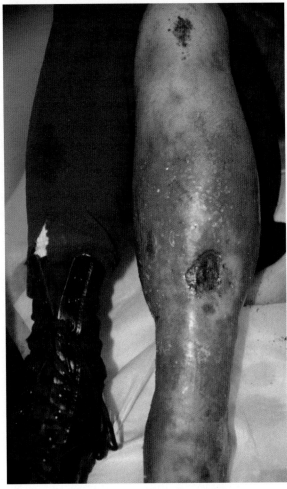

Cellulitis of the Lower Extremity. This man with COPD and chronic heart failure has intermittent edema of his lower extremities and has been hospitalized several times for severe cellulitis of his legs. Photo by James O'Connell MD

nodes that drain the area of the infection can become red, swollen, and tender. Constitutional symptoms, especially fever, can be present when the infection spreads.

Several factors can place homeless and other individuals at greater risk of developing cellulitis:

- malnutrition, exposure to the elements, lack of adequate rest, communal living with exposure to common communicable diseases, poorly-controlled chronic medical illnesses such as diabetes and peripheral vascular disease, limited access to showers and washing areas, psychiatric illness, and substance abuse are all likely to be associated with a greater risk for developing cellulitis and can hinder prevention and early treatment of this infection;

- swollen or edematous extremities are commonplace among homeless populations. This edema can lead to decreased blood flow to the extremity and cause tissue hypoxia. Changes in the integrity of the skin can result, including ulcers and chronic stasis dermatitis. Such areas of the skin are susceptible to invasion by Staphylococcus,

Streptococcus, and other bacteria that exist as normal flora of the skin;

- injection drug use can cause a chemical irritation of the skin or integument. Binswanger and colleagues assessed intravenous drug users in a San Francisco neighborhood and found that 32% had cellulitis or abscesses as a result of needle use.

Treatment

The treatment of cellulitis consists of two phases: eradication of the acute infection and preventive measures to reduce the risk of recurrence. Antibiotics are necessary to treat the acute infection. Admission to an acute care hospital is often necessary for empiric treatment with a broad-spectrum IV antibiotic, particularly for vulnerable individuals. Persons with compromised immune systems and those with chronic diseases such as diabetes are at high risk for complications from cellulitis. Other high-risk individuals include the elderly, injection drug users, and persons who are homeless.

The choice of antibiotic for the treatment of acute cellulitis depends upon the most likely organisms to be involved. *Staphylococcus aureus* and group A beta-hemolytic *Streptococcus pyogenes* (GAS) are the most common pathogens in adults, while *Haemophilus influenzae*, GAS, and *S. aureus* are seen in children. Uncommon pathogens include *Haemophilus influenzae* type b (Hib), group B streptococci (GBS) and pneumococci. Diabetics and immunocompromised persons may develop cellulitis from a variety of organisms, including *Escheria coli*, *Proteus mirabilis*, Acinetobacter, Enterobacter, and *Pseudomonas aeruginosa*. *Staphylococcus aureus* is the most common cause of cellulitis in injection drug users.

Many new antibiotics, as well as new preparations of older ones, allow once or twice a day dosing and may be good choices for homeless patients who have difficulty with TID or QID dosing regimens. These medications are more expensive than the older antibiotics and can potentially cause resistance if used frequently. We urge clinicians to use dicloxacillin (Dynapen™) or cephalexin (Keflex™) whenever possible.

Adjunctive treatment for cellulitis includes rest, hydration, proper nutrition, elevation of the affected limb, warm compresses, pain management, and the appropriate length of antibiotic treatment (usually 10 to 14 days). When the treatment is complicated by edema or excessive swelling, some clinicians have utilized a short course of diuretic therapy in order

Table 1: The Treatment of Cellulitis

ANATOMIC SITE/ MODIFYING CIRCUMSTANCES	PRIMARY REGIMEN	SECONDARY REGIMEN	COMMENTS
Extremities (not associated with venous catheter insertions, and no history of diabetes)	mild, non-toxic, can be easily monitored: dicloxacillin (Dynapen™) 500 mg PO QID X 10-14 days or cephalexin (Keflex™) 500 mg PO QID X 10-14 days	erythromycin (Eryc™, E-mycin™) 500 mg PO QID X 10-14 days or amoxicillin/clavulanate (Augmentin™) 875 mg/125 mg PO BID or 500/125 PO TID X 10-14 days or clarithromycin (Biaxin™) 500 mg PO Q12H X 10-14 days or clarithromycin ER (Biaxin XL™) 1000 mg PO QD X 10 days or azithromycin (Zithromax™) 500 mg PO QD x 1 day, then 250 mg PO QD X 4 days or clindamycin (Cleocin™) 300 mg PO Q6H X 10-14 days	With serious cellulitis requiring hospitalization: nafcillin (Nallpen™) or oxacillin (Bactocill™) 2 gm IV Q4H or cefazolin (Ancef™) 1-2 gm IV Q8H
Cellulitis in diabetics	Early and mild: 2nd or 3rd generation cephalosporins, such as cefotetan (Cefolin™) 1-3 gm IV or cefoperazone (Cefobid™) 2 gm Q12H to 4 gm Q6H		In the presence of a non-healing diabetic foot ulcer: ampicillin-sulbactam (Unasyn™) 3 gm IV Q6H or imipenum cilastatin (Primaxin™) 0.5 gm IV Q6H or meropenum (Merren™)1 gm IV Q8H
Facial cellulitis (with acute otitis media or sinusitis)	nafcillin (Nallpen™) or oxacillin (Bactocill™) 2 gm IV Q4H	ceftriaxone (Rocephin™) 2 gm IV QD or cefuroxime (Ceftin™) 1.5 gm IV Q8H	
Cellulitis in those with a serious and life-threatening allergy to penicillin allergy	Clindamycin (Cleocin™)600 mg IV Q8H or Vancomycin (Vancocin™)1 gm IV Q12H		For those with mild or non-life threatening allergies to PCN, most of the above mentioned medical regimens are well-tolerated.
For suspected or proven MRSA (methicillin-resistant S. aureus)	Vancomycin (Vancocin™) should be used		

to optimize the flow of blood and antibiotics to the affected area of the skin.

Complications

Untreated cellulitis may lead to bacteremia, endocarditis, gangrene, metastatic abscesses, and sepsis. Co-morbid conditions can impede the treatment of cellulitis and increase the likelihood of complications, such as poorly controlled diabetes, peripheral vascular disease with edema and lower extremity ulcerations, and chronic tinea pedis.

Elderly persons and homeless individuals also are at higher risk for complications.

Prevention and Control

Cellulitis can become a recurrent infection unless preventive measures are taken. Tinea pedis is often the portal of entry for the bacteria that cause cellulitis and should be aggressively treated (see chapter on Tinea Pedis). The use of support stockings can be very helpful in preventing the chronic lower extremity edema that leads to ulcers

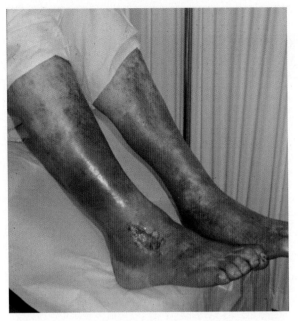

Cellulitis of the Lower Extremity. Marked swelling, redness, and warmth are characteristic of cellulitis. Photo by James O'Connell MD

and skin breakdown. Individuals with tinea pedis, chronic venous stasis dermatitis, as well as those who have undergone coronary artery bypass surgery and harvesting of the saphenous vein, should be instructed to wash their feet daily with a benzyl peroxide bar followed by an antifungal cream. All homeless individuals should receive the pneumococcal vaccine.

Special Considerations for Homeless Populations

Skin and foot problems are common among homeless people. People who live on the street are particularly prone to develop cellulitis or other skin conditions. Predisposing factors, such as onychomycosis, tinea pedis, corns, calluses, and immersion foot, are usually the result of inadequate footwear, prolonged exposure to moisture, long periods of walking and standing, and repetitive minor trauma.

Salit and colleagues compared lengths of stay and reasons for hospitalization among homeless and other low-income persons in New York City to estimate costs associated with homelessness. Skin disorders, including cellulitis, accounted for 8.4% of homeless admissions, but only 4% of admissions for poor housed patients and 3.7% of admissions to private hospitals in NYC. The mean length of stay for the homeless patients was 3.4 days more than for private patients and 1.8 days more than for the poor housed patients.

When available, medical respite care for homeless persons can be an important component of the treatment of cellulitis. Many hospitalizations can be avoided by admission to a facility where bed rest and elevation of the extremity are possible, medications can be administered, and the clinical course

carefully monitored by physicians, mid-levels, and nurses. For those homeless persons who have been admitted to the hospital for cellulitis, the length of stay can be shortened by early transfer to a respite care facility.

Summary

Cellulitis and its potential complications are seen frequently among the homeless population. Common signs of cellulitis in the lower extremities include redness, generalized swelling, pain, tenderness, and increased warmth. It can easily spread to veins, facial planes, and the lymphatics. Fever is often present if the infection spreads. Primary recommended treatment of uncomplicated infection includes either dicloxacillin (Dynapen™) or cephalexin (Keflex™). If intravenous antibiotics are needed, nafcillin (Nallpen™), oxacillin (Bactocill™), or cefazolin (Ancef™, Kefzol™) are the drugs of choice. Adjunctive treatment includes rest, hydration, proper nutrition, elevation of the affected limb, warm compresses, and pain management.

Factors that may predispose homeless persons to develop lower extremity cellulitis include chronic malnutrition, lack of adequate rest, communal living with exposure to communicable diseases, limited access to showers, and poorly controlled chronic medical illnesses. Early detection is often impeded by lack of access to health care, untreated psychiatric illness, and/or substance abuse.

Homeless persons are more often admitted to an acute care hospital for treatment, with a resultant longer length of stay than the general population. Respite facilities can aid in the timely discharge of a homeless patient or can prevent an acute care admission if the infection is noted early and treatment can be given on an outpatient basis. ▪▪

Cellulitis Medication List

Generic	Brand Name	Cost
dicloxacillin	Dynapen	$
cephalexin	Keflex	$
erythromycin	Eryc, E-mycin	$
amoxicillin-clavulanate	Augmentin	$$$
clarithromycin	Biaxin	$$$
ceftriaxone	Rocephin	$$$$$
nafcillin	Nallpen	$$$$$
oxacillin	Bactocill	$
cefazolin	Ancef, Kefzol	$$$
azithromycin	Zithromax	$$
clindamycin	Cleocin	$$
cefotetan	Cefotan	$$$$$
cefoperazone	Cefobid	$$$$$
ampicillin-sulbactam	Unasyn	$$$$$
imipenem-cilastatin	Primaxin	$$$$$
meropenem	Merrem	$$$$$
cefuroxime	Ceftin, Kefurox, Zinacef	$$$
vancomycin	Vancocin	$$$$

References

Baddour LM. Treatment of cellulitis. UpToDate; 2002. www.uptodate.com

Binswanger IA, Kral AH, Blumenthal RN, et al. High prevalence of abscesses and cellulitis among community-recruited injection drug users in San Francisco. *Clinical Infectious Diseases* 2000;30(3):579-581.

Centers for Disease Control and Prevention. Soft tissue infections among injection drug users - San Francisco, California, 1996-2000. *MMWR* 2001;50(19):381-384.

Eron LJ, Passos S. Early discharge of infected patients through appropriate antibiotic use. *Archives of Internal Medicine* 2001;161(1):61-65.

Hwang SW. Homelessness and health. *Canadian Medical Association Journal* 2001;164(2):229-233.

Johnson-Lujens LR. *Martha Rogers: the Science of Unitary Human Beings.* Newbury Park, CA: Sage Publications, Inc; 1991.

Kennedy JT, Petrone J, Deisher RW, et al. Health Care for Familyless, Runaway Street Kids. In: Brickner PW, ed. *Under the Safety Net: the Health and Social Welfare of the Homeless in the United States.* New York: W.W. Norton; 1990:82-117.

O'Connell JJ. Utilization and costs of medical services by homeless persons: a review of the literature and implications for the future. National Health Care for the Homeless Council; 1999. http://www.nhchc.org/Publications/utilization.htm

Salit SA, Kuhn EM, Hartz AJ, et al. Hospitalization costs associated with homelessness in New York City. *The New England Journal of Medicine* 1998;338(24):1734-1740.

Uphold CR, Graham MV. *Cellulitis. Clinical guidelines in adult health.* Gainesville, FL: Barmarrae Books; 1999: 207-208.

Young M. New developments in antibiotics. *Patient Care NP* 2000;8:25-47.

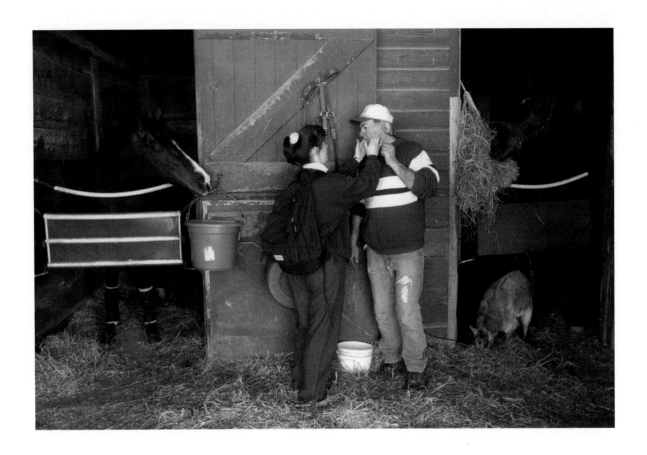

BHCHP nurse Trish Bowe offering care to
a backstretch worker outside the stables
at Suffolk Downs Racetrack in Boston.
Photo by Stan Grossfield

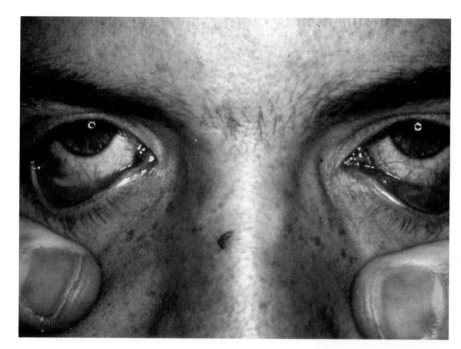

Conjunctivitis (Red Eye)

Michael S. Singer, MD, PhD
Deborah Pavan-Langston, MD, FACS
Bruce D. Levy, MD, FACP

Conjunctivitis is the most common eye condition treated by primary care providers and represents a special problem for those who live in homeless shelters or outdoors because it results from infectious or environmental exposures. The conjunctiva is a protective mucous membrane that covers the inner surface of the eyelid and extends over the eyeball to the perimeter of the cornea. This vascular tissue is a site of immune activity that responds to infection or other insults by classic inflammatory pathways, that culminate in the usual symptoms. Vasodilation renders the eye red; hypersecretion, vascular leak, and immune cells produce discharge; and inflammatory mediators provoke the patient's sense of ocular discomfort.

Prevalence and Distribution

Millions of Americans suffer from conjunctivitis every year. *Staphylococcus aureus* is the common bacterial cause in adults. *Streptococcus pneumoniae, Haemophilus influenzae,* and *Moraxella catarrhalis* are more common in children. All are readily contagious and transmitted by contact with secretions, fomites (bed linens), or contaminated surfaces. Pseudomonas is an infrequent cause. Gonococcus and Chlamydia species, which can cause serious forms of conjunctivitis, tend to spread sexually or vertically (from mother to child). Clinicians should consider these organisms in any newborn with ocular inflammation. Chlamydia is also the cause of trachoma, a cause of blindness endemic to the Middle East, North Africa, the Indian Subcontinent, and Southeast Asia; in the USA it occurs infrequently in Appalachian and Native American communities.

Mode of Transmission

Adenovirus is responsible for most cases of viral conjunctivitis. Adenovirus is endemic in emerging nations and sporadically epidemic in the industrialized world. Often associated with upper or lower respiratory tract infections, this virus is notoriously contagious and spread by direct contact, fomites, and contaminated surfaces; nosocomial infections are also common. Herpes simplex and zoster (shingles) are less common causes of viral conjunctivitis, but more serious because they can involve the cornea and cause blindness.

Noninfectious conjunctivitis is also common. Allergic conjunctivitis is evoked by seasonal or perennial allergens, including pollen, mold, dust, house mites, and animals. It is often associated with atopic conditions such as asthma, dermatitis, and rhinitis. Classically, allergic conjunctivitis develops in young adults, but severe variants can afflict

Conjunctivitis. Both eyes are reddened and tearing in this man with gonococcal conjunctivitis, one of the many infectious causes of this common eye condition. Photo courtesy of the CDC

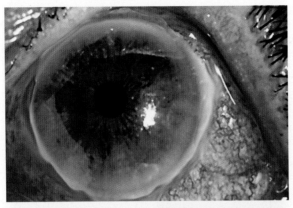

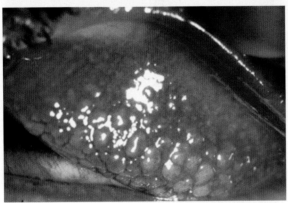

Acute Bacterial Conjunctivitis. This severe case of conjunctivitis shows engorged and reddened conjunctiva. Note the diffuse hyperemia.

Allergic Conjunctivitis. Note the papillae (raised inflammatory tissues) on the everted eyelid. Photos by Deborah Pavan-Langston MD

children or older adults. Nonspecific conjunctivitis results from dry eyes, pollution, chemical irritants, ultraviolet light, or other mechanical insults. Contact lenses, particularly when worn too much or too long, intensify the risk and repercussions of most types of conjunctivitis.

Symptoms and Diagnosis

Patients with conjunctivitis typically complain of: (1) a red eye; (2) a sensation of sand or a foreign

Table 1. When to Refer to Ophthalmology
History of ocular disease or systemic inflammatory condition
History of foreign body or other eye trauma
Neonate
Qualitative loss in visual acuity
Marked photophobia
Ciliary flush
Asymmetric or nonreactive pupil
Inability to open eye or keep it open
Copious, rapidly progressive discharge
Corneal opacity

body in the eye; and (3) a purulent, watery, or stringy discharge. Itching is the cardinal symptom of allergic conjunctivitis. Providers should bear in mind that these symptoms, particularly a red eye, also occur in less common, sight-threatening conditions. Most patients are preoccupied with discomfort and cosmetic disturbances, but the clinician's first concern should be to ensure that the patient's visual acuity is not in jeopardy (see Table 1). A brief history and exam should be done, focusing on the following areas of concern.

- *Past ophthalmic history*
  A history of eye disease, particularly keratitis, iritis, or glaucoma, often merits ophthalmic referral. The same applies for people with recurrent or refractory symptoms.
- *Past medical history*
  Patients with autoimmune, rheumatic, or vasculitic conditions can have ocular complications of systemic disease. Immunocompromised hosts or those with systemic infections require close evaluation.
- *Review of symptoms*
  Fever or upper respiratory symptoms implicate a virus. Rhinitis, asthma, or dermatitis suggest an allergic etiology. Symptoms of urethritis or cervicitis should raise suspicion for Chlamydia or gonococcus. Herpetic lesions on the face or elsewhere point to herpes virus infection. A blistering skin rash on the forehead and around the eye usually indicates zoster (shingles). History of contact with others with a red eye can be useful, especially for adenovirus. A sexual history is helpful whenever Chlamydia or gonococcus are suspected.
- *History of trauma*
  For any patient with known or suspected trauma to the eye, the provider should be careful not to diagnose conjunctivitis too hastily. Foreign body and corneal perforation should be ruled out by a fluorescein exam under cobalt blue light. The iris should be intact, and the pupils should be equally round and reactive.
- *History of chemical exposure*
  The provider should be sure not to miss any history of chemical or toxic exposure, which requires different management beyond the scope of this chapter.
- *Visual disturbances*
  Can the patient read ordinary print with

Table 2: Therapeutic Options for Conjunctivitis		
Type	**Therapy**	**Dose**
Empiric	polymyxin-bacitracin (Polysporin™)	0.5 inches QID for 7 days
	trimethoprim-polymyxin B (Polytrim™)	1-2 drops QID for 7 days
Bacterial	Polysporin™ or Polytrim™	See under Empiric
	ciprofloxacin (Ciloxan™)	1-2 drops QID for 7 days
	ofloxacin (Ocuflox™)	1-2 drops QID for 7 days
		1-2 drops QID for 7 days
Gonococcal	Ophthalmic referral necessary	Systemic
	Treat other complications and partners	
Chlamydial	Ophthalmic referral necessary	Systemic
	Treat other complications and partners	
Viral	Ocuhist™, Naphcon-A™, Visine AC™	1-2 drops QID PRN < 21 days
Allergic	Ocuhist™, Naphcon-A™, Visine AC™	1-2 drops QID PRN < 21 days
	Patanol™ or Alocril™ (2nd line)	1-2 drops BID
	Acular™ (2nd line)	1-2 drops QID PRN < 21 days
	Alomide™, Opticrom™ (3rd line)	1-2 drops QID (slow onset)
	Crolom™ (3rd line)	1-2 drops QID (slow onset)
Nonspecific	artificial tears	1-2 drops Q 1-6 hours PRN

the affected eye? Near vision should be checked in each eye with a newspaper held at a distance the patient prefers. A Snellen chart is not necessary. The patient should wear any corrective reading lenses. Low visual acuity can be described by the ability to count fingers, detect hand motions, or perceive the beam from a penlight. A discharge can cloud the patient's vision, but if it is cleansed (for example, with a damp cloth) the patient with common conjunctivitis should be able to approximate his or her baseline visual acuity. A decline in visual acuity is reason for referral to an ophthalmologist. Other visual symptoms that merit referral are photophobia, which implicates deeper inflammation, or complaints of colored halos, which suggest acute angle closure glaucoma.

The "Red Eye"

Conjunctivitis always leads to a red (hyperemic) eye, but not all red eyes imply conjunctivitis. Close inspection of the hyperemic eye shows numerous discrete, dilated blood vessels that contribute to the pink or red appearance when viewed from a distance. The dilated blood vessels spread diffusely over the mucous membrane, including the underside of the eyelid. This is in contrast to ciliary flush, where the hyperemia is concentrated within 1-3 mm of the circumference of the cornea but less on the periphery of the eye and under the eyelid. This finding, which indicates inflammation of the cornea or deeper structures, merits referral. Dilated vessels limited to a portion of the orbit usually indicate a foreign body, pterygium, episcleritis, or scleritis. A patch of blood without blood vessel definition is more consistent with subconjunctival hemorrhage; this condition is usually benign and self-limited. A layered pool of blood is called a *hyphema* and can reflect serious ocular trauma. Likewise, a layered pool of purulent fluid, or *hypopyon* implies infection of the cornea or aqueous chamber. Both hyphema and hypopyon require immediate referral.

Discomfort

The patient with conjunctivitis typically describes a foreign body sensation "like sand in the eye." This sensation is more pronounced when a virus is involved. The clinician should check to be

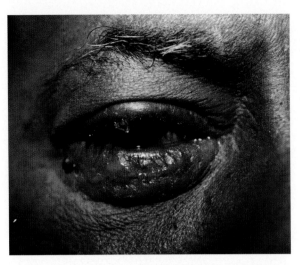

sure that the patient is able to open the eye and keep it open. If not, the cornea is likely to be involved. Corneal abrasions are caused by trauma, contact lens overuse, or vigorous eye rubbing, and should be confirmed by fluorescein exam. Otherwise, ophthalmic referral is needed to rule out bacterial keratitis (corneal infection). Itching is a classic symptom of allergic conjunctivitis. Frank pain, headache, or nausea should raise suspicion for other disorders, including uveitis or acute angle closure glaucoma.

Discharge

The quality and quantity of discharge provide clues to the type of conjunctivitis. Physical exam usually yields more reliable information than the history. An opaque discharge, with pus-like fluid pooled between the eyeball and lower lid margin, is typical of bacterial infection. A purulent discharge that is copious and rapidly progressive should arouse suspicion of a hyperacute bacterial conjunctivitis, such as gonorrhea, which requires immediate referral. A watery discharge is characteristic of viral infections. A thick, stringy discharge is more common in allergic disorders.

Preauricular nodes

A tender, inflamed preauricular node (anterior to the ear) is a clue that a virus, most likely adenovirus, is involved. Preauricular adenopathy is less common in bacterial infections.

Unilateral or bilateral symptoms

Bacterial conjunctivitis is usually bilateral. Adenoviral conjunctivitis usually starts in one eye and soon involves the other, whereas herpes is usually unilateral. Allergic conjunctivitis tends to be bilateral.

Pupil size and shape

The pupils should be equally round and reactive to light. An asymmetric, mid-dilated pupil, red eye, hazy cornea, vomiting, and patient in distress are classic signs of acute angle closure glaucoma. An asymmetric, constricted pupil and red eye are typical of uveitis.

Corneal clarity and integrity

The cornea should be examined for a white spot or other opacity, which suggests infectious keratitis. Foreign bodies can also be detected in this manner. A fluorescein exam should be done if there is any suspicion of corneal abrasion or herpes simplex or zoster keratitis; herpes will usually display a distinctive branching pattern under cobalt blue light.

Laboratory diagnosis

Discharge can be sampled for Giemsa or Gram stain and bacterial or viral culture, but in practice most conjunctivitis is treated empirically (see below). Laboratory diagnosis is preferable in suspected cases of gonococcus or Chlamydia. A tear film assay for IgE is available to diagnose allergic conjunctivitis, although history and exam are usually sufficient.

Treatment and Complications

Most conjunctivitis is self-limited. Regardless of the etiology, cold compresses can alleviate some of the symptoms. Medical therapy is summarized in Table 2.

Without treatment, bacterial conjunctivitis can require 14 days or longer to resolve or possibly become chronic. Healing is hastened with empiric therapy using polymyxin-bacitracin (Polysporin™) ophthalmic ointment, or trimethoprim-polymyxin B (Polytrim™) drops. Bacterial cases should improve within three days of treatment; if they do not, the provider should consider alternative diagnoses. Topical fluroquinolones are also available and appropriate for empiric bacterial therapy. Aminoglycosides such as tobramycin are not first-line agents for conjunctivitis.

Gonococcal conjunctivitis requires systemic treatment with ceftriaxone (Rocephin™) or ciprofloxacin (Cipro™). Empiric therapy for Chlamydia is also recommended. Chlamydia conjunctivitis requires systemic treatment with a macrolide, such as azithromycin (Zithromax™). For both conditions, treatment of sexual partners is recommended.

No specific therapy is available for non-herpetic viral conjunctivitis. Symptoms generally worsen over the first few days and then gradually resolve within 14-21 days. Some patients report relief from over-the-counter antihistamine or decongestant eye drops. Patients with suspected herpes conjunctivitis should be referred to specialty care.

Contact lenses should not be worn until bacterial or viral infection has resolved.

The mainstays in treating allergic conjunctivitis are: (1) avoidance of allergens, such as animals, dust, or pollens; (2) ophthalmic or systemic antihistamines or mast cell stabilizers; and (3) lubricating drops. Patients should be instructed not to rub their eyes. A cold wet compress (facecloth) provides some symptomatic relief. For isolated allergic conjunctivitis, the first line of therapy is an over-the-counter antihistamine or decongestant; however, rebound can result if these are used more than a month. The second line of therapy is a mast cell stabilizer, e.g. olopatadine (Patanol™), nedocromil (Alocril™), or NSAID ketorolac (Acular™). A third line is available in more potent mast cell stabilizers, e.g. cromolyn sodium (Crocom™) or ledoxamide tromethamune (Alomide™). Many patients with allergic conjunctivitis suffer from concurrent rhinitis or dermatitis, for which they will often take systemic antihistamines. While these agents tend to quell the ocular inflammatory reaction, they also reduce eye secretions and lead to dryness, which aggravates allergic conjunctivitis. Solutions to this problem include non-prescription artificial tears or non-sedating antihistamines, which are less likely to dry the eye.

Nonspecific conjunctivitis is treated with lubricating eye drops. Topical antihistamines or decongestants can provide some relief.

Topical steroids are rarely indicated for conjunctivitis, with the exception of some severe allergic conditions. Steroids carry significant risk and should not be prescribed by primary care providers. Topical anesthetics, such as tetracaine, facilitate the eye exam but should never be prescribed because they inhibit the eye's protective reflexes.

The long-term complications of acute conjunctivitis are relatively few. Occasionally there is dry eye or residual corneal haze, which resolves over time. Chronic conjunctivitis in its most severe form can lead to blood vessel growth over the cornea (pannus) and lasting visual impairment.

Prevention and Control
Bacterial and viral conjunctivitis
Prompt treatment of bacterial conjunctivitis

minimizes the transmission of this infection. Infected persons should be instructed to wash their hands frequently and try not to touch their eyes. They should not share towels, linens, handkerchiefs, clothes, sunglasses, makeup, or eyedrops. Anyone with a concurrent upper respiratory tract infection should take steps to minimize airborne droplets. Gonococcal and Chlamydial transmission can be minimized by safe sex practices and careful handwashing.

Allergic conjunctivitis
Patients should be educated on how to avoid pollens, animals, dust, or other known allergens. Artificial tears, which dilute allergens in the tear film, can be beneficial. Patients should be instructed to avoid rubbing the eye, which can introduce more allergens, aggravate the inflammatory response, and increase the risk of long-term corneal complications.

Special Considerations for Homeless Populations
Adenoviral conjunctivitis is highly contagious. Outbreaks occur frequently in schools, hospitals, and other shared facilities. Since homeless shelters are at similar risk, staff and guests should be sure to follow infection control guidelines outlined in this chapter and elsewhere in this book. Allergic conjunctivitis is a special problem for homeless people, who have less control over the air quality in their surroundings. Special arrangements should be made to keep sleeping quarters free from dust and animal dander. Linens should be laundered frequently in hot water. A plastic bag between pillow and pillowcase forms a barrier to dust mites. Staff should be aware that significant amounts of cat and dog dander can be delivered on the clothing of other guests. For patients with seasonal allergies, shelters should provide a space indoors, particularly in the morning, on days when pollen counts are high. ■

The authors of this chapter gratefully acknowledge the invaluable contribution of the late Thomas Bennett, MD, who authored this chapter in the original Manual.

Conjunctivitis Medication List

Generic	Brand	Cost
polymyxin B + bacitracin	Polysporin	$
polymyxin B + trimethoprim	Polytrim	$
ciprofloxacin	Ciloxan	$$
ofloxacin	Ocuflox	$$
olopatadine	Patanol	$$$
nedocromil	Alocril	$$
ketorolac	Acular	$$$
lodoxamide	Alomide	$$$
cromolyn sodium	Crolom, Opticrom	$$$
artificial tears	Hypotears, Tears Naturale	$

References

Leibowitz HM. The red eye. *New England Journal of Medicine* 2000;343(5):345-351.

Pavan-Langston D. *Manual of Ocular Diagnosis and Treatment.* Philadelphia: Lippincott, Williams, and Wilkins; 2002. Also available in Spanish.

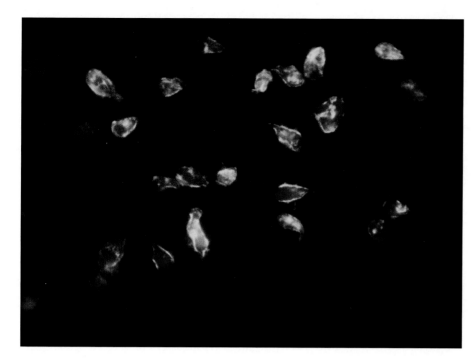

Diarrhea

Joel Bass, MD

Diarrhea can be a persistent problem in any crowded setting, especially with diapered children, communal bathrooms, and shared eating facilities. Shelters are particularly prone to outbreaks of diarrhea because food management may involve many different people with varying degrees of training in safe food handling. Shelters commonly receive donations of prepared food without any information about the management of the food prior to its arrival. Helpful strategies for handling such food donations are discussed in Part VI on Food Management.

Fortunately, many steps to prevent and control the incidence of diarrhea can be taken if the staff understands how the illnesses are spread and all those in the shelter follow a few simple guidelines.

Causes

Dozens of infectious agents can cause diarrhea, including:

- viruses (Norwalk, Norwalk-like, and rotovirus);
- bacteria (Campylobacter, Salmonella, Shigella, Staphylococcus, Yersinia and *E.coli*);
- parasites (Giardia, Cryptosporidium).

Furthermore, any child or adult recovering from infectious diarrhea may have damaged the lining of the intestine to such a degree that chronic diarrhea results. At this point, the infection is no longer the primary concern, and focus should shift to the malabsorption of dietary carbohydrates that can lead to malnutrition.

Symptoms

Infectious agents in all three categories can cause diarrhea of varying degrees of severity and duration. Symptoms often overlap from one type of diarrhea to another. Diarrhea caused by viruses tends to be more self-limiting than that resulting from either bacteria or parasites. Parasites are apt to produce subacute or chronic diarrhea, while bacterial diarrhea is often an acute illness. Needless to say, exceptions to these generalizations are common.

Gastrointestinal infection may produce a range of symptoms from mild to life threatening. Mild symptoms include an increase in the frequency of stools, a softening or liquefying of the texture of stools, abdominal cramping, gas, nausea, vomiting, weakness, and fever. Severe diarrhea produces watery, voluminous, or explosive stools, which can lead to dehydration. Stools may contain blood or mucous depending on the specific cause of diarrhea.

*Giardia.
A photomicrograph of a positive indirect immunofluorescence test checking for the presence of Giardia lamblia. This protozoan organism causes the disease Giardiasis, a diarrheal disorder of the small intestine. Photo courtesy of the CDC*

Campylobacter	
Symptoms:	Diarrhea, fever, abdominal pain, sometimes blood in stool, nausea and vomiting
Onset:	1 to 7 days after exposure, but can be longer
Infectious period:	2 to 3 weeks without treatment; 2 to 3 days with therapy
Source:	Contact with feces of infected persons, exposure to feces of infected household pets or wild animals, including birds; improperly cooked or stored foods of animal origin
Treatment:	Erythromycin (shortens course of illness), ciprofloxacin (not in children) Treat 5 to 7 days
Infected person:	Special precautions for all those who are symptomatic No food handling until the symptoms have resolved and 2 stool cultures taken 48 hours apart are negative
Close contacts:	Not infectious after 2 to 3 days Treating close contacts may limit spread of disease

Complications

Young children and infants are at the greatest risk of rapid deterioration because of the dehydration brought on by acute diarrhea. Caregivers should closely monitor any young child with diarrhea to guard against dehydration.

The signs of severe dehydration are:
- decrease in the production of tears;
- no urine output for 8 hours;
- depressed fontanel (in infants);
- dry mouth, tongue, and skin.

Anyone with these signs, particularly an infant or child, needs medical attention immediately.

Young children, the elderly, and those chronically ill also risk systematic infection from certain infectious diarrheas such as Salmonella and *E. coli*.

Prevalence

Although scant information in known about the prevalence of diarrheal illness in shelters, experience suggests that it is widespread. One study of shelters for battered women and their children found that 9 of the 73 facilities reviewed had outbreaks of diarrhea involving more than 10 people.

Transmission

Infectious diarrhea spreads directly or indirectly from person to person. If staff and guests do not wash their hands carefully after using the toilet or changing a diaper, an infected person can easily contaminate food, surfaces, or objects with stool that then contacts the hands or mouths of others. The amount of stool needed to cause disease varies with the different organisms.

Diarrheal germs commonly spread when people are preparing and serving food and when children, particularly those in diapers, play together.

Areas within shelters conducive to the spread of organisms include:
- communal bathrooms;
- kitchens;
- changing tables.

Some persons with bacterial or parasitic infections may remain asymptomatic. However, these "carriers" can still transmit the disease to others.

Food Management

The primary focus of this chapter is the spread of diarrhea from an infected person to other people.

Cryptosporidium	
Symptoms:	Frequent, watery diarrhea Can be prolonged (up to 20 episodes per day) and lead to weight loss and malnutrition Can become chronic and/or disseminate in persons with poor immune systems
Onset:	2 to 14 days
Infectious period:	Unknown
Source:	Animals, humans (easily spread in day care centers), and water
Treatment:	Usually supportive in otherwise healthy persons In immuno-compromised persons, IV hyperglobulin therapy
Infected person:	No food handling until all symptoms are gone
Close contacts:	Evaluate stool of all who are symptomatic Avoid food handling until asymptomatic

Giardia	
Symptoms:	Often none May have intermittent bouts of diarrhea, chronic diarrhea with malabsorbtion, and/or anemia Children may show failure to thrive
Onset:	1 to 4 weeks
Infectious period:	Variable; until all cysts are gone
Source:	Infected humans, animals, contaminated water Commonly spread in day care May also be spread through oral-anal sexual practices
Treatment:	Quinicrine (Atabrine™) is 85 to 95% effective but bitter and difficult to give to children. Can cause GI upset and occasionally jaundice. Metronidazole (Flagyl™) is 90% effective but not approved for use in Giardiasis in the USA. Possibly carcinogenic. Little data available on safety in children. Causes a metallic taste as well as nausea, dizziness, and headache. Use with alcohol can cause a disulfiram-like (Antabuse™) reaction. Furazolidone (Furoxone™) is 80% effective. Liquid suspension is available. Generally the treatment of choice for young children. Can cause GI distress, headache, and dizziness. Can likewise cause a disulfirim-like reaction when taken with alcohol. Paramomycin (Humatin™) is 50 to 70% effective. Has been used for pregnant women because the drug is not measurably absorbed from the intestines. All of the above drugs may have to be repeated in 2 weeks in the event of therapy failure
Infected person:	Special precautions for all those who are symptomatic All family members should be evaluated with stool smears for ova and parasites regardless of symptoms
Close contacts:	In a family shelter, an initial smear for ova and parasites should be done on persons who are symptomatic. If the problem persists, smears for ova and parasites should be done on all persons living or working in the shelter. Infected persons should not handle food until symptoms have resolved and 2 stool cultures taken 48 hours apart are negative. Kitchen workers, regardless of symptoms, with contact to an infected person, should avoid food handling until 2 stool cultures taken 48 hours apart and after the last possible exposure are negative.

Salmonella	
Symptoms:	Diarrhea, cramping, fever, headache, nausea, sometimes vomiting May be complicated by bacteremia and/or focal infection, or a multisystem disorder called enteric fever Asymptomatic in some, constipation in some, especially with enteric fever
Onset:	6 to 72 hours; 3 to 60 days with enteric fever; usually 7 to 14 days
Infectious period:	Until the organisms are no longer excreted; can be weeks or even years in chronic carriers Antibiotic therapy can prolong carriage
Source:	Humans, household and farm animals, improperly prepared or stored foods, contaminated water and food
Treatment:	Usually none for uncomplicated cases of gastroenteritis Children less than 3 months old, people at risk for invasive disease (such as immunocompromised), and persons with *Salmonella typhii* should be treated with ampicillin or trimethoprim-sulfamethoxazole (Bactrim™, Septra™) (if the organism shows sensitivity in cultures) Ciprofloxacin should be used for strains resistant to ampicillin and trimethoprim-sulfamethoxazole (Bactrim™, Septra™), although this antibiotic should be avoided in children
Infected person:	Special precautions for all who are symptomatic No food handling until symptoms have resolved and 2 stool cultures taken 48 hours apart are negative
Close contacts:	No food handling by symptomatic close contacts until symptoms have resolved and 2 cultures taken 48 hours apart are negative In addition, kitchen workers (regardless of symptoms) with contact to an infected person should avoid food handling until 2 cultures taken 48 hours apart and after the last possible exposure are negative Can return if asymptomatic

Shigella

Symptoms:	Mild to severe diarrhea, the latter being associated with sudden onset of fever, headache and possibly vomiting Stools may contain blood or mucous
Onset:	1 to 7 days, usually 2 to 4 days
Infectious period:	Until no longer passed in the stool, usually no longer than 4 weeks Antibiotics can shorten this period to less than 1 week
Source:	Humans are the only known source Crowding, particularly in setting with few handwashing facilities, can promote spread Eating contaminated food or water or mouthing infected objects can also spread Few organisms are needed to cause infection
Treatment:	Antibiotics are recommended in most cases. Treat for 5 days. Generally trimethoprim-sulfamethoxazole (Bactrim™, Septra™), ampicillin, or ciprofloxacin (Cipro™) (not in children) are effective However, it is important to check the sensitivity pattern of the organism. Resistant strains use ceftriaxone (Rocephin™), or cefotaxime (Claforan™).
Infected person:	Special precautions for all those who are symptomatic No food handling until symptoms have resolved and 2 stool cultures taken 48 hours apart are negative

Staphylococcus

Symptoms:	Abrupt onset of severe cramps, vomiting and diarrhea Fever is not usually associated with this infection
Onset:	Very short, 30 minutes to 6 hours
Infectious period:	Unable to be transmitted by the sick person Can be spread to food by staphylococcal carriers until organisms have cleared from site of colonization
Source:	Usually by food handlers with staphylococci colonized in sites including normal skin, lesions (often on the face or hands), nose and throat
Treatment:	Supportive; no antibiotics needed
Infected person:	No control measures necessary Review of foods eaten within 8 hours of onset should occur. If eaten in shelter, evaluate food handlers for lesions, poor hygiene.
Close contacts:	No restrictions

Many foods, particularly dairy and meat products, are inherently prone to bacterial growth and can cause diarrheal outbreaks. If food is properly bought, stored, prepared, and served, the risk of illness is minimal. Please see Part VI on Food Management.

Diagnosis

Different causes of diarrhea are indistinguishable by observation alone. To determine the specific cause of illness, a stool culture or smear is necessary. Diarrhea happens very frequently in crowded settings, and the decision to culture the stool is based on several factors. In adult shelters, symptoms of diarrhea that have lasted three days or more, or are severe enough to risk dehydration, warrant a stool culture to rule out common bacteria such as Campylobacter or Salmonella.

Family shelters are comparable to day care settings, which often experience Shigella and Giardia infections. In family shelters, health providers should collect stool specimens for both bacteria and parasites in symptomatic people. Once a child or an adult has been diagnosed with a bacterial or parasitic

Yersinia	
Symptoms:	Fever, headache, watery diarrhea (blood, mucous, WBCs commonly in stool), abdominal pain Can cause a syndrome resembling acute appendicitis in children Arthritis, ostromyelitis, septicemia, abcesses of the liver and spleen, and skin rashes have been reported in certain types (Y. enterocolitica).
Onset:	4 to 6 days typically; range 1 to 14 days
Infectious period:	For as long as the organism is excreted (up to 6 weeks)
Source:	Household and wild animals, contaminated water and food
Treatment:	Trimethoprim-sulfamethoxazole (Bactrim™, Septra™), chloramphenicol (Chloromycetin™), aminoglycosides, tetracycline (not in children less than 8 years old)
Infected person:	Special precautions for all those who are symptomatic No food handling until symptoms have resolved and 2 stool cultures taken 48 hours apart are negative
Close contacts:	No food handling by symptomatic close contacts until 2 stool cultures taken 48 hours apart are negative and symptoms have resolved Kitchen workers (regardless of symptoms) with close contact to an infected person should avoid food handling until 2 stool cultures taken 48 hours apart and after the last possible exposure are negative

illness, all other symptomatic people in the shelter who share toilet facilities or have a common food source should have specimens sent for analysis.

Treatment

Specific treatment of diarrhea will vary depending on culture results. People with bacterial or parasitic diarrhea always need medical supervision. Some general observations about supportive care follow.

Infants and children

An infant with diarrhea can dehydrate rapidly and the condition may become life threatening. Any child under 12 months of age with more than three episodes of diarrhea or unusually loose stools per day, especially if accompanied by vomiting and/ or fever, or who seems very weak or sick, requires a prompt medical evaluation. Any child with no urine output for 8 hours also requires a medical evaluation.

Most cases of diarrhea are mild. In these cases the child should continue a regular diet with an emphasis on starchy foods that are better absorbed. Fluids should also be encouraged, except for fruit juices and soft drinks that can make the diarrhea worse. Commercial oral solutions (e.g., Pedialyte™, Enfalyte™) are preferable to traditional clear liquids. Lactose intolerance can commonly follow a diarrheal illness and last from 2 to 6 weeks. Soy-

based, lactose-free formula may be recommended as a substitute for infants who develop this problem.

Prevention and Control

In Massachusetts, as in many other states, the law requires that outbreaks of diarrhea or episodes of infectious diarrhea be reported to the local health department.

Specific prevention and control measures will depend upon the population in the shelter and the physical arrangements of the building. In the unusual situation where resources and circumstances permit, screening of all shelter residents for stool pathogens prior to entry may be helpful. Shelter residents with poor immune systems may be at special risk during outbreaks and should see a health provider.

Summary

Diarrhea can be a common problem in crowded places such as shelters. The presence of diapered children, the use of shared bathrooms and kitchens, and inappropriate food management heighten the likelihood of diarrheal outbreaks in shelters. While an episode of diarrhea is usually short-lived, it can be very serious, particularly in young children and people with other chronic illness.

Diarrhea is spread when a person gets infected feces on the hands and then touches other hands, food, or mouthed objects. Some people can carry germs that cause diarrhea but have no symptoms themselves.

Careful hand washing with soap and warm water after using the bathroom or diapering a child is the best way to prevent the spread of diarrhea. Questions regarding episodes of diarrhea should be brought to a health provider. The local board of health and appropriate health agencies are also sources of information regarding the control of diarrhea.

Contact a health provider whenever:
- an adult has had diarrhea lasting three or more days;
- a child has diarrhea accompanied by vomiting or fever;
- a person with diarrhea appears dehydrated;
- more than two people from a family shelter have diarrhea simultaneously;
- the same organism has been identified in two different cases of diarrhea within two weeks in the same shelter. ▦

References

Bass JL, Brennan P, Mehta KA, et. al. Pediatric problems in a suburban shelter for homeless families. *Pediatrics*1990;85(1):33-38.

Donowitz LG ed. *Infection Control in the Child Care Center and Preschool.* Williams and Wilkens;1996.

Gross TP, Rosenberg ML. Shelters for battered women and their children: an under-recognized source of communicable transmission. *American Journal of Public Health* 1987;77(9):1198-1201.

Isolation and quarantine regulations. (Massachusetts Department of Public Health). 2004.

Pickering LK, Peter G, Baker CJ, et al., eds. *The 2003 Red Book: Report of the Committee on Infectious Disease.* Elk Grove Village, Illinois: American Academy of Pediatrics; 2003.

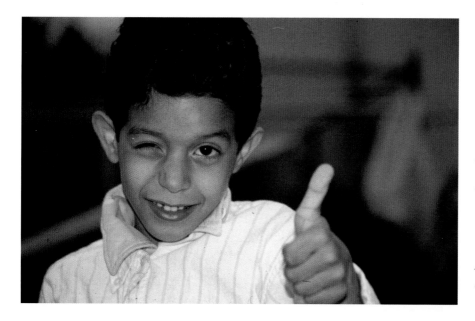

Haemophilus Influenza Type b (Hib)

Melinda Thomas, PA-C
Stacy Kirkpatrick, NP

Haemophilus influenzae type b (Hib) is a bacterium capable of causing serious infection, primarily in children. These bacteria exist in two forms: non-encapsulated and encapsulated.

- Non-encapsulated forms of the bacteria are commonly carried in the upper respiratory passages and can cause ear infections, acute exacerbations of chronic obstructive pulmonary disease (COPD), and a number of other infections that are generally not life threatening.

- Encapsulated *Haemophilus influenzae* comes in six types designated by letters "a" through "f". Type b (Hib) causes 95% of serious invasive infections, including blood infections, meningitis, epiglottitis, cellulitis, pneumonia, arthritis, osteomyelitis (infection of the bone), and pericarditis (infection of membrane surrounding the heart). Children from the ages of 2-4 months to 2-3 years are most susceptible to these infections. Native American and Alaskan children have a 10-fold increase of invasive Hib disease.

Hib Infection in Children

Meningitis

Approximately two-thirds of all cases of invasive Hib disease present as meningitis, an infection of the membrane surrounding the brain and spinal cord. Initial symptoms of meningitis may be similar to a common upper respiratory infection and can progress to include fever, a stiff neck, headache, nausea, vomiting, and a change in mental status such as confusion or disorientation. Infants may have a bulging fontanel or "soft spot". Occasionally these symptoms can progress very rapidly, leading to death in only a few hours. For this reason anyone suspected of having meningitis must be promptly evaluated by a medical professional. People suspected of having meningitis will undergo lumbar puncture (spinal tap) for inspection and culture of cerebrospinal fluid so the exact bacterial cause can be identified. Meningitis causes death in 2-5% of all cases, even with treatment. Permanent neurological damage occurs in 15-30% of all children with meningitis, including hearing loss, mental retardation, vision loss, seizure disorders, and speech and motor delays.

Epiglottitis

Epiglottitis is an infection of the upper airway that causes swelling of the tissue that covers and protects the larynx when swallowing. This infection is seen most often in children between the ages of 2-5 years. Symptoms of fever and sore throat develop quickly, followed within hours by difficulty with speech, swallowing, and breathing. Airway obstruction can cause children to make harsh, high-pitched breathing sounds known as stridor. A child with epiglottitis appears quite ill and often leans forward with mouth opened and jaw thrust forward in an effort to open the blocked airway.

This young boy plays in a motel near Boston while his mother is seen by the BHCHP pediatrician and nurse practitioner. Photo by James O'Connell MD

Cellulitis

Cellulitis or infection of the skin due to Hib is seen most often in children less than two years of age. Infection occurs most often on the face and especially on the cheeks or around the eye.

Other Infections

Other less common infections caused by Hib include: pneumonia; septic arthritis, or joint infection; osteomyelitis, or bone infection; and pericarditis, or infection of the membrane surrounding the heart.

Hib in Adults

Hib vaccines were not developed until the 1980s. Most adults are immune to infection with Hib, probably because they formed protective antibodies to the bacterium after childhood exposure.

Adults considered at increased risk of serious infection for Hib include:
- individuals who have had their spleens removed;
- persons with compromised immune systems due to HIV or AIDS, cancer, organ transplant, etc.;
- those with diabetes and chronic respiratory disease;
- the elderly;
- persons institutionalized or living in crowded situations, such as shelters or dormitories.

Transmission

Hib is thought to spread via respiratory droplets (coughing) and nasal secretions (sneezing). Some people, known as carriers, have no symptoms and never become sick, but are still capable of spreading Hib. Sharing drinking glasses, cigarettes, infant toys, bottles, and other objects that have been in contact with the mouth and saliva may spread Hib.

Bacteria enter the body through the nose and throat and can spread to the skin, lungs, ears, joints, blood, and brain. 2-5% of unimmunized children are carriers of Hib. The highest rates of Hib are found in children aged three to five years, people in crowded conditions (shelters, daycare, etc.), and persons in direct contact with an Hib case. Hib is not considered to be highly contagious since only a small percentage of people exposed to the disease actually become ill. However, household contacts are 500-600 times more likely to develop infection from exposure to an infected household member. Newborns are somewhat protected from Hib because of maternal antibodies but this wanes after two months.

Diagnosis

The first step in the diagnosis of Hib infection is the recognition of the common signs and symptoms of this infection. A careful history is very important, including when, where and how the symptoms started. Clinicians should inquire about close contacts of the patient who are sick. If Hib is suspected, testing should be done which includes blood cultures as well as Gram stain and cultures of the infected body fluid (e.g. CSF, middle ear, pleural, joint).

Treatment

Delaying the start of antibiotic therapy can lead to poor outcomes. Therefore anyone suspected of having invasive Hib disease needs prompt evaluation by a doctor or health care professional and treatment in the hospital. Patients with suspected or known invasive Hib disease are placed under precautions for 24 hours in an attempt to prevent the spread of disease. Hib is treated using a third-generation cephalosporin. Rifampin (Rifadin™) is then used to remove any remaining organisms that may have colonized the upper respiratory tract. Persons with Hib meningitis may also receive treatment with an IV steroid to prevent hearing loss.

The issue of antibiotic resistance is important to consider because strains of Hib resistant to ampicillin, the drug once considered first-line therapy, are now common in the United States. Rates of resistance vary by region.

Prevention and Control

Vaccination

Vaccination is the best way to prevent and control Hib and is responsible for a 99% decrease in the disease from 1989 to 1997 among children under five years of age. Before the vaccine was developed, about 20,000 persons in the USA developed invasive Hib disease annually (meningitis, bacteremia, epiglottitis, pneumonia, cellulitis, arthritis, osteomyelitis, pericarditis). One in 200 children experienced invasive disease before age five. Meningitis was the most common manifestation of infection, occurring in about 60% of young children who experienced invasive disease and resulting in about 600 deaths per year. Hib was the most important cause of invasive bacterial disease in young children before the introduction of an effective Hib vaccine in 1990.

The first vaccination for Hib, designed to be given to children 18 months of age and older, was introduced in 1985 but was not very effective. In the same year a more effective vaccine for children ages 15 months and older was introduced. In 1990 a vaccine for infants was approved.

In 1991 the American Academy of Pediatrics Committee on Infectious Diseases and the Advisory Committee on Immunization Practices recommended that all children should be immunized with the vaccine beginning at two months of age. A four-dose schedule for most Hib vaccines is recommended (at 2, 4, 6, and 12-15 months). The dose at six months is not needed if PRP-OMP vaccine is used. Children over the age of seven months who have not been immunized can start with an abbreviated schedule because of their age. Vaccination is generally not recommended for healthy children age 5 and over, as the majority of these children have developed immunity through previous asymptomatic infection. Immunocompromised children and adults who have not been immunized in the past can follow an abbreviated schedule based on their particular medical conditions.

Two combination vaccines are available in the USA. TriHIBit combines DTaP (diphtheria, tetanus, and acellular pertussis) and Hib, but is only recommended as a booster shot. COMVAX combines hepatitis B and Hib, but must not be used in infants whose mothers are hepatitis B surface antigen positive.

Although all of the vaccines have an excellent safety record and do not interfere with other vaccines given at the same time, adverse reactions have occurred. These reactions are uncommon, short lived, and include fever, irritability, swelling, redness, and pain at the injection site. Vaccination should be delayed in individuals with moderate or severe acute illness, and no Hib vaccines should be given to children less than six weeks old.

Although the incidence of Hib is low, illness and death still occur among infants who have not completed the primary series of Hib vaccination. Certain situations have been documented that hinder people from completing the vaccination schedule: families with younger mothers (under 30 years of age); families with large numbers of children; and having multiple vaccination providers. Families in shelters experience frequent changes in address, health care providers, daycare centers, and schools, making it difficult to coordinate and follow a tight immunization schedule. At every early childhood health care visit, providers should conduct a thorough assessment of vaccination status in order to help with vaccination compliance.

Post-Exposure Prophylaxis

Another method of controlling Hib is to treat individuals who have been exposed to Hib infection. Prophylaxis for household contacts is no longer indicated if all contacts under age four are fully vaccinated against Hib disease. A child is considered fully immunized under the following conditions:

- at least one dose of conjugate vaccine at 15-59 months of age; or
- one dose of conjugate vaccine at 12-14 months of age, followed by booster at 15 months; or
- two or more doses of conjugate vaccine before 12 months of age, followed by a booster at age 12-15 months.

Following a case of Hib infection in a family member, household contacts should receive rifampin (Rifadin™) if there is at least one inadequately vaccinated child less than four years old. Prophylaxis is also indicated if there are any immunocompromised children in the household. Prophylaxis of contacts in daycare/preschool/shelter settings is controversial, but is generally indicated if there have been at least 25 hours of exposure by incompletely immunized children under age two years. Prophylaxis is also indicated after two or more cases have occurred within a 60-day period in any facility with incompletely immunized children. In these cases all children and staff should be treated. If all children under four years of age are fully vaccinated, then no treatment is indicated.

Treatment includes the antibiotic rifampin (Rifadin™), administered once daily for four days in a dose of 20 mg/kg (maximum daily dose is 600 mg) or 10 mg/kg in infants younger than one month. Treatment should be implemented quickly since efficacy declines after 14 days.

Summary

Haemophilus influenzae type b infection can be very serious and cause severe, long-term complications. Thanks to the development of a vaccine, the incidence of disease has declined dramatically since the first edition of this manual in 1991. From 1989 to 1997, disease attributable to Hib among children under five years of age declined 99%. Invasive Hib infections are now reportable to state health departments, which in turn help local public health professionals understand and track current disease prevalence and patterns.

Bacterial resistance to antibiotic therapy in the treatment of Hib infection is on the rise and rapidly becoming a major concern. Moreover, homeless individuals have an increased risk of developing Hib because of the crowded living conditions of shelters. Homeless families who move and change medical providers frequently are less likely to finish the immunization schedule. Thus the importance of taking a vaccination history from every child can not be underestimated. One of the objectives of Healthy People 2010 is the elimination of all invasive diseases among children under the age of five by the year 2010. The availability of vaccines, the tracking of disease patterns by state and federal health departments, and prophylactic post exposure treatment should help attain this goal. ▪

The authors of this chapter gratefully acknowledge the invaluable contribution of George Alliegro, MD, who authored this chapter in the original Manual.

Haemophilus Influenzae (Hib) Medication List		
Generic	Brand	Cost
rifampin	Rifadin, Rimactane	$$$

References

Burns IT, Zimmerman RK. Haemophilus influenza type B disease, vaccines and care of exposed individuals. *Journal of Family Practice* 2000;49(9 Suppl):S7-13.

Centers for Disease Control and Prevention. Progress towards elimination of Haemophilus influenza type B invasive disease among infants and children -- United States. *MMWR* 2002;51(11):234-237.

Luman ET, McCauley MM, Stokely S, et al. Timelines of childhood immunizations. *Pediatrics* 2002;110(5):935-939.

Meissner HC, Pickering LK. Control of disease attributable to Haemophilus influenzae type B and the national immunization program. *Pediatrics* 2002;110(4):820-823.

Pasternack MS. Bacteriology and epidemiology of Haemophilus influenza. UpToDate; 2000. www.uptodate.com

World Health Organization. Vaccines, immunization and biologicals, Haemophilus influenzae type B vaccine. World Health Organization; 2002. http://www.who.int.com

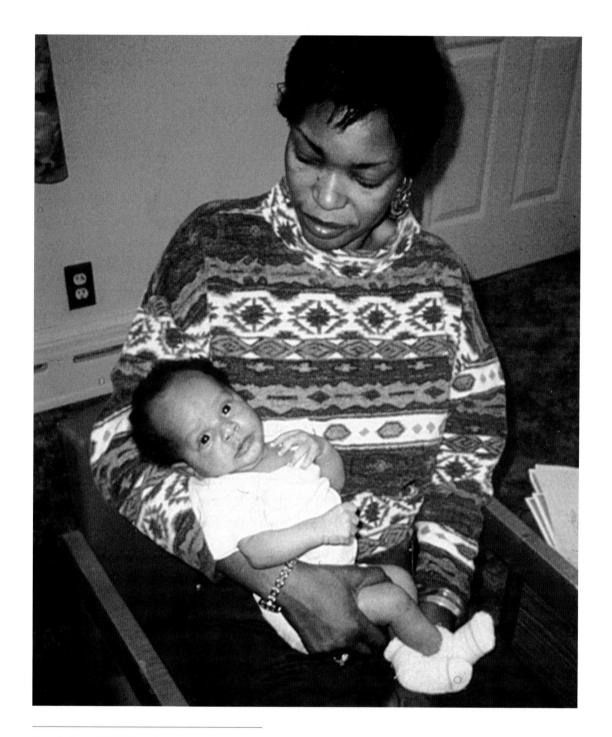

Betty Latham, BHCHP's senior case manager, cares for a child in a motel while the mother receives care from the medical team.
Photo by James O'Connell

Overview of Viral Hepatitis

	A	B	C	D	E
Virus Family	Picornaviridae	Hepadnaviridae	Flaviviridae	N/A	Appears to be member of Caliciviridae
Transmission	Fecal-oral, permucosal	Percutaneous, permucosal	Percutaneous, permucosal	Percutaneous, permucosal	Fecal-oral (especially contaminated water)
Chronicity	None	6%-10% of adults	75%-85%	Average 6%	25%-50% of children age 1-5 years; 70%-90% of infants
Onset	Usually abrupt	Usually insidious	Insidious	Usually abrupt	Usually abrupt
Incubation	Average 28 days; range 15-45 days	Average 60-90 days; range 45-180 days	Average 6-7 weeks; range 2-26 weeks	21-90 days	Average 40 days; range 15-60 days

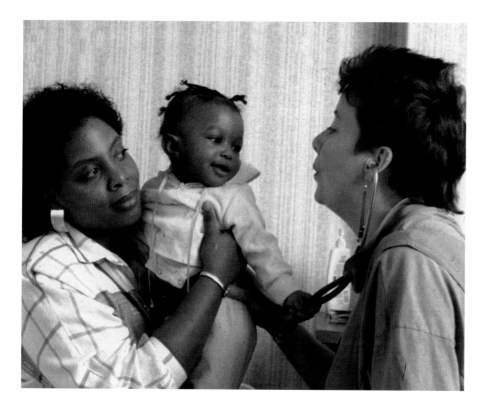

Hepatitis A

Lori Fantry, MD, MPH

Hepatitis A, once called "short incubation" or "infectious" hepatitis, is a viral infection that involves the liver. Infection with hepatitis A leads to symptoms that are very similar to other types of hepatitis. Unlike hepatitis B and C, hepatitis A is rarely fatal and does not lead to chronic liver disease. Nonetheless, hepatitis A is a significant cause of illness and suffering in many parts of the world, including the USA.

Prevalence and Distribution

Hepatitis A is common throughout the world. In the developing countries, the incidence of hepatitis A is very high due to overcrowding and poor sanitation. The highest rates in the USA are in Arizona, Alaska, Oregon, New Mexico, and Utah. Approximately 33% of persons living in the USA have been infected with hepatitis A.

Mode of Transmission

Hepatitis A virus is spread primarily by the fecal-oral route, either through person-to-person contact or ingestion of contaminated food or water. Transmission is often facilitated by poor personal hygiene, lack of sanitation, and oral-anal sexual contact. Common sources of contaminated food include shellfish, frozen raspberries and strawberries, and milk.

Hepatitis A virus can also be directly transmitted through transfusions of blood or blood products, although this is much less common due to the brief period of time that hepatitis A virus

remains in the blood of an infected person. The increased risk for hepatitis A infection among drug users is primarily due to poor hygiene rather than transmission through blood.

Children born to mothers with past or present hepatitis A infection are not at risk for infection in utero or at birth unless the mother is jaundiced at the time of delivery. Breastfeeding is not a mode of transmission. Urine and saliva do not transmit hepatitis A virus.

About half the time, the person transmitting hepatitis A virus cannot be identified. Often the source identified is a young child with no or minimal symptoms. Stools of infected persons are infectious from approximately 2 weeks before until about 1 week after the appearance of yellow skin (jaundice). The most infectious period is before jaundice appears.

Symptoms and Diagnosis

The clinical course of hepatitis A varies from person to person. Some people, especially infants

BHCHP nurse practitioner Jennifer Burroughs and family advocate Jocelyn Beverly perform a well-child examination at the Milner Hotel. Photo by David Comb

less than two years old, never develop symptoms after infection. Older people have a higher frequency of symptoms and tend to get a more severe illness. Symptoms usually develop within 28 days after exposure. This period of incubation may be as short as 15 days or as long as 50 days. Initial symptoms usually include fever, fatigue, poor appetite, nausea, and vomiting. Diarrhea occurs more commonly in children (see Table 1). Cough, sore throat, coryza (runny nose and eyes), and arthralgias (joint aches) have been reported in some outbreaks. As with other types of hepatitis, hepatitis A can alter taste and smell.

After several days to a week, the initial symptoms usually begin to diminish (see Figure 1). At this point, the infected person may develop yellow skin and eyes, dark urine, light stools, itching, and abdominal pain. Weight loss may continue throughout the illness. In most cases, symptoms of hepatitis A resolve within 1 to 2 months.

Once infected with hepatitis A virus, a person is immune from further infection with hepatitis A for life. There is still a risk, however, from other types of hepatitis.

Hepatitis A cannot be differentiated from other types of hepatitis by symptoms alone. A blood test, the immunoglobulin M antibody to hepatitis A (IgM anti-HAV), is obtained to diagnose acute hepatitis A. This test becomes positive 5-10 days before the onset of symptoms and remains positive for up to 6 months after infection. IgG anti-HAV also becomes positive early in the course of infection, but usually remains positive for life and thus cannot be used to differentiate present from past infection. However, IgG anti-HAV is useful in determining whether or not a person is a candidate for hepatitis A vaccination.

Treatment and Complications

No specific treatment is available for hepatitis A. Certain measures can alleviate the symptoms. Bed rest may provide some comfort. If the person is having frequent vomiting, caregivers should watch for signs of dehydration.

Infected people should avoid alcohol and drugs, legal and illegal, that are metabolized or broken down by the liver. For this reason, aspirin is a safe alternative to acetaminophen (Tylenol™) for fever and muscle aches except in children less than 18 years old who are at risk for a liver-brain disorder called Reye syndrome.

Although most people with hepatitis A recover completely within 1 to 2 months, 10-15% have a prolonged or relapsing disease. In addition, about 100 persons per year in the United States die from acute liver failure due to hepatitis A. This most commonly occurs in persons over 50 years old and those with chronic liver disease.

Prevention and Control
Basic Precautionary Measures

All states require that each case of hepatitis A be reported to the local or state health department. The early symptoms of hepatitis A are similar to many other diseases and are hard to recognize until jaundice appears. As noted above, jaundice may never arise in some cases.

Thorough hand washing is an essential part of preventing the spread of any infection, including hepatitis A. Hand washing is especially important before preparing or serving food and after diapering and using the bathroom. Caregivers should always wear gloves when handling stools and should wash hands after removing the gloves.

Persons with hepatitis A do not require any

Symptoms of Hepatitis A in Children and Adults. Modified from Lemon, SM. Type A viral hepatitis. New developments in an old disease. New England Journal of Medicine, 1985.

Table 1: Symptoms of Hepatitis A in Children and Adults		
Symptom	**Children 2-5 years old (day-care center outbreak)**	**Adults 18-26 years old (U.S. Army soldiers)**
Nausea/vomiting	11(65%)	5(26%)
Jaundice/yellow eyes	11(65%)	16(88%)
Diarrhea	10(58%)	3(18%)
Dark urine	10(58%)	12(68%)
Light-colored stools	10(58%)	10(58%)
Abdominal pain	8(48%)	7(37%)
Malaise/fatigue	8(48%)	11(63%)
Fever/chills	7(41%)	6(32%)
Decreased appetite	7(41%)	8(42%)

Figure 1:

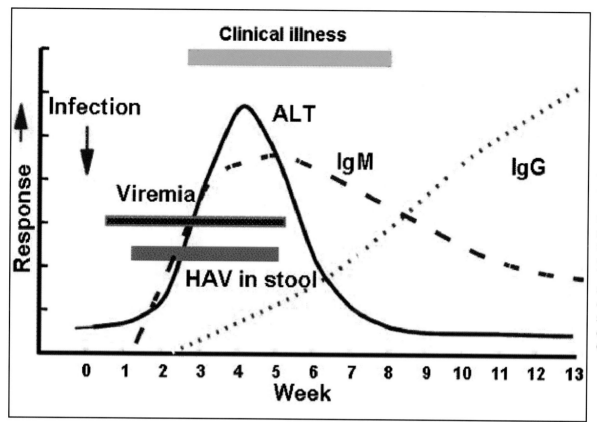

The Clinical Signs and Serology of Hepatitis A Infection. Viral shedding of hepatitis A virus is present in the stool about two weeks after initial exposure. The timing of clinical symptoms and various serological markers are shown here. Courtesy of the CDC

special type of isolation unless they are incontinent of stool. Infected people who regularly handle food should avoid tasks that require direct contact with food until 1 week after the appearance of jaundice.

Post-Exposure Immunization

An immunization containing antibodies, called immunoglobulin or IG, against the hepatitis A virus can limit the spread of the virus. When given within 2 weeks of exposure, the immunization will lessen the severity of illness and totally prevent clinical signs and symptoms in some cases.

Those who should receive IG include:

- household contacts of the infected person (see Special Considerations for Homeless Populations);
- sexual contacts of the infected person;
- persons who have shared illegal drugs with the infected person;
- staff or day care centers with at least one infected child;
- other food handlers at the same establishment of a food handler known to be infected.

Table 2: States with ≥ 20 Cases per 100,000 Population of Hepatitis A

State	Rate (per 100,000)
Arizona	48
Alaska	45
Oregon	40
New Mexico	40
Utah	33
Washington	30
Oklahoma	24
South Dakota	24
Idaho	21
Nevada	21
California	20

Prevalence of Hepatitis A. These states have ≥ 20 cases of hepatitis A per 100,000 population. Modified from Prevention of hepatitis A through active or passive immunization. Recommendations of the Advisory Committee on Immunization Practices (ACIP). MMWR 1999;48 (RR-12):1-37.

The recommended dose of IG for postexposure prophylaxis is 0.02 mL/kg. Side effects from IG other than pain and tenderness at the injection site are extremely rare. IG has never been reported to transmit other viruses, including human immuno-deficiency virus (HIV), hepatitis B, or hepatitis C.

Pre-Exposure Immunization

Persons who are at increased risk for developing infection or have increased risk of severe disease should receive hepatitis A vaccination. These include:

- sexually active men who have sex with men;
- drug users (injection and non-injection);
- persons with chronic liver disease;
- children living in states, counties, or communities where the average annual hepatitis A rate during 1987-1997 was greater than or equal to 20 cases per 100,000 population (see Table 2);
- persons who have clotting factor disorders;
- persons traveling to or working in countries with high or intermediate rates of hepatitis A;
- persons who work with HAV-infected primates or with HAV in a research laboratory setting.

The two vaccines approved for active immunization against hepatitis A virus (HAVRIX™ and VAQT™) are both inactivated vaccines. Both vaccines are given in two doses at least 6 months apart. The doses differ depending on the age of the patient and which product is used. Present data suggest that immunity may be lifelong and repeat vaccination after the initial series is not recommended. About 50% of persons receiving the hepatitis A vaccine experience soreness at the injection site, but other side effects are extremely rare.

Special Considerations for Homeless Populations

Homeless people are often at high risk for hepatitis A due to overcrowded and unsanitary living conditions. In addition, homeless persons may use illegal drugs or have chronic liver disease. Homeless persons with these risk factors should receive active immunization against hepatitis A.

Hepatitis A can spread rapidly through a shelter if certain precautions are not followed. The local or state public health department should be informed of any cases of hepatitis A as soon as possible. They can evaluate the situation and determine who should be immunized with IG. Whenever a child still in diapers develops hepatitis A in a family shelter, all children, parents, and staff should receive IG.

Summary

Hepatitis A is a viral infection of the liver that may cause a short-term sickness but generally does not cause prolonged liver disease. Both children and adults are affected. Adults tend to have a more severe course of illness. In fact, many children are infected but never show signs of hepatitis. A person can only become infected once in his or her lifetime. An infected person may develop cold- or flu-like symptoms from 15-50 days after exposure to the virus. The typical signs of hepatitis appear a few days later: yellowing of the skin and eyes, dark urine, itching, and abdominal pain. The illness usually lasts 4 to 8 weeks.

Hepatitis A usually spreads by direct contact with an infected person and less commonly through fecal contamination of food or water. Those at highest risk include travelers or persons from developing countries, children (and secondarily staff and parents) in day-care centers, men who have sex with men, injection drug users, hemophiliacs who have received pooled blood products, and persons in institutions.

Persons at risk for hepatitis A can receive active immunization with a formalin-inactivated vaccine to prevent infection. In addition, persons who have recently been exposed to hepatitis A and have not been vaccinated can receive IG. This will provide passive immunization that can lessen or completely abort the symptoms and manifestations of the disease.

No specific treatment exists for hepatitis A, but certain measures can ameliorate the symptoms. Bed rest, high calorie foods, and aspirin can help with the symptoms of muscle aches, abdominal pain, and fevers. Remember that aspirin should be avoided in children under the age of 18 because of the risk of Reye syndrome. Prescription medications can relieve itching. ▪

References

Centers for Disease Control and Prevention. Prevention of hepatitis A through active or passive immunization. Recommendations of the Advisory Committee on Immunization Practices (ACIP). *MMWR* 1999;48(RR-12): 1-37.

Dienstag JL, Isselbacher KJ. Acute viral hepatitis. In: Braunwald E, Fauci AS, Kasper DL, et al., eds. *Harrison's Principles of Internal Medicine.* New York: McGraw-Hill; 2001:1721-1737.

Hoofnagle JH, Lindsay KL. Acute viral hepatitis. In: Goldman L, Bennett JC, eds. *Cecil Textbook of Medicine.* Philadelphia: WB Saunders Company; 2000:783-790.

Lemon S. Type A viral hepatitis. New developments in an old disease. *New England Journal of Medicine* 1985;313(17): 1059-1067.

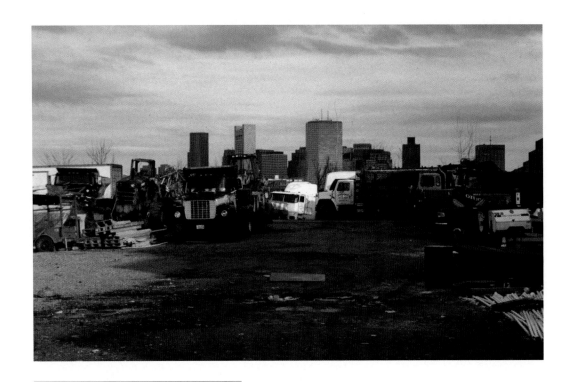

Several street folks seek refuge each night in
this South Boston junkyard for abandoned or
demolished trucks and buses. The city's skyline
is in the background.
Photo by James O'Connell MD

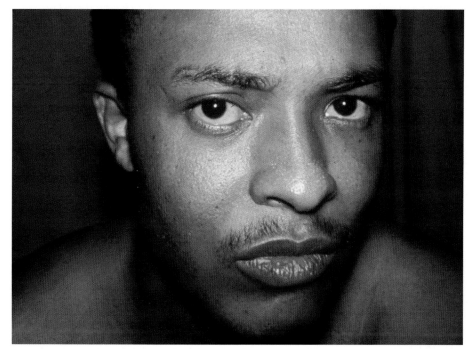

Hepatitis B

Lori Fantry, MD, MPH

Hepatitis B is a viral infection that primarily affects the liver. Earlier names for this disease were "long incubation" and "serum" hepatitis. Those infected with the hepatitis B virus may show no symptoms, have a self-limited acute illness, progress to acute liver failure, or develop chronic liver disease.

Prevalence and Distribution

Hepatitis B is found throughout the world and is most common in Southeast Asia, sub-Saharan Africa, Micronesia, and China. Even though hepatitis B is far less common in the USA than in these endemic countries, 0.5% of Americans are chronically infected, and hepatitis B virus is the second most common cause of acute hepatitis. There are over 5,000 new cases of hepatitis B diagnosed each year in the USA.

Mode of Transmission

The spread of hepatitis B depends on the contact of blood, semen, or saliva with open skin or mucous membranes (mouth, eyes, vagina, or rectum). Blood has the highest concentration of the hepatitis B virus. Researchers have found hepatitis B virus in almost every other body fluid as well, including urine, feces, tears, breast milk, and menstrual fluids. However, their roles in the transmission of the virus are not clearly known.

The most common modes of transmission in the USA are through injection drug use and sexual contact. A pregnant woman can also transmit the

virus to her unborn child, which is a common mode of transmission in endemic countries while an infrequent occurrence in the USA.

Symptoms and Diagnosis

The incubation period can range from 50 to 180 days, but most commonly is 70-80 days.

Cold- or flu-like symptoms characterize the first stages of the acute illness. These symptoms include headache, runny nose, cough, weakness, fatigue, poor appetite, nausea, vomiting, sore throat, and aches in the muscles and joints. The patient may have a mild fever. Some people lose their taste for cigarettes or coffee. Rarely, a person can develop arthritis or a rash. This early phase lasts between 1 and 28 days.

The second stage of the acute illness, the "icteric" phase, is characterized by yellow skin (jaundice) and eyes (scleral icterus), dark urine (often Coca-Cola or tea colored), and light or tan stools. Nausea and vomiting can continue and grow worse while other symptoms found in the first stage usually diminish. Some people complain of mild right-sided abdominal pain or itching. As in other

Jaundice. This African-American man developed hepatitis A from contaminated shellfish. Note the yellow hue to his eyes (called scleral icterus). Photo courtesy of the CDC

Table 1: Hepatitis B Serology

Clinical Status	HBsAg	Anti-HBc	Anti-HBs
Susceptible. Never infected or vaccinated	Negative	Negative	Negative
Immune due to prior infection	Negative	Positive	Positive
Immune due to prior vaccination	Negative	Negative	Positive
Acute infection	Positive	Positive	Negative
Chronic Carrier	Positive	Positive	Negative

types of hepatitis, young children are less apt to show symptoms of illness or jaundice. However, infection without symptoms can happen at any age.

The diagnosis of acute hepatitis B is made by finding hepatitis B surface antigen (HBsAg) and IgM anti-hepatitis B core antibody (anti-HBc) in the blood of an infected person. Clinical symptoms may be suggestive of hepatitis but are not unique enough to determine the type of hepatitis. Blood tests for anti-hepatitis B surface antibody (anti-HBs) and HbsAg can determine if a person is immune to hepatitis B (anti-HBs positive) or a chronic carrier (HbsAg positive and anti-HBc and anti-HBs negative).

Treatment and Complications

Most cases of acute hepatitis B do not call for hospitalization. There are no specific treatments that have been proven to decrease the length or severity of acute hepatitis B. However, certain measures do provide symptomatic relief. Most people prefer bed rest. No set rules exist about how many days or hours in a day a person should rest. People with hepatitis B should follow a high calorie diet. The diet should supply most of the calories early in the day, because nausea and vomiting tend to be worse later. Cholestyramine (Questran™), a prescription medicine, helps relieve itching. Patients should avoid substances metabolized or broken down by the liver, such as acetaminophen (Tylenol™), alcohol, and many illegal drugs.

In rare instances, the acute phase of hepatitis B can be fatal. However, most people recover clinically within 2 or 3 months. The HBsAg usually disappears from the blood in about 6 months, although in some persons it will persist for a few years. About 5% of persons infected with hepatitis B will never clear HbsAg and are called chronic carriers. Men and immunosuppressed persons are more likely to

become chronic carriers. All chronic carriers can infect others with the virus. In addition, some chronic carriers develop chronic hepatitis, cirrhosis, and hepatocellular carcinoma, all of which may lead to death. Hepatitis B virus is the most important cause of liver cancer in the USA. Chronic carriers may also have extra-hepatic disease with joint pain, arthritis, and skin rashes.

Chronic hepatitis B can be treated with interferon alfa-2b (Intron A™) or antiviral agents such as lamivudine (Epivir™, 3TC) or famciclovir (Famvir™). Exactly how best to use these medications to prevent resistance and result in long-lasting cure is still being evaluated. Therapy is monitored by PCR measurement of the amount of hepatitis B DNA in the blood.

Prevention and Control
Basic Precautionary Measures

All cases of hepatitis B should be reported to the local or state health department.

Persons with hepatitis B are most infectious prior to the time of diagnosis, and many persons with hepatitis B are either chronic carriers or have asymptomatic infection. Hence the best precaution against all diseases transmitted through body fluids, including hepatitis B, is to follow basic preventive measures with all people, regardless of what is known about their medical problems.

Hands should always be washed thoroughly, especially before preparing or serving food and after diapering or using the bathroom. Gloves should always be used when handling body fluids and hands should be washed after removing the gloves.

Persons with hepatitis B do not require any special type of isolation. However, they should be instructed not to have unprotected sex. Injection drug users should not share needles and should seek help for their addiction.

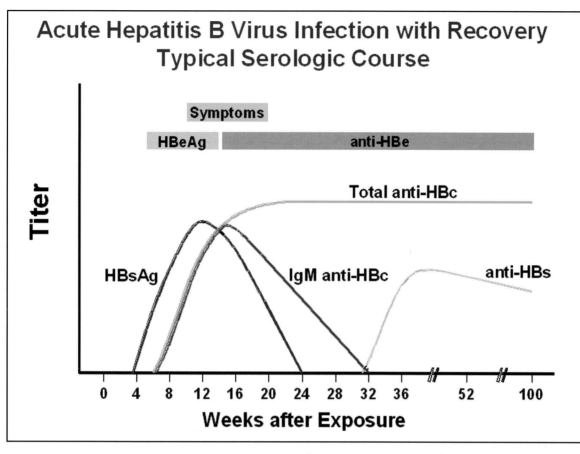

Acute Hepatitis B Virus Infection with Recovery
Typical Serologic Course

The Clinical Signs and Serology of Hepatitis B Infection. Flu-like symptoms usually appear 70-80 days after exposure to HBV. The timing of other clinical symptoms and serological markers is depicted here. Courtesy of the CDC

Post-Exposure Immunization

An immunization containing antibodies against hepatitis B virus, called hepatitis B immune globulin (HBIG), can prevent or lessen the severity of hepatitis in persons who have been recently exposed and are not immune. Non-immune persons who should receive HBIG include infants born to mothers with hepatitis B, sexual contacts of infected people, and those exposed directly by accidental needle stick injury. In all cases, the hepatitis B vaccine series should be started at the same time that HBIG is given.

Pre-Exposure Immunization

Active hepatitis B vaccine, which allows the body to make antibodies against hepatitis B, offers the best method of prevention. The two formulations of the vaccine available in the USA, Energix-B and Recombivax, are synthetic vaccines made from recombinant techniques using yeast. Both preparations are extremely safe. The most common side effects are pain at the injection site and mild fever. The vaccine is given intramuscularly in the deltoid muscle in a series of 3 shots, with the second and third given at 1 and 6 month intervals after the

first. Since most people respond to vaccination, post-vaccination testing for immunity is not recommended. In addition, booster doses are not usually recommended since most persons vaccinated remain immune for life.

All children and adolescents are recommended to receive the hepatitis B vaccine. The vaccine is also recommended for adults who have an increased risk for hepatitis B infection. These include:
- injection drug users;
- medical, dental, laboratory workers, and others with exposure to human blood;
- men who have sex with men;
- persons with multiple sexual partners or with sexually transmitted diseases;
- populations, such as Alaskan natives, in which hepatitis B is endemic;
- travelers to highly endemic areas if there is anticipated human blood contact or sexual or household contact with locals;
- household contacts of HbsAg-positive individuals;
- hemophilia patients;
- hemodialysis patients;
- patients for whom multiple blood transfusions or blood products are anticipated;

Table 2: Post-Exposure HBIG

Exposure	Dose	Timing
Infant born to HbsAg positive mother	0.5 mL	Within 48 hours of birth
Adult with sexual contact	2 mL	Within 14 days of last sexual contact
Adult with parental exposure	2 mL	Within 7 days of exposure, preferably 48 hours

Table 3: Hepatitis B Pre-Exposure Vaccination

Age of Person (years old)	Number of Doses	Dosing Schedule (months)*	Recombivax-HB	Energix-B
Infant (< 1)	3	0, 1, and 6	.25 mL	0.5 mL
Child (1-10)	3	0, 1, and 6	.25 mL	0.5 mL
Adolescent (11-19)	3	0, 1, and 6	0.5 mL	1.0 mL
Adults (>19)	3	0,1, and 6	1.0 mL	1.0 mL

*If a dose is missed it should be given as soon as possible. However, repeat dosing or repeating the schedule is not necessary.

- prison inmates and staff; and
- staff and patients of institutions for the mentally disabled.

Most employee health departments provide the vaccine for workers who are at risk of exposure.

Special Considerations for Homeless Populations

Homeless people who inject drugs or have frequent sexual contacts are at high risk for hepatitis B if they are not vaccinated. Persons immunocompromised by conditions such as HIV/AIDS have a higher risk of becoming chronic carriers. All homeless children, adolescents, and adults with risk factors should receive three doses of hepatitis B vaccine to prevent hepatitis B.

Summary

Hepatitis B is a viral infection of the liver that can cause either short- or long-term illness. Initial symptoms often begin 70 to 80 days after exposure and are similar to those of a cold or flu. In the second phase, a person may develop yellow skin and eyes, dark urine, light-colored stools, and itchy skin. Complete recovery takes 2 to 3 months.

An infected person may become a "chronic carrier". Although chronic carriers may show no symptoms of the disease, they can infect others with the virus for the rest of their lives. Chronic carriers can also develop chronic hepatitis, cirrhosis, and hepatocellular carcinoma.

Hepatitis B spreads most commonly by blood or semen. Sharing needles or having sex without using condoms transmits the virus very effectively. A person does not have to look ill or have symptoms to be able to spread hepatitis B.

There is no specific treatment for acute hepatitis B. Bed rest, high calorie food, and aspirin can help the aches and fevers. Aspririn should be avoided in children under 18 because of the risk of Reye syndrome. Prescription medications are available to relieve itching. Alcohol and drugs such as acetaminophen (Tylenol ™) that are broken down by the liver should be avoided. Chronic hepatitis B can be treated with interferon-α and antiviral agents.

Prevention of hepatitis B is now possible with universal vaccination of children, adolescents, and high-risk adults. Good general infection control principles should be routinely followed to prevent further spread of infection. In addition, there is a vaccine available for persons who are not immune and have had recent exposure. ∎

Table 4: Interpretation of the Hepatitis B Panel

Test	Results	Interpretation	
HBsAg anti-HBc anti-HBs	Negative Negative Negative	Susceptible	anti-HBc = hepatitis B core antibody anti-HBcIgM = IgM antibody against HBc anti-HBs = hepatitis B surface antibody HBV = hepatitis B virus HBsAg = hepatitis B surface antigen
HBsAg anti-HBc anti-HBs	Negative Positive Positive	Immune due to natural infection	
HBsAg anti-HBc anti-HBs	Negative Negative Positive	Immune due to hepatitis B vaccination	
HBsAg anti-HBc anti-HBc IgM anti-HBs	Positive Positive Positive Negative	Acutely infected	
HBsAg anti-HBc anti-HBc IgM anti-HBs	Positive Positive Negative Negative	Chronically infected	
HBsAg anti-HBc anti-HBs	Negative Positive Negative	Four interpretations possible: May be recovering from acute HBV infection May be distantly immune and test is not sensitive enough to detect very low level of anti-HBs in serum May be susceptible with a false-positive anti-HBc May be an undetectable level of HBsAg present in the serum and the person is actually a carrier	

The Interpretation of HBV Serology. This figure is designed to help clinicians interpret the often confusing results of the serological tests for hepatitis B. Courtesy of the CDC

Hepatitis B Medication List

Generic	Brand Name	Cost
cholestyramine	Questran	$$$
famciclovir	Famvir	$$$
interferon alfa-2b	Intron A	$$$$$
lamivudine	Epivir, 3TC	$$$$$

References

Centers for Disease Control and Prevention. Hepatitis B: A comprehensive strategy for eliminating transmission in the United States through universal childhood vaccination: Recommendations of the Advisory Committee on Immunization Practices (ACIP). *MMWR* 1999;40(RR-13):1-19.

Dienstag JL, Isselbacher KJ. Acute viral hepatitis. In: Braunwald E, Fauci AS, Kasper DL, et al., eds. *Harrison's Principles of Internal Medicine*. New York: McGraw-Hill; 2001:1336.

Hoofnagle JH, Lindsay KL. Acute viral hepatitis. In: Goldman L, Bennett JC, eds. *Cecil Textbook of Medicine*. Philadelphia: WB Saunders Company; 2000:783-790.

Robinson WS. Hepatitis B virus and hepatitis D virus. In: Mandell GL, Bennett JE, Dolin R, eds. *Mandell, Douglas, and Bennett's Principles and Practices of Infectious Disease*. Philadelphia: Churchill Livingston Company; 2000:1645-1685.

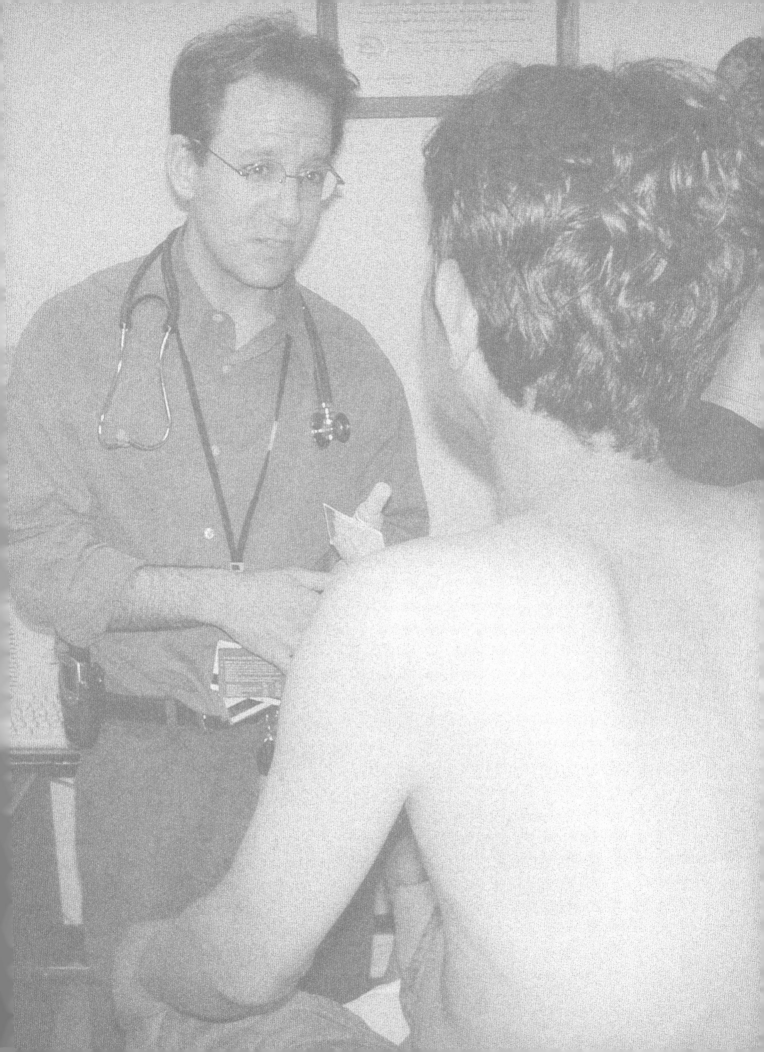

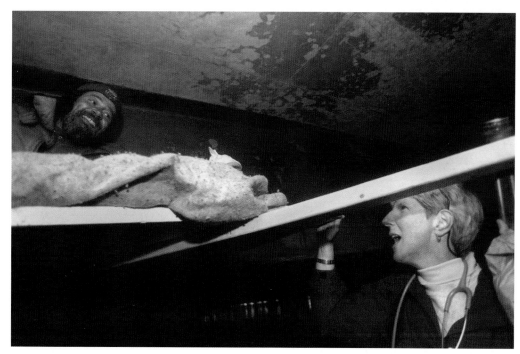

Hepatitis C

Pedro Jose Greer, MD

T he hepatitis C virus (HCV) was identified in 1989 and found to account for the majority of those patients with "non-A, non-B hepatitis". HCV is now the most common blood-borne infection in the USA and a leading cause of chronic liver disease. Almost 4 million Americans have been infected with HCV, and 2.7 million are chronically infected. Many of those who are chronically infected are unaware because they have no signs or symptoms. By conservative estimates, 35,000 new hepatitis C infections occur each year in the USA. The world wide burden of chronic hepatitis C infection is estimated to range from 140-170 million individuals.

Hepatitis C is a small enveloped RNA virus belonging to the Flaviviridae family and the genus hepacivirus. HCV replicates rapidly in the liver and has marked sequence heterogeneity with 6 genotypes and over 90 subtypes. In the USA, 75% of individuals infected with HCV have genotypes 1a and 1b, 15% have genotypes 2a and 2b, and 7% have genotype 3. Genotype 1a is common in Europe, while 1b is found frequently in southern Europe and around the world. Genotypes 2a and 2b are common in Italy, North Africa, and Spain. Genotype 3 is common in Northern Europe.

After infection with HCV, 55-85% of individuals fail to clear the virus and develop chronic hepatitis C infection. This infection is usually asymptomatic, although persistent or fluctuating elevations in the liver enzyme ALT are common. However, 30-40% of persons with chronic HCV infection will have normal ALT levels. The consequential hepatic

sequelae of hepatitis C include progressive hepatic fibrosis, cirrhosis, and hepatocellular carcinoma. The extra-hepatic manifestations include sicca syndrome, cryoglobulinemia, glomerulonephritis, porphyria cutanea tarda, as well as all the extra-hepatic manifestations of chronic liver disease.

Transmission

The known risk factors for infection with HCV have evolved as understanding of the pathogenesis has progressed. Blood transfusions received before 1991 accounted for a substantial portion of those infected prior to that time. Improved testing of blood supplies has resulted in a dramatic decline in the number of new HCV infections due to transfusions. Rather, intravenous drug use (IVDU) now accounts for 60% and sexual exposure for 20% of new HCV infections. Occupational exposure, hemodialysis, household contacts, and perinatal

Cheryl Kane, a nurse on BHCHP's Street Team, brings medication to a man living under a bridge near the Charles River. Photo by Stan Grossfeld

Figure 1:

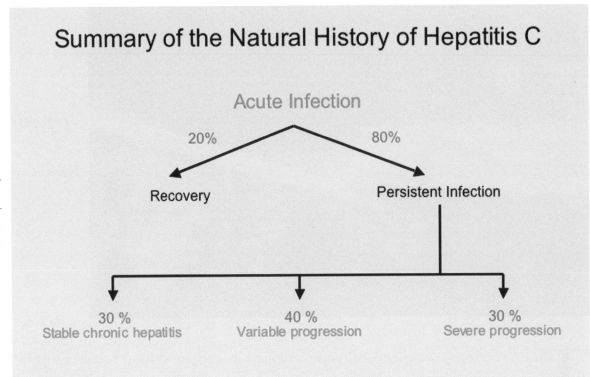

exposure account for another 10%. The remaining 10% of HCV infections have no recognized source, although low socio-economic status appears to be common in this group. Other risk factors include: intranasal cocaine use; tattooing with contaminated needles or ink; extensive body piercing; and a history of military service, especially during the Vietnam era. Certain occupations have a higher risk of hepatitis C, including health care providers, emergency medical personnel, and public safety workers (firefighters, law enforcement officials, and correctional facility personnel).

Using a computer cohort simulation model, Wong and his colleagues estimate that HCV will cause the loss of 1.83 million years of life in individuals younger than 65 and cost society $54.2 billion during the decade 2010-2019. Their model predicts 165,900 deaths from chronic liver disease and 27,200 deaths from hepatocellular carcinoma during that period.

Prevalence of HCV among Homeless Populations

Given our understanding of the risk factors for HCV and the silent and aggressive nature of this infection, one should not be surprised that studies have found the prevalence of HCV to be 10-20 times higher in some sub-groups of the homeless population than in the general population. The

USA population has a prevalence of 1.8%, while one study of homeless veterans showed an overall prevalence of 44%. The prevalence increases with age among homeless populations that have been studied. A study of homeless adolescents published in 2003 found that 12% tested positive for HCV. Rates among sub-groups of homeless adults have ranged from 22% to 80%, with the latter number found among those with a history of IVDU. Studies have shown higher HCV prevalence rates among recent daily users of intravenous drugs than those who were non-users or less frequent users. Co-infection with the human immunodeficiency virus (HIV) increases the risk of mortality from HCV.

With such high prevalence rates among homeless populations, clinicians caring for homeless individuals should maintain a high index of suspicion for HCV infection. Because this disease is indolent and often asymptomatic yet can have dire consequences, we feel strongly that all patients in homeless clinics should be offered HCV testing whenever treatment is a viable and accessible option.

Diagnosis and Evaluation of HCV Infection

The initial test in the evaluation of at-risk individuals and those with clinical liver disease should be an antibody against the HCV. An initial enzyme immunoassay (EIA) can detect the presence of anti-HCV antibody, which is present from 6-16 weeks after the acute infection. The positive predictive value of this test is low in populations with low incidences of HCV infection, and therefore the CDC recommends a confirmatory test with a higher specificity, such as recombinant immunoblot assay (RIBA). This test can be performed on the same sample of blood used for the EIA. HCV antigens from the core and non-structural genes are utilized in both techniques. The newer third generations EIAs have a sensitivity of greater then 99% and specificity of 99% in immuncompetent patients. The use of these tests will eliminate the need for a confirmatory immunoblot assay except in certain situations, such as individuals who are immunocompromised or undergoing hemodialysis. These patients rarely have false-negative results. Conversely, false positives can occur in patients with autoimmune disorders.

The diagnosis of HCV may also be made by the detection of HCV RNA using gene amplification techniques such as polymerase chain reaction (PCR) or transcription mediated amplification (TMA). These tests are expensive but allow the diagnosis of HCV to be made within 1-2 weeks of HCV infection. Many clinicians advocate the early treatment of acute HCV in order to prevent chronic disease, and many studies are underway to evaluate this approach. These tests are qualitative and detect the presence of HCV RNA but do not measure the amount or level of the virus in the blood. These tests can detect viral levels as low as 50-100 IU/ml, and the latest generation TMA can now detect levels as low as 5-10 IU/ml. This type of qualitative testing is very helpful in establishing the diagnosis of HCV infection but is not useful in the management of patients who are being treated for HCV.

The HCV RNA level (or viral load) can be measured with quantitative assays that utilize PCR or branched DNA signal amplification. The viral load provides important information on the likelihood of response to antiviral treatment, although it should be noted that disease severity is not correlated with the level of the viral load. The viral load is measured regularly during and after treatment to determine success or failure. The goal is to maintain a sustained viral response (SVR) after treatment.

The Treatment of HCV Infection

The current standard treatment for chronic HCV infection is interferon alfa in combination with ribavirin. The length of treatment is from 24-48 weeks. Interferon alfa is given subcutaneously three times a week; pegylated interferon alfa is now available, which is given once a week. The side effects of interferon alfa include flu-like symptoms (which usually occur early in therapy and then improve), fatigue, bone marrow suppression, and psychiatric problems. Ribavirin can cause hemolytic anemia (in persons with a pre-existing anemia), bone marrow suppression, and renal failure. Ribavirin is teratogenic and contraindicated during pregnancy.

All individuals with HCV infection should be vaccinated against hepatitis A, which is more virulent in persons who have HCV. HCV patients who are seronegative for hepatitis B virus (HBV) should be vaccinated against HBV.

The Importance of Genotype to Treatment Response

Persons with known HCV who are candidates for treatment should be tested for genotype. The most common genotypes in the USA are 1a and 1b, followed by 2a and 2b, and then genotype 3. The genotype is a major factor in determining the length of treatment and amount of ribavirin needed. The standard treatment regimen of genotype 1a and 1b lasts 48 weeks, with SVRs from 47-54%; genotypes 2 and 3 require only 24 weeks of treatment, with SVRs of 73% and 82% respectively.

Liver Biopsy

Individuals with HCV who are candidates for antiviral therapy should have a liver biopsy performed in order to establish the degree of injury to the liver. Treatment can be deferred for those with stage 0-1 fibrosis. The necessity and the timing of a follow-up biopsy remain controversial and must be determined on an individual basis.

Who is a Candidate for Treatment?

A past history of alcohol abuse is not a contraindication to treatment. Alcohol accelerates the progression of HCV liver disease to cirrhosis and hepatocellular carcinoma, and continued alcohol use during therapy adversely affects response to treatment.

HIV infection is not a contraindication to treatment. Treatment for HCV does not appear to compromise antiretroviral treatment for HIV/AIDS. This should be approached on a patient by patient basis and requires specialty referral.

Homeless populations and substance abusers have higher rates of depression then the general population. The prevalence of depression is also more common in persons with HCV. Depression is also a very common complication of our current therapies for HCV and occurs in 12-44% of persons who are treated with interferon and combination therapy with interferon and ribavirin. Therefore the identification of homeless patients with HCV and a history of depression is very important prior to the initiation of treatment. The potential neuropsychiatric side effects of HCV treatment should be carefully explained to each patient and are an important consideration in each patient's decision to undergo treatment. Several years ago, when the treatment response (SVR) was less then 15%, moderate to severe depression was a relative contraindication to treatment. With overall SVR rates now in excess of 50%, and as high as 80% in selected populations, depression is no longer considered a reason to withhold treatment. The SSRIs have proven effective for pre-existing depression as well as treatment-induced depression. Most patients have been able to tolerate and finish treatment. Whenever the antidepressant therapy is not successful, the interferon dose is reduced. If the depression persists, then the HCV treatment is terminated.

Active injection drug use is not a contraindication for the treatment of HCV. Since IVDU is the most common risk behavior for new HCV infection in the USA, any successful treatment modality will help to reduce transmission of the virus within this population. Management is enhanced by linking these patients to drug treatment programs, including methadone maintenance programs. All patients with drug and alcohol abuse should be offered these programs.

Several individuals are **not** good candidates for treatment with interferon and ribavirin:
- pregnant or nursing mothers, because of the teratogenicity of these medications;
- unmonitored psychiatric disease or untreated depression;
- active substance abuse;
- decompensated liver disease, since HCV treatment can cause thrombocytopenia, neutropenia, and progression of liver disease;
- severe co-morbid illnesses, which can be exacerbated by HCV treatment.

Who Should Start and Monitor Treatment?

Ideally, all patients with HCV who are potential candidates for treatment should be referred to a hepatologist. In today's world, the waiting times in academic and public hospital settings are often unacceptably prolonged. Homeless patients face enormous obstacles to specialty and other health care clinics, including language barriers and a lack of insurance, transportation, and housing. Health care professionals trained in the monitoring and treatment of HCV should ideally be available at health care for the homeless clinics. While the management of HCV treatment is not difficult, the time commitment is significant, particularly in monitoring the side effects of antiviral therapy.

Complications of Treatment

(1) Depression is the principal side effect and cause of termination of therapy. Thus, optimal treatment for depression in patients with a prior history of depression is essential before and during therapy. Identification of mood disturbances in treated patients is of utmost importance.

(2) Hematologic consequences of HCV therapy are significant and require careful monitoring. Anemia occurs in 9-23% of patients, neutropenia in 18-21%, thrombocytopenia in 1-4%, and any adverse hemodynamic event in 32-42% of treated patients. The anemia can be caused by bone marrow suppression from interferon alfa-2b (both pegulated and non-pegulated interferon), while ribavirin can cause hemolysis. The decline in hemoglobin can be 2-4 grams and occur in the first two weeks of therapy. Anemia can be treated by reducing the dose of both interferon and ribavirin and by using epoetin alfa. The hematological consequences can be life-threatening, and patients must be carefully monitored. When patients fail to appear for scheduled visits, this becomes a contraindication to either the initiation or the continuation of HCV treatment.

(3) Fatigue and viral like symptoms are the most frequently reported complications. These are treated symptomatically, usually with acetaminophen and hydration. Virtually all patients experience fatigue, but this generally lessens with time.

(4) Other possible side effects include dermatologic problems, hair loss, and thyroid dysfunction.

Summary

The key lessons from this chapter are the following:
1) homeless populations are at extremely high risk for infection with HCV;
2) the consequences of HCV infection are significant and long term;
3) all patients in a homeless clinic should be screened for exposure to HCV;

4) all HCV patients should be vaccinated against hepatitis A and B;

5) a careful and thorough medical and neuro-psychiatric evaluation is necessary for all potential candidates for anti-viral therapy, as many relative and absolute contraindications to treatment remain;

6) regular attendance at clinic visits and adherence to therapy are essential for treatment;

7) active IVDU is not a contraindication to treatment, but compliance is;

8) active alcohol use is a strong contraindication to treatment;

9) side effects from HCV treatment are significant and appropriate management is essential;

10) much work remains to be done, especially in screening and in the development of appropriate systems to care for this disease in the homeless population. ▪

Hepatitis C Medication List

Generic	Brand Name	Cost
interferon alfa-2a	Roferon - A	$$$$$
interferon alfacon-1	Infergen	$$$$$
peginterferon alfa-2a	Pegasys	$$$$$
interferon alfa-2b	Intron A	$$$$$
peginterferon alfa-2b	PEG-Intron	$$$$$
ribavirin	Rebetol, Copegus	$$$$$
interferon alfa-2a + ribavirin	Rebetron (each kit contains 2-week supply of each)	$$$$$

References

Alter MJ. Epidemiology of hepatitis C. *Journal of Hepatology* 1997;26(Supplement 1):S62-S65.

Beech BM, Myers L, Beech DJ. Hepatitis B and C infections among homeless adolescents. *Family and Community Health* 2002;25(2):28-36.

Beech BM, Myers L, Beech DJ, et al. Human immunodeficiency syndrome and hepatitis B and C infections among homeless adolescents. *Seminars in Pediatric Infectious Diseases* 2003;14(1):12-29.

Desai RA, Rosenheck RA, Agnello V. Prevalence of hepatitis C virus infection in a sample of homeless veterans. *Social Psychiatry and Psychiatric Epidemiology* 2003;38(7):396-401.

Hoofnagle JH. Course and outcome of Hepatitis C. *Journal of Hepatology* 2002;36(5 Supplement 1):S21-29.

Hunt CM, Dominitz JA, Bute BP, et al. Effect of interferon-alpha treatment of chronic hepatitis C on health-related quality of life. *Digestive Diseases and Sciences* 1997;42(12):2482-2486.

Manns MP, McHutchison JG, Gordon SC, et al. Peginterferon alfa-2b plus ribavirin compared with interferon-2b plus ribavirin for initial treatment of chronic hepatitis C: a randomised trial. *The Lancet* 2004;358(9286):958.

Martins RM, Porto SO, Vanderborght BO, et al. Short report: prevalence of hepatitis C viral antibody among Brazilian children, adolescents, and street youths. *American Journal of Tropical Medicine and Hygiene* 1995;53(6): 654-655.

Miyaoka H, Otsubo T, Kamijima K, et al. Depression from interferon therapy in patients with hepatitis C. *American Journal of Psychiatry* 1999;156(7):1120.

National Institutes of Health. NIH Consensus Statement on Management of Hepatitis C. *NIH Consensus and State-of-the-Science Statements.* June, 2002.

Nyamathi AM, Dixon EL, Robbins W, et al. Risk factors for hepatitis C virus infection among homeless adults. *Journal of General Internal Medicine* 2002;17(2):134-143.

Raoult D, Foucault C, Brouqui P. Infections in the homeless. *The Lancet Infectious Diseases* 2001;1(2):75.

Renault PF, Hoofnagle JH, Park Y, et al. Psychiatric complications of long-term interferon alfa therapy. *Archives of Internal Medicine* 1987;147:1577-1580.

Simmonds P. Viral heterogeneity of the hepatitis C virus. *Journal of Hepatology* 1999;31(Supplement 1):54-60.

Thomas DL. Hepatitis C and human immunodeficiency virus infection. *Hepatology* 2003;36(5B):S201-S209.

Wong JB, McQuillan GM, McHutchison JG, et al. Estimating future hepatitis C morbidity, mortality, and costs in the United States. *American Journal of Public Health* 2000;90:1562-1569.

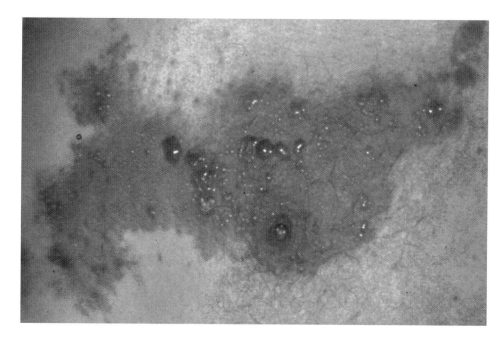

Herpes Zoster (Shingles)

Jessie McCary, MD

Infection with varicella-zoster virus (VZV) causes two distinct clinical syndromes: primary varicella infection (chickenpox) and herpes zoster (shingles). Herpes zoster will be discussed in this chapter. Varicella infection is discussed in a separate chapter.

Once a person has had chickenpox, VZV lies dormant in the human body for decades before reactivating to cause a localized skin eruption in the distribution of one or two dermatomes. The typical lesions of shingles are painful red blisters (or vesicles) that occur on one side of the body and do not cross the midline. The zoster lesions erupt for several days and go through stages of healing over the course of 2-4 weeks.

The likelihood of occurrence and severity of this illness are related to each person's underlying health status. Elderly and immunosuppressed (people are at highest risk of VZV reactivation, and the resulting illness is often more severe. Antiretroviral medications, if given early in the course of illness, can decrease the severity and duration of symptoms and reduce the complications of herpes zoster.

Prevalence and Distribution

The cumulative lifetime incidence of herpes zoster is estimated to be 10-20% of the population. The majority of cases occur in the elderly, with both sexes affected equally. This infection seems to occur less often in African-American people than white populations, as evidenced by a study of elderly people in North Carolina. Approximately 4% of patients who develop herpes zoster will experience a recurrence.

Immunocompromised individuals, including transplant recipients, HIV-infected patients, and patients receiving long term steroids, are at higher risk of developing herpes zoster than the general population, and these patients are more likely to have disseminated disease and recurrence of shingles.

Mode of Transmission and Pathogenesis of Disease

During an episode of primary varicella infection (chickenpox), VZV is highly contagious and spread both by respiratory droplets (sneezing and coughing) and direct contact. Infection with VZV occurs when the virus comes into contact with the mucosa of the upper respiratory tract or the conjunctiva of the eye. The virus travels in the bloodstream via mononuclear cells to the skin, resulting in the generalized rash of chickenpox. The virus also infects human cells in the dorsal root ganglia of the spinal column and cranial nerve ganglia, where it becomes latent. Essentially protected from the human immune system, VZV typically remains dormant in the ganglia for decades.

Herpes zoster occurs when the virus subsequently reactivates, initially causing pain and soon

Herpes Zoster (Shingles) of the T5 Dermatome. The lesions are red, raised, fluid-filled vesicles or blisters that contain varicella-zoster virus. Note that these lesions are confined to a very specific area on one side of the chest. Photo by Howard Koh MD

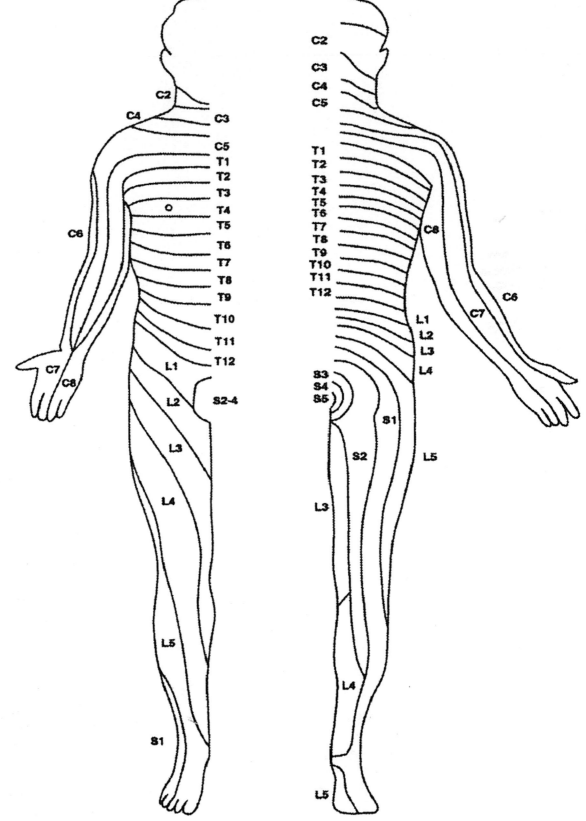

*Dermatomes.
A dermatome is a
segmental area of
the skin innervated
by fibers from a
single dorsal
nerve root of the
spinal cord.
Helpful hints:
C6 (thumb),
T10 (umbilicus),
L5 (top of foot),
S1 (bottom of foot).
Courtesy of MGH*

afterwards a vesicular rash in the distribution of one or two contiguous dermatomes. Herpes zoster is less contagious than varicella. Zoster generally spreads only by direct contact with open, draining lesions and not via airborne droplets. This fragile virus can live for short periods of time on fomites such as towels, linens, and clothes. These items must be viewed as potential sources of transmission. Once

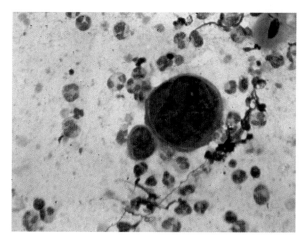

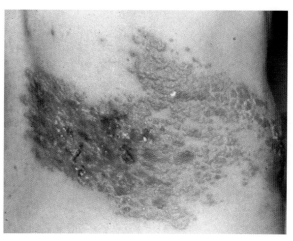

the lesions of shingles have crusted over and are no longer draining, the patient is no longer infectious.

Remember that a person with shingles cannot transmit zoster or shingles to others. However, contact with drainage from zoster lesions can cause chickenpox in individuals who have no history of prior varicella infection and have never had chickenpox.

Immunocompromised patients with zoster are at risk of developing widespread infection with VZV, called disseminated herpes zoster. This potentially serious illness may result in skin lesions over the entire body and infection of internal organs. This infection is thought to be more contagious than typical herpes zoster and may be spread by airborne droplets, as in primary varicella infection. For this reason, any patient with disseminated zoster, as well as those at risk for this infection, should be hospitalized with strict respiratory isolation.

Symptoms and Diagnosis

A prodrome of fever, malaise, and headache often precedes the vesicular eruption. Many patients experience pain and dysesthesias in the distribution of a sensory dermatome several days or weeks before the rash appears.

In immunocompetent individuals, the typical rash begins with groups of fluid-filled vesicles on a red or erythematous base. These are on one side of the body and limited to one or two dermatomes. The most commonly involved dermatomes are those innervated by the thoracic and lumbar nerves, and the ophthalmic branch of the trigeminal nerve. Crusting of the lesions usually occurs within ten days but may take as long as one month.

The diagnosis of herpes zoster is made clinically by the history of the prodrome, often with localized pain, and followed by the typical rash. Shingles can usually be differentiated from chickenpox and herpes simplex on the basis of these characteristic symptoms and findings. Laboratory confirmation is necessary only in cases in which an atypical rash renders the diagnosis uncertain. Vesicular fluid can be examined by Tzanck smear, culture, polymerase chain reaction, or fluorescence microscopy.

Treatment

The goal of treatment of acute herpes zoster is to accelerate the healing of painful lesions and to prevent complications such as those mentioned in the next section. Many studies have examined the effects of antiviral therapy with acyclovir (Zovirax™), valacyclovir (Valtrex™), and famciclovir (Famvir™), all three of which are FDA-approved for the treatment of herpes zoster infection. The use of oral steroids in combination with antiviral therapy has also been studied. The evidence that any of these therapies is effective in preventing complications is limited, and no formal consensus for the use of these agents exists.

An acceptable approach is to withhold antiviral therapy from healthy adults under the age of 50 unless there is ophthalmic involvement or severe pain. Patients over the age of 50 should be treated with an antiviral agent. Antiviral agents are more effective if begun within 72 hours of the onset of symptoms. Some clinicians consider initiating therapy after this 72 hour window if new skin lesions continue to emerge. The mainstay of antiviral therapy for normal adults has been a 7-10 day course of acyclovir (Zovirax™) 800 mg PO five times per day. Valacyclovir (Valtrex ™) 1000 mg PO TID and famciclovir (Famvir ™) 500 mg PO TID have simpler dosing regimens and may be preferred for this reason.

Oral antiretrovirals are also effective in HIV positive patients with localized zoster infection. Because of the increased risk of relapse, treatment should continue until all lesions have completely resolved. If dissemination occurs, intravenous therapy is indicated.

The addition of steroids to an antiviral regimen has not been proven to prevent post herpetic neuralgia, but should be considered in patients with severe pain in order to reduce the duration of acute symptoms. Steroids should not be used in patients with relative contraindications such as diabetes mellitus, gastritis, osteoporosis, or glaucoma.

Amitriptyline (Elavil ™), a tricyclic antidepressant that has also been used to treat neuropathic pain, may decrease the risk of post herpetic neuralgia. A dose of 25 mg nightly, started within a couple days of the onset of the rash and continued for 90 days, has not been widely studied.

Pain control is a very important aspect in the treatment of this illness as well as zoster's most common complication, post herpetic neuralgia. Potential treatments to control pain include capsaicin ointment (Zostrix™), tricyclic antidepressants, gabapentin (Neurontin™), topical lidocaine, narcotics, and even regional nerve blocks.

Complications

Post herpetic neuralgia is the most common complication of herpes zoster, occurring in 10-15 percent of all patients. The risk of this complication increases with age. Post herpetic neuralgia is defined as sensory symptoms (usually pain or numbness) that exist in the distribution of the previously involved dermatome more than 30 days after the initial rash.

Herpes zoster ophthalmicus is another common complication. Caregivers should be aware that involvement of the ophthalmic branch of the trigeminal nerve is potentially sight-threatening. Evidence of this complication may include unilateral eye pain, vesicular eruption around the eye, conjunctivitis, episcleritis, iritis, or lid droop. Referral to an ophthalmologist must be made immediately.

Health care providers should monitor patients for signs of bacterial superinfection of skin lesions, which may require antibiotic therapy. Change in mental status, spread of skin lesions beyond two dermatomes, or involvement of the eyes should prompt immediate referral to specialists.

Prevention and Control

Herpes zoster is not as contagious as primary varicella infection (chickenpox). People who have had chickenpox in the past are considered immune and are not at risk of developing shingles or chickenpox if exposed to a patient with shingles.

Persons who have never had primary varicella infection are at risk of developing chickenpox if they are exposed directly to the draining vesicles of shingles. For this reason, several precautions should be taken to decrease the risk to non-immune persons. Caregivers should wear gloves when examining the patient. Draining vesicles should be covered with a dressing until they have crusted over. Fomites, such as linens and clothes, may harbor the virus and should be handled with gloves. Once crusting of the vesicles occurs, there is no longer a risk of infectivity. If these precautions are taken, the risk to others in a shelter is minimal.

Pregnant women who are susceptible to VZV (have never had chickenpox) and are exposed to a patient with shingles should be referred for administration of varicella zoster immune globulin (VZIG) to decrease potential risk to the fetus.

Immunocompromised patients with herpes zoster are at high risk of developing disseminated disease, in which airborne spread is possible in addition to direct contact. Therefore, hospitalization and respiratory isolation should be considered in immunocompromised patients with localized or disseminated zoster.

Varicella vaccine is a live, attenuated vaccine against VZV that was licensed in 1995. It is contraindicated during pregnancy and is currently not recommended in HIV-infected individuals, although its safety in this population is under evaluation. Vaccination against VZV is currently recommended for the following susceptible adults (without a reliable history of chickenpox or a serologic test indicating immunity): health care workers, those with close contact to immunocompromised individuals or young children, and women who could become pregnant.

Special Consideratons for Homeless Populations

While not proven by research studies at this time, psychological stress may be a risk factor for the development of herpes zoster. Although the prevalence of herpes zoster in homeless populations has not been specifically determined, the profound psychological stresses of homelessness may be associated with an increased risk of this condition in homeless persons, especially the elderly.

Summary

Herpes zoster results from reactivation of VZV, the same virus that causes chickenpox. The illness is generally less severe than chickenpox, with painful skin lesions that are typically limited to one or two dermatomes.

Early treatment of localized zoster infection with antiretroviral medication is indicated in patients over the age of 50 or any patient with either ophthalmologic involvement or severe pain. Steroids, in addition to anti-retrovirals, may decrease the severity and duration of pain. Analgesia is an important aspect in the treatment of this painful infection.

Serious complications may arise from herpes zoster, including disseminated disease, ophthalmologic involvement, and infection of various organs. Immunocompromised individuals are at particular risk of complications. Immediate referral to infectious disease specialists is indicated in these situations.

Patients with herpes zoster can transmit VZV to others via direct contact with draining skin lesions. Only people who have never had chickenpox are at risk, and the resulting illness is primary varicella infection (chickenpox). This risk becomes minimal in shelters if skin lesions are covered with dressings and gloves are worn when clothes and linens are handled. ▪▪

The author of this chapter gratefully acknowledges the invaluable contribution of Janet Groth, RN, MS, who authored this chapter in the original Manual.

Herpes Zoster Medication List

Generic	Brand Name	Cost
acyclovir	Zovirax	$
amitryptyline	Elavil	$
capsaicin	Zostrix	$
famciclovir	Famvir	$$$
gabapentin	Neurontin	$$$$$
valacyclovir	Valtrex	$$$$

References

Albrecht MA. Clinical features of varicella-zoster infection: herpes zoster. UpToDate; 2002. http://uptodate.com

Abrecht MA. Treatment and prevention of herpes zoster. UpToDate; 2002. http://www.uptodate.com

Alper BS, Lewis PR. Does treatment of acute herpes zoster prevent or shorten postherpetic neuralgia? *Journal of Family Practice* 2000;49(3):255-264.

Buchbinder SP, Katz MH, Hessol NA, et al. Herpes zoster and human immunodeficiency virus infection. *Journal of Infectious Diseases* 1992;166(5):1153-1156.

Cohen JI, Brunell PA, Straus SE, et al. Recent advances in varicella-zoster virus infection. *Annals of Internal Medicine* 1999;130(11):922-932.

Glesby M, Moore RD, Chaisson RE. Clinical spectrum of herpes zoster in adults infected with human immunodeficiency virus. *Clinical Infectious Diseases* 1995;21(2):370-375.

Gnann JW, Whitley RJ. Clinical practice. Herpes zoster. *New England Journal of Medicine* 2002;347(5):340-346.

Straus SE, Ostrove JM, Inchauspe G, et al. Varicella-zoster virus infections. Biology, natural history, treatment, and prevention. *Annals of Internal Medicine* 1988;108(2):221-237.

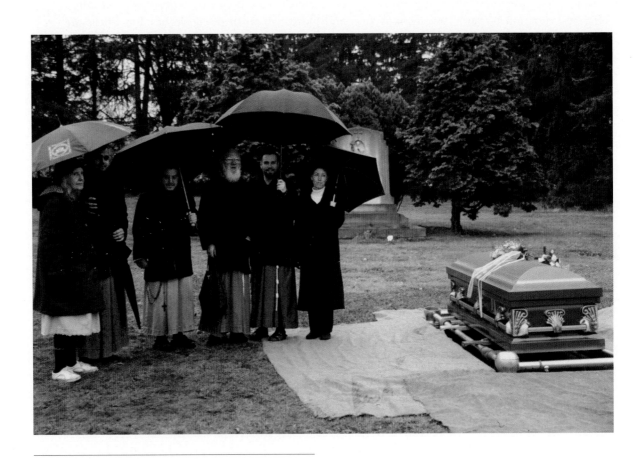

*Quiet Burial. The death and burial of a beloved homeless man
is quietly celebrated in the rain. This pauper's field in Boston is
the final resting place of hundreds of poor and homeless persons.
Photo by James O'Connell MD*

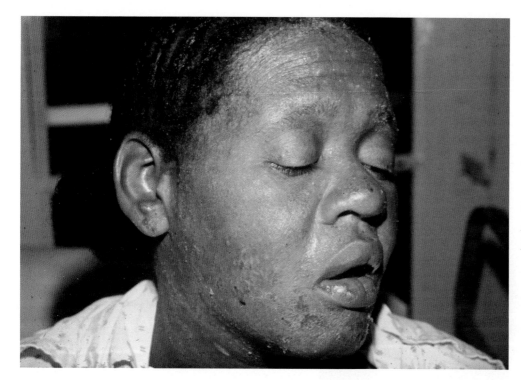

HIV / AIDS

Carole Hohl, PA-C
Phillip E. Pulaski, MD
Robin K. Avery, MD

W hen the first case of AIDS was reported in the USA in 1981, no one could have foreseen the impact of the HIV epidemic throughout the world. The prevalence of HIV/AIDS in homeless populations is unknown. Various studies have shown an incidence of HIV/AIDS to be from 3-20%. Homelessness itself is not a risk factor for HIV infection, although many homeless individuals are at risk because survival on the streets can include unprotected sex and injection drug use.

HIV stands for the Human Immunodeficiency Virus. This virus severely damages a person's immune system and impedes the body's ability to fight certain infections, cancers, and other diseases. When this virus progresses and causes enough damage, the person develops AIDS, or Acquired Immune Deficiency Syndrome. At this stage the immune system has been compromised and can no longer fight off life-threatening infections and cancers.

As the HIV/AIDS epidemic spreads throughout the USA and the world, the number of homeless persons diagnosed with HIV continues to grow. More than 790,000 cases of AIDS have been reported in the USA since 1981, and as many as 900,000 Americans may be infected with the virus. The epidemic is growing fastest among minority populations and is the leading cause of death among African-American men aged 25-44.

Although many advances have been made in treatment, HIV/AIDS remains a serious illness that presents difficult challenges to persons infected, especially to those without safe and stable homes. The medications available for treatment are complicated and have many side effects. Shelter personnel have an important role in providing medical and social support to people infected with the virus. Understanding, patience, and compassion from the shelter staff are absolutely essential.

In addition to dealing with often overwhelming medical complications, a person infected with HIV must live with the stigma of the disease while coping with other psycho-social issues, such as child custody, partners who may or may not be infected, substance use, mental illness, and keeping a roof over their heads. Confidentiality, which is never easy in a shelter setting, is particularly important around this diagnosis.

Transmission

HIV is transmitted through person-to-person contact with blood or other body fluids such as semen, vaginal secretions, and breast milk. Common ways to transmit the virus include: sexual

Seborrheic Dermatitis in HIV/AIDS. This woman presented to a shelter clinic with weight loss and this flare of seborrheic dermatitis. Subsequent studies showed her to be HIV positive with a CD4 count of 25. Photo by Jon Fuller MD

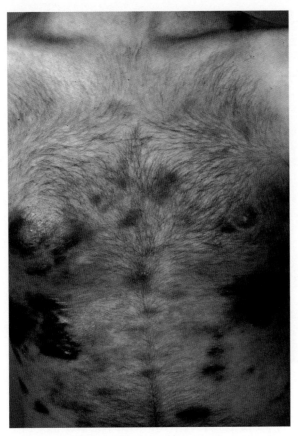

Women who are HIV infected can transmit the virus to the baby, both during the pregnancy and during delivery. HIV can also be transmitted to the baby through breast-feeding. In the USA, pregnant women with HIV infection are now treated with medications during pregnancy, and the babies are treated after delivery. The babies of women who take HIV medications during pregnancy have much less risk of getting infected, but the risk is still present.

HIV is not transmitted through casual or household contact. Neither is HIV transmitted through sweat, tears, urine, or feces. While HIV can be found in saliva, scientists have found no evidence of transmission through saliva. There should be no risk to shelter workers or guests if men or women with HIV live or eat at the shelters.

Prevention and Control

Prevention is the key to control of HIV/AIDS. Significant advances have been made over the past two decades in the prevention of the spread of this virus, but this momentum should not be lost.

The role of shelter staff in the prevention of HIV is critical and cannot be underestimated. Education and prevention materials are available to shelters through local agencies and some Internet sites, e.g. www.thebody.com and Project Inform (www.projectinform.org). These materials are useful tools to educate both shelter staff and guests about ways to prevent the spread of HIV and are usually available in both Spanish and English. Shelters should make these educational materials readily available along with easily accessible condoms, dental dams, and bleach kits. Educational materials should be provided in multiple languages and should be easily understood by those with limited literacy skills.

contact; sharing needles or other drug paraphernalia; and mother to child during pregnancy, birth, or breast-feeding. Before donated blood was tested and treated, many people (especially individuals with hemophilia) contracted HIV from blood transfusions.

Unsafe sexual practices allow for transmission of the virus through the lining of the vagina, vulva, penis, rectum, or mouth during sex. HIV can be spread to a sexual partner whether the partner is of the same sex or opposite sex. HIV medications do not eliminate the transmission of the virus from one person to another. Even if a person has a low level of virus in the blood stream, there can be a high level in other parts of the body and therefore the virus can still be spread through sexual contact and through sharing needles.

In the USA all blood products are treated and screened so that the risk of transmission is extremely low. In other countries, where the blood may not be screened as carefully, HIV can still be spread through blood transfusions

Injection drug users can transmit HIV through needles or syringes that have been used by someone who has the virus. Cocaine users who share contaminated drug paraphernalia can transmit the virus through the breakdown in the lining of the nose.

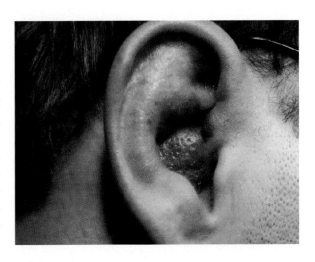

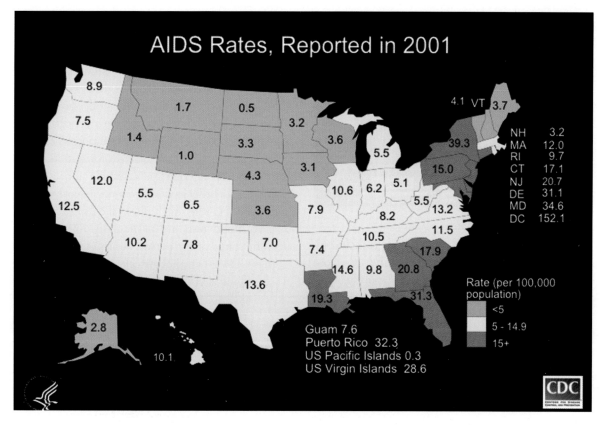

AIDS Rates, Reported in 2001

NH	3.2
MA	12.0
RI	9.7
CT	17.1
NJ	20.7
DE	31.1
MD	34.6
DC	152.1

Rate (per 100,000 population)
<5
5 - 14.9
15+

Guam 7.6
Puerto Rico 32.3
US Pacific Islands 0.3
US Virgin Islands 28.6

The AIDS Epidemic in the USA. AIDS cases per 100,000 persons in each state as of December, 2001. Courtesy of the CDC

Safer Sex

Abstinence is the only sure way to avoid passing HIV or other sexually transmitted diseases (STDs) to a partner. No sexual contact is completely safe even with the use of condoms and other barriers. Even oral sex has some risk of spreading the HIV virus. Condoms can break or fall off. For these reasons, HIV counselors use the term "safer sex" rather than "safe sex".

In order to decrease the risk of passing HIV or other STDs to partners, everyone engaging in any sexual act is urged to use a barrier such as a condom, female condom, or dental dam. Condoms are placed over the penis during penetrating sex – oral, vaginal, or anal. A woman can use a female condom if her partner will not use a male condom. A dental dam is a piece of plastic used to prevent contact during oral sex performed on a woman. Any piece of plastic that is a barrier can be used. If a dental dam is not available, Saran Wrap™ or similar products can be used. Nonoxynol 9, a very commonly used spermicidal agent, is no longer recommended. Studies have shown that this agent irritates the lining of the vagina or anus and can lead to an increased risk of HIV transmission. Safer sex should be practiced whether or not a partner is known to have HIV. Unfortunately, many individuals are unaware of their HIV infection.

Safer Needle Use

Sharing needles is a very common mode of transmission of this virus. Any individual who shares needles or other drug "works" with a person infected with HIV has a very high risk of HIV infection. While the best prevention is undoubtedly the treatment of addiction, the reality is that substance abuse is a chronic and relapsing illness and not all injection drug users will become drug free. Therefore, good public health practice should emphasize the education of injection drug users about needle exchange programs whenever available in the community. In more and more communities, programs have been developed that will exchange used syringes for clean ones in order to help reduce the spread of HIV and other diseases. A growing body of evidence has shown that such programs are very effective in reducing the transmission of HIV among injection drug users.

Use of Other Drugs

People who use cocaine must be aware that they can spread HIV by sharing straws or other tools with someone infected with the virus. Cocaine, alcohol, methamphetamines, and other drugs can affect a person's ability to make clear decisions and easily lead to unsafe sex and sharing of drug works.

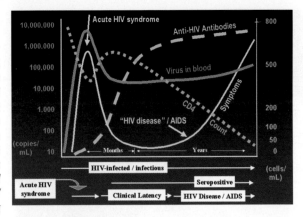

Daily Activities

HIV is not spread by casual contact, including touching, hugging, and even sleeping in close quarters. People infected with HIV can share in all normal activities in a shelter without the risk of infecting staff or other guests. Shelter personnel should use universal precautions whenever cleaning spills of bodily fluids. Individuals should not share razors, toothbrushes, or any sharp object that could have come in contact with blood.

Diagnosis

Over the years, remarkable advances have been made in the technology involved in the testing for HIV. Prior to 1985, no blood test was available for HIV and the diagnosis of AIDS was a strictly clinical one. Otherwise "healthy" individuals who became ill with Kaposi's sarcoma, *Pneumocystis carinii* pneumonia, or other illnesses that occurred only in severely immunocompromised patients, were said to have an "acquired immunodeficiency syndrome" or AIDS.

In addition to the routine blood tests for HIV that have been available since the mid-1980s, an individual's saliva can now be checked for antibodies to the virus. Both of these tests can take up to 2 weeks for results to be returned. If the initial test is positive, the blood or saliva is sent to a reference lab for a confirmatory test. These laboratory tests indicate whether an individual has been exposed to HIV but cannot determine how sick an individual is or how advanced the HIV disease has become. Other tests, as well as a thorough history and complete physical examination, are necessary to determine the status of the HIV infection.

The Centers for Disease Control and Prevention have approved another test that can get results to the person as quickly as 20 minutes after testing. This finger stick requires a very small drop of blood for the test to be performed. This result is considered preliminary until a confirmatory test is done.

Counseling, both before testing and after giving the results, is critical and must be given the highest priority. Pre-test counseling helps to educate the person being tested about prevention of future infection, even if the test result is negative; post-test counseling offers needed support and education to individuals who test positive, as these individuals must cope with a chronic and often devastating illness.

Any person who tests positive for antibodies to HIV should be referred for accessible and available medical care in order to undergo more extensive evaluation, including tests and a physical examination.

Two blood tests are particularly important to assess the status of the person's immune system:

(1) CD4 T-lymphocyte cell count. These white blood cells are a subset of T lymphocytes and one of the body's main immunologic tools to prevent certain types of infection and cancer. HIV targets these cells and gradually destroys them. By measuring the number of these cells in the blood, health care practitioners can tell how much damage has been done to the immune system;

(2) HIV "viral load" directly measures the amount of virus circulating in the bloodstream. This test is utilized to measure the effectiveness of antiretroviral medications, and the goal is to reduce the viral load as much as possible.

Clinical Signs and Symptoms

"Acute HIV infection" is a syndrome that develops a few days to a few weeks after exposure to the virus. This non-specific syndrome is typically a "flu-like illness" accompanied by fevers, headache, sore throat, and enlarged lymph nodes. Any person with this syndrome who has a history of recent high-risk behavior, such as injection drug use or unsafe sex, should immediately receive a thorough medical evaluation. Important studies over the past few years have demonstrated that prompt treatment with antiretroviral medications may improve the ability of the body's immune system to control HIV and favorably alter the course of the disease.

Persons with acute HIV syndrome are highly infectious and have a large burden of virus in the bloodstream. The HIV viral load is elevated, but the tests for HIV antibodies are usually negative at this early stage of infection when the body has not yet had time to generate an immune response and form these antibodies. The signs and symptoms of acute HIV infection usually disappear within a week to a month.

After the initial infection, the person with HIV may have no signs or symptoms of illness for months or years, sometimes as long as 10 years. Even though an individual does not feel sick, the virus continues to multiply and gradually kills certain T lymphocytes, known as CD4 cells, that are important to the body's immune system. Since these cells often decrease before any signs or symptoms are present, the measurement of the CD4 cell count has become a mainstay in monitoring and treating HIV disease. The normal CD4 count is greater than 500 cells/ml³ (per cubic milliliter of blood). Some early signs and symptoms may be present as HIV infection progresses, including: lack of energy; fevers and night sweats; weight loss; frequent yeast infections (oral or vaginal); flaky scaly skin; memory loss; and recurrent herpes virus infections of the mouth or genital or anal area. Shingles or herpes zoster virus can also be an early sign of HIV progression.

More serious infections can ensue as the CD4 count falls and the immune system becomes more compromised. These "opportunistic" infections (OIs) take advantage of the person's damaged immune system. Some examples include the following:

- *Pneumocystis carinii* pneumonia (PCP) is one of the most common and most dangerous of these OIs. *Pneumocystis carinii* can cause a very serious pneumonia when the CD4 cell count falls below 200 cells/ml³. The typical signs and symptoms of PCP include a cough accompanied by high fevers and shortness of breath;
- Toxoplasmosis is a single-celled parasite that can be found in cat feces (cat litter) or in partially cooked pork, lamb, or venison. In persons with poorly functioning immune systems, it can infect the brain and cause severe headaches, seizures, fevers, and stroke-like symptoms. People with HIV are at risk for this infection when their CD4 cell counts fall below 100;
- *Mycobacterium avium* complex (MAC) is due to a bacteria related to tuberculosis that causes weight loss, fevers, weakness, and gastrointestinal symptoms. It may infect persons with CD4 cell counts less than 50;
- *Mycobacterium tuberculosis* (TB), both pulmonary and extra-pulmonary, is more easily contracted by persons with HIV than those with normal immune systems.
- As HIV progresses, people can develop many infections caused by viruses, bacte-

ria, and parasites. They are also at greater risk of developing some cancers, such as lymphoma (cancer of the lymph nodes), Kaposi's sarcoma, and cervical and anal cancer.

Diagnosis

The diagnosis of AIDS in a person with HIV infection is made when: (1) the CD4 cell count has dropped below 200; or (2) the individual has developed one of the many infections or cancers associated with HIV infection.

Treatment

The treatment of HIV disease involves education, prevention, and medications. The optimal treatment for HIV requires a multidisciplinary team approach in which doctors, nurse practitioners, physician assistants, mental health clinicians, nurses, substance abuse counselors, nutritionists, and case managers work together to care for each patient.

Infected individuals must be educated to avoid high-risk behaviors and prevent the spread of the virus to others. In addition, infected individuals who continue to engage in high-risk behaviors can receive repeated inoculums of virus and risk infection with another strain of HIV.

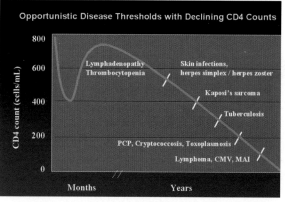

Opportunistic Disease Thresholds with Declining CD4 Counts. This chart shows the types of opportunistic infections that can occur as HIV destroys the immune system and the number of CD4 cells falls. Courtesy of Jon Fuller MD

Living with HIV without safe and stable housing creates an emotional roller coaster, especially for those persons also coping with substance abuse and mental illness. Virtually all individuals struggle with the stigma of HIV in our society and homeless persons already face a profound social isolation. Rejection by a partner often follows the diagnosis of HIV infection. Many persons infected with HIV have struggled with childhood and adult sexual and physical abuse, and coping with this infection often rekindles those memories. All persons with HIV infections should have ready access to sensitive mental health clinicians.

The relationship between the person infected with HIV and the health care clinician (or team) is paramount. This relationship must be based on mutual respect and trust, and the treatment plan must be mutually agreed upon and reflect the individual's social, cultural, racial, economic, and spiritual background.

Medications for the Treatment of HIV/AIDS

The advances in the treatment of HIV/AIDS have been dramatic, although we still have no cure for this virus. The advent of highly active anti-retroviral therapy (HAART, or simply ART) in the mid-1990s has revolutionized the treatment of HIV/AIDS, but it is very expensive and requires each individual to take several medications (usually 3-4) from one to three times each day. These medications also have several potentially serious side effects. The other danger is that the virus can develop resistance to one or more of the HAART medications.

Each patient who begins ART must become thoroughly familiar with each of the prescribed medications, including the proper timing and frequency of administration, as well as the common side effects. Some important considerations are:

- social supports – does the person have a supportive family or friends? Does the person's spouse or partner know of the diagnosis? Is the partner able to help with the treatment?;
- commitment – does the person understand that taking medications for HIV/AIDS will probably be a lifelong commitment necessary for the control of this chronic disease?;
- "medical home" – does the person have a medical clinician, or health care team, skilled in the treatment of HIV/AIDS? Is there someone on the team with whom

the person feels comfortable and safe when talking about personal health and other issues?;
- safety and privacy – does the person have a safe place for the storage of medication? Is there sufficient privacy for taking the medications? Many homeless persons fear that just being seen with these medications allows others to know about their HIV infection.

These issues are all very important for clinicians to address with their homeless patients. ART therapy should be considered lifelong and requires many lifestyle changes that can be very challenging for those without homes. Proper administration of the medications is critical, as the virus can more easily develop resistance if doses are skipped or individuals take "drug holidays". Once the virus develops resistance to a medication, the person may not be able to use that medication again. Whenever side effects appear, persons should notify the clinician immediately. The medications should not be discontinued unless instructed by the clinician. Fortunately, most side effects resolve over time. Thousands of people take the medications without developing side effects.

During the last ten years, researchers and scientists have developed many new medications to treat HIV infection. Used in combination, these medications are very potent and can lead to remarkable improvements in a person's immune function and overall health. Nucleoside reverse transcriptase inhibitors (NRTI's) prevent viral replication within the cell. Non-nucleoside reverse transcriptase inhibitors (NNRTI's) work in a similar way to the nucleoside inhibitors. A third class of medications prevent viral replication at a later stage and are called protease inhibitors (PI's). A recently approved class of drugs called fusion inhibitors keeps the HIV virus from entering the cell.

Some of the most frequently used HIV medications are listed in the table at the end of this chapter.

Combivir™ is a combination of zidovudine and lamivudine. Trizivir™ combines zidovudine, lamivudine and abacavir.

Doctors and medical providers should be aware of the patient's homelessness and prescribe drugs appropriate for those struggling to live in shelters or on the streets. For example, drugs that require refrigeration or require food for absorption should be avoided whenever possible. Regimens that involve several pills taken multiple times per day

Oral Hairy Leukoplakia. This lesion of the tongue is usually asymptomatic and indicates immunocompromise and a poor prognosis. The white, irregular lesions can appear as columns on the lateral surface of the tongue.
Photo by Irwin Freedberg MD

are very difficult for homeless persons, and the goal should be to prescribe medications that involve few pills that can be taken once or twice a day. Newer medications have made this possible, and many regimens involve medications taken twice a day, while at least one ART therapy is taken once a day. Some communities offer directly observed therapy of HIV medications in drop-in centers, methadone clinics, or medical clinics.

When to Start Medications

Federal guidelines recommend offering medical treatment for HIV infection when the CD4 count is between 200 and 350. The goal is to control the replication of the virus and delay the onset of opportunistic infections.

Translating this recommendation into reality is often complicated, as each treatment plan must address the special needs of each individual. Is the person ready and able to take medications every day at scheduled times? Does the person suffer from an underlying mental illness or abuse substances that hinder the ability to take 3 or more different medications? Does the HIV infected person have access to clinicians and support staff who will be available in the event of side effects of medications? Does the person have a safe place to store medicines? The medical team and the person with HIV infection should carefully discuss all these issues and make a mutual and informed decision concerning the best time to start taking medications.

The importance of offering HIV medications to pregnant women cannot be overemphasized. This practice has significantly decreased the number of babies born with HIV infection.

Prevention of OIs and AIDS-Related Cancers

Individuals with CD4 counts below certain levels must take medications to prevent the most common opportunistic infections. For example:
- CD4 = 200 or less, individuals should take trimethoprim-sulfamethoxazole (Bactrim™, Septra™) or dapsone (Avlosulfon™), or atovaquone (Mepron™) to prevent *Pneumocystis carinii* pneumonia (PCP);
- CD4 = 100 or less, medication should be taken to prevent toxoplasmosis. The preferred medication is trimethoprim-sulfamethoxazole (Bactrim™, Septra™). If the person cannot tolerate that medication, then dapsone (Avlosulfon™) with pyrimethamine (Daraprim™) and folinic

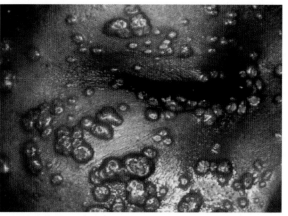

Molluscum Contagiosum. The papules are pearl-colored with central umbilications, and often involve the eyelids. This rash resolved three months after the initiation of ART.

Reprinted with permission from Cotell, R. Molluscum contagiosum in a patient with the Acquired Immunodeficiency Syndrome. New England Journal of Medicine 1998;338:888. ©Massachusetts Medical Society. All rights reserved.

acid (Leukovorin™), or atovoquone (Mepron™) with pyrimethamine (Daraprim™) and folinic acid (Leukovorin™) can be used.
- CD4 = 50 or less, medication to prevent mycobacterium avium complex (MAC), a bacteria related to tuberculosis is added. The preferred medication is azithromycin (Zithromax™) once a week or clarithromycin (Biaxin™) daily.

The federal guidelines for treatment of HIV and opportunistic infections are available online at www.aidsinfo.nih.gov.

Summary

Human immunodeficiency virus is a retrovirus that infects humans through sexual contact, shared drug paraphernalia, mother-to-child transmission, and blood transfusions (primarily in less developed countries). The virus attacks the immune system, damaging cells that fight infections and cancers.

Blood tests are available to diagnose the presence of antibodies to the virus, and these tests indicate that a person is infected with the virus. Further tests can assess how advanced the disease is. These tests are called CD4 counts and HIV viral load measurements. These tests are critical because early involvement in medical care can lead to greatly improved outcomes.

Although HIV medications are difficult to take and can cause side effects, they can allow a person to live a much longer life. Much like diabetes or high blood pressure, HIV has become a chronic disease that, with diligence, can be managed. Homeless people have a particular challenge in managing this disease, but success is very possible with support from their health care providers and others. Everyone infected with this virus, regardless of income or housing status, deserves the best that medicine has to offer.

Shelter personnel play an important role in providing counseling and support, as well as facilitating access to medical, psychosocial, and supportive care. ▪

HIV Medication List

Generic	Brand	Cost
NRTI's		
zidovudine	Retrovir, AZT	$$$$$
stavudine	Zerit, d4T	$$$$$
lamivudine	Epivir, 3TC	$$$$$
didanosine	Videx, ddl	$$$$$
abacavir	Ziagen, ABC	$$$$$
tenofovir	Viread, TDF	$$$$$
abacavir+lamivudine+zidovudine	Trizivir	$$$$$
emtricitabine	Emtriva, FTC	$$$$$
lamivudine+zidovudine	Combivir	$$$$$
zalcitabine	Hivid, ddC	$$$$$
NNRTI's		
nevirapine	Viramune, NVP	$$$$$
efavirenz	Sustiva, EFV	$$$$$
delavirdine	Rescriptor	$$$$$
Protease Inhibitors		
nelfinavir	Viracept, NFV	$$$$$
saquinavir	Fortovase, Invirase, SQV	$$$$$
indinavir	Crixivan, IDV	$$$$$
ritonavir	Norvir, RTV	$$$$$
amprenavir	Agenerase, APV	$$$$$
lopinavir+ritonavir	Kaletra, (LPV/r)	$$$$$
atazanavir	Reyataz	$$$$$
fosamprenavir	Lexiva	$$$$$
Fusion Inhibitors		
enfuvirtide	Fuzeon, T-20	$$$$$

References

Bamberger JD, Unick J, Klein P, et al. Helping the urban poor stay with antiretroviral HIV drug therapy. *American Journal of Public Health* 2000;90(5):699-701.

Bangsberg D, Tulsky J, Hecht F, et al. Protease inhibitors in the homeless. *Journal of the American Medical Association* 1997;278(1):63-5 1997 Jul 2.

Bartlett JG, Gallant JE., ed. *Medical Management of HIV Infection.* Baltimore: Lighthouse Point; 2003.

Centers for Disease Control and Prevention, Division of HIV/AIDS Prevention. Surveillance Reports, Year-end 2001. *MMWR* 2002;13(2).

Commonwealth of Massachusetts Department of Public Health. HIV/AIDS in Massachusetts: An epidemiologic profile. November, 2002.

Conanan B, London K, et al. *Adapting Your Practice: Treatment and Recommendations for Homeless Patients with HIV/AIDS.* Nashville: Health Care for the Homeless Clinicians' Network, National Health Care for the Homeless Council, Inc., 2003.

Peiperl L. Antiretroviral treatments to reduce mother-to-child transmission of HIV. *HIV Clinical Trials* 2001;2(1): 46-55.

Susser E, Valenci E, Concver S. Prevalence of HIV infection among psychiatric patients in a New York City men's shelter. *American Journal of Public Health* 1993;83(4):568-570.

U.S. Public Health Service. 2001 USPHS/IDSA guidelines for the prevention of opportunistic infections in persons infected with human immunodeficiency virus. November, 2001.

For useful references, please refer to these CDC web sites:
http://www.cdc.gov/hiv/prevtools.htm
http://www.cdc.gov/hiv/testing.htm

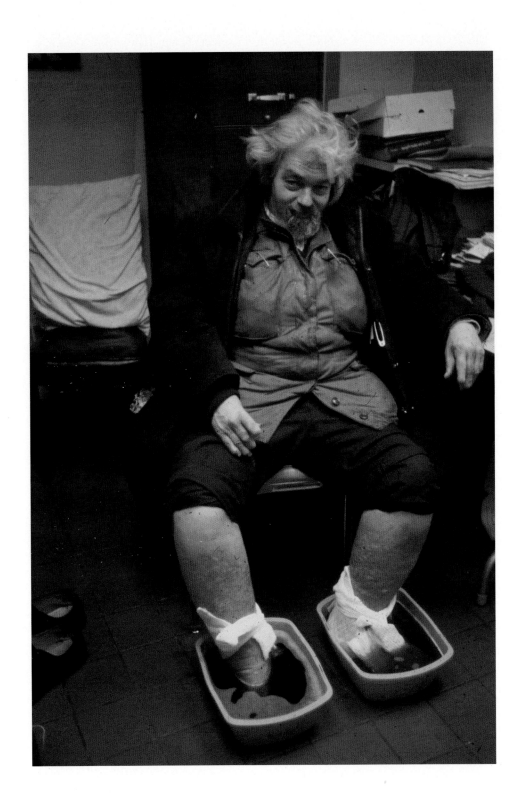

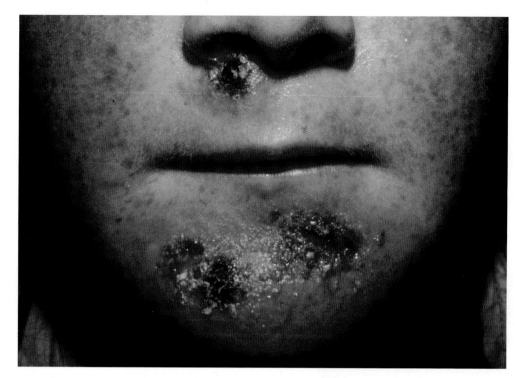

Impetigo

Sarah McSweeney-Ryan, MD
Megan Sandel, MD

Impetigo is a very contagious bacterial infection of the superficial layer of the skin. The bacteria usually infect skin that has been damaged by scratching an insect bite or picking a scab. The lesions may cause mild soreness and itching, but are typically painless. Fever or other symptoms of systemic illness are not seen with impetigo.

The two types of bacteria that cause impetigo are group A, beta-hemolytic streptococci and *Staphylococcus aureus*. Impetigo is classified as bullous, or non-bullous based on the presence or lack of large blisters, called bullae.

Bullous Impetigo

Bullous impetigo is characterized by bullae, large thin-walled blisters that contain clear or cloudy yellow fluid and measure up to 5 cm in diameter. Bullae are caused by staphylococcal infections, not by streptococci. A certain type of staphylococcal bacteria produces a toxin that causes the large blisters to form. These blisters easily rupture and leave behind a moist area of eroded skin surrounded by a thin ring of the remaining blistered skin. This lesion dries and crusts over, creating a light brown appearance that resembles "varnish". The lesions are discrete, with little redness or inflammation surrounding them. These large blisters typically occur on the face but may quickly spread to different areas of the skin. A mix of bullous and non-bullous skin lesions may occur.

Non-Bullous Impetigo

This is the more common type of impetigo and is characterized by reddened sores with honey-yellow crusting on them. The sores may initially appear as small blisters that rupture, ooze, and lead to the layer of crusting. The crust typically appears to be "stuck on". The infection does not disappear easily with topical cleaning. The lesions are painless, often occur around the mouth and nose or on the arms and legs, and resolve without scarring.

These non-bullous lesions are caused by either Streptococcus or Staphylococcus, and in some cases both types of bacteria may be present.

Prevalence and Distribution

Impetigo can affect people of any age. However, the disease most commonly affects children ages 2 to 5 years. Children in crowded settings, such as in day care centers and shelters, have higher rates of infection with impetigo. Warm humid weather and poor hygiene promote the development and spread of impetigo.

Impetigo. Yellow-gold crusts that glisten and have a "stuck-on" appearance. Note the oozing from many areas. Photo by Irwin Freedberg MD

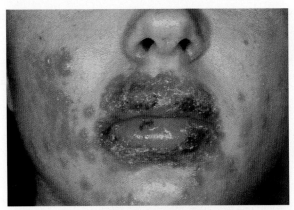

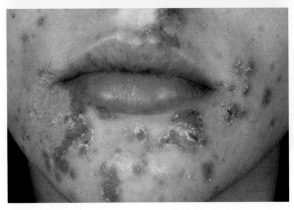

Transmission

Impetigo spreads easily and most commonly by direct contact to infected skin. Infection may also spread through contaminated clothing. People who begin treatment with topical or oral antibiotics are no longer infectious after 24 to 48 hours.

Breakdowns in skin integrity, such as cuts, scratched insect bites, burns, and other chronic skin conditions (most commonly eczema), provide sites of entrance for bacteria.

Diagnosis

The diagnosis of impetigo is usually based on the clinical appearance, as described above. A culture from the infected area may sometimes be necessary to differentiate between Streptococci and Staphylococci, although both bacteria are often present. Most infections can be treated without obtaining cultures. A culture is necessary when the infection has not responded to antibiotics, which may suggest an infection with methicillin-resistant *Staphylococcus aureus*.

Treatment

Children infected with impetigo should be encouraged not to touch the lesion or pick the scabs. Trimming children's fingernails and encouraging frequent washing with antibacterial soap may help.

Impetigo can be treated with either oral or topical antibiotics. Topical treatment may be selected if the area of impetigo is localized. Treatment is with mupirocin (Bactroban™), which is effective against both Staphylococcus and Streptococcus. An allergy or sensitivity to mupirocin is the only contraindication. Stinging and burning of the skin can rarely occur. While costly, mupirocin is as effective as oral antibiotic agents and is less apt to cause resistance to develop in the organisms. Mupirocin (Bactroban™) ointment should be placed on the lesions three times each day, for a total of five days. At the initiation of treatment the crusty scabs should be removed after softening with wet compresses. The lesions should be washed with an antibacterial soap twice daily.

Oral, or systemic, antibiotics are usually used when lesions are bullous or when non-bullous lesions appear to be spreading over a person's body or from one person to another. The use of oral antibiotics accelerates healing and diminishes the period of infectivity. Because the risk of transmission of impetigo is high in shelters, we recommend the use of oral rather than topical antibiotics whenever possible.

The appearance of a typical non-bullous impetigo lesion is similar for infections caused by either Streptococcus or Staphylococcus. Initial cultures are usually not necessary, since health care professionals commonly prescribe dicloxacillin (Dynapen™), oxacillin (Bactocill™), azithromycin (Zithromax™), or cephalexin (Keflex™), all of which are effective treatments for the common types of Streptococci and Staphylococci that cause impetigo.

A culture should be obtained if there is no resolution of the lesion after one week of conventional therapy. If an organism grows from this culture, a laboratory can then measure sensitivity patterns to determine the best antibiotic treatment for the bacteria. If there are signs of increased redness, warmth, fullness, or pain in the skin surrounding the lesions, then patients should seek medical attention to be sure that the infection has not worsened and developed into a skin infection, called cellulitis.

The risk of transmission of impetigo is high in shelters, and we recommend the use of systemic or oral antibiotics rather than topical antibiotics whenever possible.

Prevention and Control

Caregivers should encourage all guests and staff to seek medical care for new rashes or draining wounds.

When impetigo arises in a shelter, staff should

watch for similar eruptions on other guests, especially those in close contact with the infected person(s). Mupirocin (Bactroban™) or other antibiotic ointments can be applied to open cuts and insect bites in an attempt to prevent infection.

Residents of the shelter should be reminded of the importance of contact precautions in preventing the spread of this contagious infection.

The towels and clothes used by an infected person should not be shared with others.

Infected people should keep their lesions covered with bandages or clothing during the first 48 hours of antibiotic therapy. Children should not go to daycare or be in crowded shelter areas until 24 hours after starting antibiotic therapy.

If an infected person is taking oral antibiotics, all of the recommended therapy should be completed even though the rash will usually clear within 2 to 3 days.

Summary

Impetigo is a very contagious bacterial infection of the skin, often seen around the mouth and nose or the arms and legs. Impetigo is common in young children.

Impetigo spreads very easily during hot weather and in crowded settings. Spread can occur when a person has direct contact to the infected skin of another person. Infection is more likely when there is damage to skin, such as burns, abrasions, and scratched insect bites.

There are two types of impetigo, bullous and non-bullous. Bullous lesions are large, thin, fluid-filled blisters. Both types have reddened sores that will ooze, causing either a yellow or varnish-colored crust to form.

Antibiotics are needed to eliminate impetigo. Left untreated, this infection can spread very quickly in a shelter. If impetigo is suspected, consult a health provider. ▓

The authors of this chapter gratefully acknowledge the invaluable contribution of Ben Siegel, MD, who authored this chapter in the original Manual.

Impetigo Medication List

Generic	Brand Name	Cost
azithromycin	Zithromax	$$
cephalexin	Keflex	$
dicloxacillin	Dynapen	$
mupirocin	Bactroban	$$
oxacillin	Bactocill	$

References

Habif TP. *Clinical Dermatology.* St Louis: Mosby-Year Book Inc.; 1996:236-242.

Jain A, Daum RS. Staphylococcal infections in children: part 1. *Pediatrics in Review* 1999;20(6):183-191.

Pickering LK, Peter G, Baker CJ, et al. eds. *The 2000 Red Book: Report of the Committee on Infectious Diseases.* Elk Grove Village, Illinois: American Academy of Pediatrics; 2000:526-527, 532-533.

Stulberg DL, Penrod MA, Blatny RA. Common bacterial skin infections. *American Family Physician* 2002;66(1): 119-124.

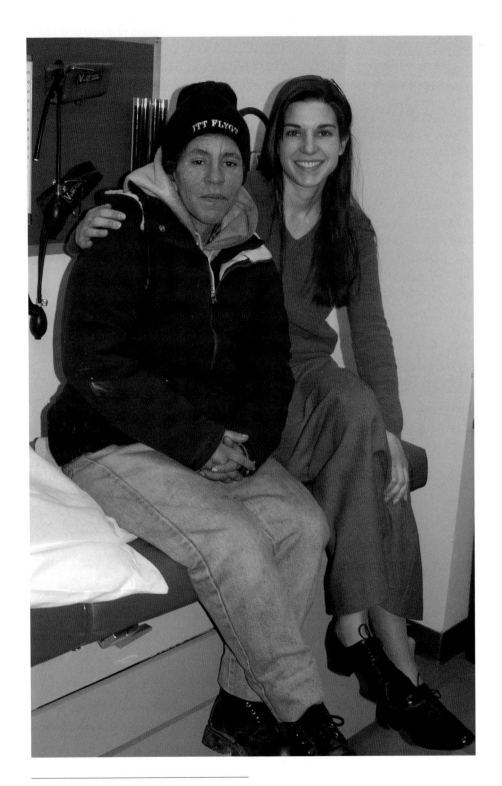

BHCHP physician assistant Jill Roncarati with a patient in the exam room during the Thursday Street Clinic at Massachusetts General Hospital. Photo by James O'Connell MD

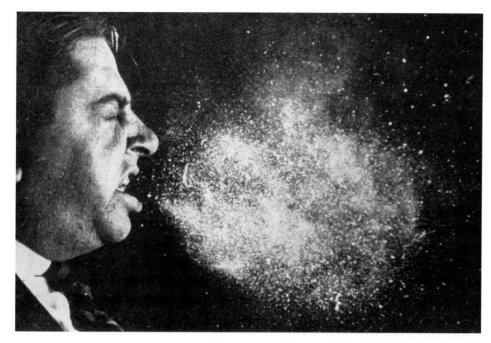

Influenza

Marisa A. Rogers, MD, MPH
Jennifer Gordon Wright,
DVM, MPH
Bruce D. Levy, MD, FACP

Influenza is a respiratory illness caused by either influenza A or influenza B viruses. Sporadic cases or outbreaks of influenza can occur at any time during the year, but epidemic activity peaks during the winter months in temperate climates. Influenza is usually a self-limited illness; however, elderly persons and those with pre-existing chronic cardiac and pulmonary disease are at higher risk for developing severe complications from influenza. Vaccination is the most effective means of preventing influenza and its complications.

Prevalence and Distribution

The timing of influenza activity differs by zone. The onset of influenza activity in temperate climates typically occurs in late fall, although the timing if individual influenza seasons can vary substantially from year to year. In the northern hemisphere, peak influenza activity typically occurs between December and March, while in the southern hemisphere influenza peak activity typically occurs between May and August. Outbreaks of influenza often occur in unvaccinated populations.

Rates of infection are highest in children, but elderly persons and persons with certain medical conditions which predispose them to complications from influenza have the highest rates of serious morbidity and mortality. Millions are infected with influenza each year in the United States and over 100,000 individuals on average are hospitalized annually for influenza or its complications. Influenza is estimated to cause an average of 36,000 deaths per year in the United States.

Influenza A viruses are divided into subtypes based on two proteins on the surface of the virus:

the hemagglutinin and the neuraminidase. Minor changes in the hemagglutinin are referred to as "antigenic drift" and facilitate seasonal epidemics. Replacement of the hemagluttinin with a new hemagluttinin is known as "antigenic shift". Such changes are associated with the development of influenza pandemics.

Mode of Transmission

Influenza virus is primarily spread from person to person through coughing and sneezing of virus particles in respiratory secretions. On average the incubation period lasts two days, but can range from one to four days. The period of infectivity for adults begins about 1 day prior to the development of symptoms and typically lasts for 3 to 5 days after the onset of symptoms.

Symptoms and Diagnosis

The classic symptoms of influenza include the abrupt onset of fever accompanied by chills, myalgias, headache, malaise, nonproductive cough and sore throat. Rhinitis may also be present. The

"The Sneeze". Sneezing is a very efficient way to spread many airborne diseases, such as influenza. The virus is contained in the many small droplets shown by backlighting in this photograph. Photo courtesy of the CDC

Table 1: Drugs Used in Prevention and Treatment of Influenza

Drug	Type of influenza	Effectiveness in prevention	Side effects
amantadine (Symmetrel™)	A	70-90%	CNS (dizziness, jitteriness, insomnia, anxiety), CHF, anticholinergic effects
rimantadine (Flumadine™)	A	70-90%	CNS (less than amantadine)
oseltamivir (Tamiflu™)	A and B	82%	Nausea, vomiting
zanamivir* (Relenza™)	A and B	84%	Bronchospasm

*zanamivir is not approved for the prevention of influenza

symptoms of influenza are difficult to distinguish from many other viral upper respiratory infections that occur during the winter months and the predictive value of these symptoms for diagnostic purposes reflects the degree of co-circulation of other respiratory pathogens and influenza viruses. When influenza viruses are circulating, fever and cough are the most useful diagnostic symptoms, with reports of sensitivity ranging from 63-73% and reports of specificity ranging from 55-71%. A fever of 100°F/37.7°C (or 99°F/37.2°C in the elderly) and cough within 48 hours of symptom development in one study had a positive predictive value of 79%. The positive predictive value increases to greater than 80% if the fever increases to 100.4°F (38°C). Since influenza cases can occur year-round, health care providers must remain alert to the possibility of influenza throughout the year, especially when outbreaks of respiratory illness occur.

The physical examination is usually unrevealing in uncomplicated influenza infection. Confirmatory testing can be very helpful in making a diagnosis of influenza. The gold standard for laboratory testing is viral culture. Other diagnostic tests include rapid antigen testing, polymerase chain reaction and immunofluorescence. Serology requires the collection of an acute and convalescent serum sample. The sensitivity and specificity of these tests vary greatly depending on the lab performing the test, the type of test and the specimen type. Rapid antigen tests have become widely used in outpatient clinics because results can be obtained within 30 minutes or less. When interpreting the results of rapid tests, one should take into account the community prevalence of influenza and the pre-test probability of disease.

Treatment and Complications

Influenza is usually a self-limited illness that resolves after several days, although cough and malaise may persist for 2 weeks or longer. The treatment of uncomplicated influenza is supportive, with analgesics to treat fever and myalgias, and antitussives for cough when needed. Aspirin should be avoided in children with fever. Fever can increase insensible losses, and fluids are necessary to prevent dehydration. Influenza can exacerbate pre-existing medical conditions such as asthma or chronic obstructive pulmonary disease (COPD), and these patients should be monitored closely for exacerbation of underlying conditions.

Antiviral medications can reduce the duration of illness by 1 day when started within 48 hours of illness onset (Table 1). They have not been shown to be effective at preventing serious influenza-related complications such as bacterial pneumonia. The adamantanes, amantadine and rimantadine, are older drugs that are effective only against influenza A. Side effects of the adamantanes include central nervous system disturbances such as jitteriness, insomnia, and anxiety. These side effects occur more frequently with amantadine and are more pronounced in the elderly. Neuraminidase inhibitors, oseltamivir (Tamiflu™) and zanamivir (Relenza ™), are approved for the treatment of both influenza A and B, and have fewer side effects than amantadine or rimantadine.

Antivirals can be useful for prophylaxis of unvaccinated persons or those at high risk for influenza related complications, as well as for treatment of ill individuals.

Pneumonia is the most common secondary bacterial complication of influenza. Less often influenza may lead to primary viral pneumonia, which is usually severe and should be suspected in a patient with progression of fever and respiratory symptoms beyond what would be expected from uncomplicated infection. Secondary bacterial pneumonia is more common and should be suspected when symptoms associated with pneumonia appear after initial improvement of influenza illness. One case series reported that *Streptococcus pneumoniae* and *Staphylococcus aureus* are the most common pathogens, occurring in 48% and 19% of secondary bacterial pneumonia cases, respectively.

Myositis and rhabdomyolysis are infrequent complications of influenza, occurring more often in children. Aspirin should not be used in treating children with suspected influenza because of the association with Reye syndrome, a rare illness marked by central nervous system disturbance and hepatic dysfunction. Central nervous system complications of influenza are uncommon, but influenza should be considered in the differential diagnosis of encephalitis/encephalopathy in children

Prevention and Control

Vaccination is the best way to prevent influenza and is indicated for persons at increased risk of complications from influenza, as well as close contacts of those at increased risk (Table 2). The most widely used influenza vaccine is a trivalent inactivated vaccine and consists of two A viruses and one B virus. Vaccine effectiveness depends on the match between the vaccine and circulating virus, as well as the age and immune status of the host. In years when the match between the vaccine and the circulating virus has been good, vaccination has prevented influenza in 70-90% of vaccinated, healthy adults under the age of 65, and 58% of vaccinated elderly persons. Vaccination is 30-70% effective in preventing hospitalization for pneumonia and influenza in persons aged 65 years. The vaccine is less effective in preventing primary influenza illness in nursing home residents, but can be 50-60% effective in preventing pneumonia and hospitalization, and 80% effective in preventing death in this high-risk population.

Recently, a live, attenuated trivalent influenza vaccine (LAIV) was approved by the Food and Drug Administration (FDA) for intranasal administration. Efficacy is similar to the inactivated influenza vaccine in healthy adults and children. Currently LAIV is approved only for healthy persons aged 5-49 years.

Influenza vaccine can be cost-effective in some circumstances. Savings in the elderly population are related to decreased hospitalization and death. In those younger than 65, savings are due to a decrease in direct medical costs, as well as indirect costs associated with a decrease in work absenteeism.

The ideal time to vaccinate in the northern hemisphere is October and November, as most influenza infections occur in late December through March. Peak antibody protection occurs two weeks after vaccination. Antibody levels begin to fall in the elderly within 4 months, but data are not available to support a second administration of the vaccine to boost immunity. A new vaccine, updated to cover

---

Table 2: Indications for Influenza Vaccination

Increased Risk of Complications

♦ Age ≥ 65

♦ Residents of nursing homes and chronic care facilities

♦ Chronic cardiovascular and pulmonary disease, including asthma

♦ Chronic metabolic diseases (diabetes), renal disease, hemoglobinopathies, or immunosuppression (chronic steroids, HIV)

♦ Children receiving long-term aspirin therapy

♦ Women who will be pregnant during influenza season

♦ All children aged 6 -23 months

Age 50-64 years

♦ Exposure to high risk persons

♦ Health care workers

♦ Employees of nursing homes and chronic care facilities

♦ Household contacts of high risk persons

newly circulating strains, must be given annually.

Individuals with hypersensitivity to eggs should not receive the vaccine without consultation with a physician. Vaccination generally should be deferred in patients with an acute febrile illness.

The most common side effect of influenza vaccination is soreness at the injection site, occurring in 10-64% of patients and lasting <2 days. Fever, malaise and myalgias may also occur after vaccination. These side effects usually begin within 6-12 hours of inoculation, persist for 1-2 days and are more common in first time recipients of the vaccine. Influenza vaccine cannot cause influenza.

Despite its effectiveness and safety, influenza vaccine remains underutilized. Only 64% of the elderly and 32% of those aged 50-64 were vaccinated in the 2000-2001 season. Vaccination rates are lower in African-Americans and Latinos than in Caucasians.

Antiviral agents are effective in the prevention of influenza, but vaccination remains the primary means for prevention. Amantadine and rimantadine are 70-90% effective in preventing influenza A infection. The newer antivirals, oseltamivir (Tamiflu™) and zanamivir (Relenza™) are 82% and 84% effective in preventing influenza, respectively. Chemoprophylaxis may be warranted in populations such as residents of chronic care facilities during outbreaks of influenza In addition to vaccination and antiviral agents, hand washing is important for decreasing transmission rates of respiratory infections.

Special Considerations for Homeless Populations

Influenza infection rates, morbidity, mortality, and vaccination coverage in homeless populations are unknown. The crowded living conditions and poor ventilation in many shelters, as well as the high incidence of chronic medical conditions, may place homeless persons at increased risk for contracting influenza. Homeless shelters offer a unique opportunity to administer influenza vaccines to both residents and staff. Vaccination may be provided to all residents and staff who do not have specific contraindications. Since homeless populations are often mobile, a coordinated effort to vaccinate all staff and residents during the same day or week in a particular area may be attempted. This effort should include outreach efforts to vaccinate homeless populations not living in shelters to maximize coverage.

Summary

Influenza is a contagious respiratory illness that occurs primarily during the winter months in temperate climates. The illness is usually self-limited, but the elderly and persons with chronic medical conditions are at increased risk for serious complications. Vaccination is the most effective way to prevent influenza and its complications. To prevent the spread of influenza, residents of shelters and homeless persons should consider receiving annual influenza vaccination. The optimal time for vaccination is in the fall, and vaccination of all homeless persons on the same day or within the same week may be an effective strategy. ■

The authors of this chapter gratefully acknowledge the invaluable contribution of Noreen A. Hynes, MD, MPH, who authored this chapter in the original Manual.

Influenza Medication List

Generic	Brand Name	Cost
amantadine	Symmetrel	$
oseltamivir	Tamiflu	$$$
rimantadine	Flumadine	$$
zanamivir	Relenza	$$

References

Gubareva LV, Kaiser L, Hayden FG. Influenza virus neuraminidase inhibitors. *Lancet* 2000;355(9206):827-835.

Centers for Disease Control and Prevention. Influenza and pneumococcal vaccination levels among persons aged >= 65 years - United States, 2001. *MMWR* 2002;51(45):1019.

Centers for Disease Control and Prevention. Neuraminidase inhibitors for treatment of influenza A and B infections. *MMWR* 1999;48(RR-14):1.

Centers for Disease Control and Prevention. Prevention and control of influenza. Recommendation of the advisory committee on immunization practices (ACIP). *MMWR* 2003;52(RR-8):1.

Couch RB. Prevention and treatment of influenza. *New England Journal of Medicine* 2000;343(24):1778.

Monto AS, Gravenstein S, Elliott M, et al. Clinical signs and symptoms predicting influenza infection. *Archives Internal Medicine* 2000;160(21):3243-3247.

O'Connell JJ. Nontuberculous respiratory infections among the homeless. *Seminars in Respiratory Infections* 1991;6(4): 247.

Wenzel RP. Expanding the treatment options for influenza. *Journal of the American Medical Association* 2000;283(8): 1057-1059.

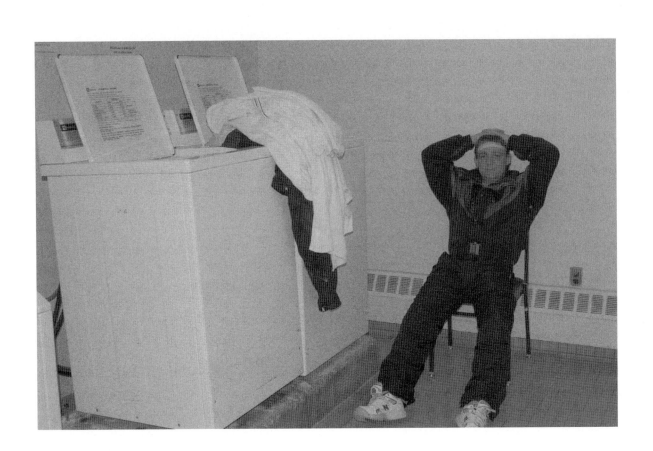

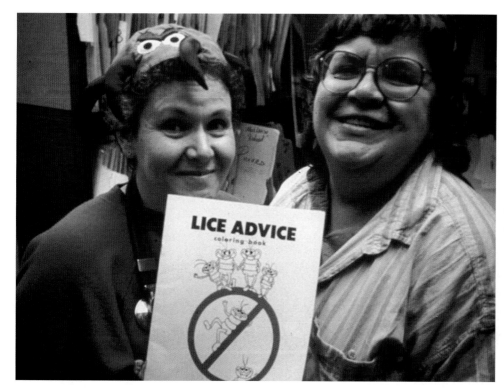

Lice

Keith Williams, MD, MS
Alison May, MD

O f more than 200 species of 'sucking lice', only two infest humans: (1) *Pediculus humanus*, which is subdivided into two variants, head lice and body lice (*capitis* and *corporis*, respectively); and (2) *Phthirus pubis*, or pubic "crab" lice.

Lice are wingless, obligate blood-leeching ecto-parasites. Lice cause significant cutaneous disease, but also are important medically as the vectors (via the body louse) for several infectious diseases:

- epidemic typhus (*Rickettsia prowazekii*);
- trench fever (*Bartonella quintana*); and
- relapsing fever (*Borrelia recurrentis*).

Head and body lice are morphologically similar, 2-4 mm in length, and grayish-white in color. Pubic lice are 1-2 mm in length (with an even greater transverse dimension) and have a 'crab' like appearance. Of note, head and body lice are capable of traveling at a rate of 23 cm/min, whereas the pubic louse travels at a rate of only 10 cm/day. All species produce oval eggs (nits) that are attached firmly to the base of a hair shaft (head and pubic lice) or to clothing (body louse-nits are viable up to one month and hatch when they encounter warmth of a host when clothes are worn again). Nits are difficult to remove without the use of tweezers or a fine-toothed nit comb. Nymphs emerge from the nits after 7-10 days and must feed within twenty-four hours to survive. After 2-3 weeks and three successive molts,

the adult lice mate. Fertilized females may produce 250-300 eggs over the 20-30 days prior to death.

Head lice infest primarily scalp hair, usually in the temporal and occipital areas, and rarely involve facial or pubic hair. Body lice live on clothing (especially in seams), and leave clothing only to obtain a blood meal from the host. Pubic lice most commonly infest the genital area but also can involve the axilla, hair of face, eyelashes, eyebrows, other areas where coarse hair exists such as the legs and torso of men, and occasionally even scalp hair. Up to one third of those with pubic lice may have another sexually transmitted infection.

Prevalence and Distribution

Infestations occur in essentially every area of the world inhabited by humans. Major epidemics have occurred during times of war, overcrowding, or widespread inattention to personal hygiene.

Head lice infest individuals of all social and economic backgrounds. Infestations may reach epidemic proportions, especially among school children. In general, infestations are more common in white people than black people, females than males,

Lice Patrol.
Pine Street Inn nurses Betsy Kendrick and Barbara McInnis found that humor is often the best approach to controlling unwanted infestations.
Photo by James O'Connell MD

Body Lice. This gentleman seen at the Boston Night Center was infested with many generations of body lice. Body lice live on clothing, especially in the seams, and leave only to feed on the human host. Photo by James O'Connell MD

and children than adults. Of note, hair length is not an important risk factor for infestation.

Body lice infestations occur primarily in settings with low income, poor hygiene, and overcrowded living conditions (as seen with homeless individuals and refugees). Children are rarely infested except in colder climates in which clothing is not changed on a regular basis.

Pubic lice infestations are usually seen in adolescents. Occasionally, small children will have infestations of eyelashes, which, as some sources suggest, should warrant an investigation into the possibility of child sexual abuse. As noted in the introduction, pubic lice infestations often exist concurrently with other sexually transmitted infections.

Mode of Transmission

Head lice are transmitted via close personal (head-to-head) contact and sharing of hats, grooming implements (e.g. combs, brushes), and towels.

Body lice spread via contact with skin, clothing, or bed linens.

Pubic lice are transmitted primarily via sexual or skin contact, or contact with clothing or other fomites. There is a 95% chance of transmission with one sexual exposure.

Symptoms and Diagnosis

Pediculosis is diagnosed by visualizing viable nits, nymphs, or adult lice and is often aided by the use of a hand magnifier or microscope. Nits may simulate the scale of seborrheic dermatitis, hair casts, or artifact (e.g. hair spray), but they are very difficult to remove from the hair shaft.

Nits initially attach to the base of the hair shaft. As the hair grows, the length of infestation can be estimated by the distance of the nit from the base of the hair shaft. The bites of lice are painless, but the injected saliva causes intense itching and irritation. Individuals who are sensitized by previous infestations can develop urticaria and a maculopapular rash.

Severe pruritis or itching is the hallmark of all forms of lice infestation. This usually leads to repeated scratching of the skin, which leaves the skin excoriated and allows secondary bacterial infections. Lymphadenitis and fever may occur with chronic infestation.

Head lice. As noted earlier, head lice are typically confined to the scalp. Severe pruritis leads to excoriation and secondary bacterial infection manifested by weeping and crusting of the scalp, matting of hair, tender occipital and cervical lymphadenopathy, and fever. Alopecia may accompany pyoderma.

Body lice. This type of louse is usually not seen until a person has been heavily infested. Numerous nits are typically found in clothing seams, especially around the crotch, armpits, belt line, and collar. Body lice cause a pruritic dermatitis that primarily involves the trunk or torso and consists of small erythematous macules and papules. As with other types of lice, repeated scratching leads to excoriation of the skin and secondary bacterial infection. Fever, malaise, and fatigue can occur with severe infestations. Post-inflammatory hyper-pigmentation is common. Left untreated, infestation with body lice may result in multiple hyperpigmented plaques with scaling skin, a condition known in the past as "vagabond's disease".

Pubic lice. Pubic lice are unique among sexually transmitted diseases (STDs) because the diagnosis can be made from physical examination alone. These lice most commonly infect the pubis and usually do not move far from the initial site of contact. However, these lice may infest other places on the body that have short and thick hair, such as the thighs, truck, perianal area, as well as the beard and mustache. Children may rarely have pubic lice on the eyelashes and the periphery of the scalp.

In a study by Meinking and Taplin, sixty percent of homeless individuals with pubic lice had lice in areas in addition to or exclusive of the pubis. Involvement of extragenital areas may complicate the diagnosis of pubic lice. As with head and body lice, marked pruritis causes scratching that leads to excoriation of the skin and secondary bacterial infection. This can lead to pyoderma, lymphadenopathy, and fever. The cutaneous findings of pubic lice are usually less severe than with head and body lice. Characteristic but uncommon, maculae cerulae are asymptomatic transient blue- or slate-colored macules (less than 1 cm in diameter) on the torso, thighs, or upper aspect of the arms (possibly related to hemoglobin degradation products of the host or to anticoagulant secretions from the louse). Eyelash infestation may simulate seborrheic, infectious, or eczematous blepharitis.

Treatment and Complications

The treatment of lice infestation requires the treatment of clothing and other fomites. This includes bed linens, towels, and hair care utensils such as brushes and combs. These objects should be laundered with hot water, dry cleaned, isolated for 1-2 weeks, or treated with pediculocides.

Individuals infested with lice are treated with one of several agents able to destroy the lice:

- permethrin cream rinse, although the ovicidal activity is incomplete;
- lindane (gamma benzene hexachloride) (Kwell™);
- natural pyrethrins with piperonyl butoxide.

Neither lindane nor the natural pyrethrins are ovicidal and therefore require retreatment in 7-10 days in order to kill the hatching nymphs.

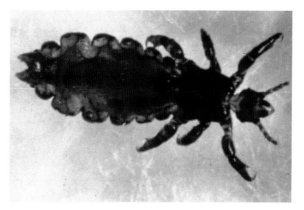

Pediculus capitis. Under the microscope this adult head louse resembles a prehistoric creature. Photo courtesy of the National Pediculosis Association

Head Lice

Head lice infestations may be treated with 1% permethrin (a synthetic pyrethroid, e.g. Nix™) cream rinse. The hair should first be washed with shampoo. Then the hair and scalp should be saturated with the permethrin cream rinse. Allow this to sit for 10 minutes before rinsing with water. Such treatment is sufficient in 90% of cases. After treatment, the nits should be removed with a fine-toothed comb. Permethrin cream rinse has been shown to be equally, if not more, effective than lindane in controlled studies and has much lower toxicity. If adult lice are observed after 7-10 days, the treatment should be repeated.

Infestations may also be treated with natural pyrethrins containing piperonyl butoxide (extracts of the plant chrysanthemum, e.g. RID™). RID™ is applied undiluted to the scalp until saturated for a total of ten minutes. Hair is washed with shampoo and towel dried, and nits are removed with a nit comb. A second treatment may be applied in 7-10 days to kill nymphs hatched from eggs that survived the first treatment. Natural pyrethrins have low mammalian toxicity but may cause a reaction in those allergic to chrysanthemums or ragweed. Also, they may contain refined kerosene or petroleum distillates that cause eye irritation. Eyes should be flushed thoroughly with tap water in the case of contact. Synthetic pryethroids have greater pediculocidal activity than the natural agents.

Lindane 1% shampoo (e.g. Kwell™) is the only agent requiring a prescription. After a ten minute application to the scalp, the hair is rinsed and towel dried leaving the hair tangled and difficult to comb. Nevertheless, nits should be removed with a fine-toothed comb. Again, if adult lice are observed within 7-10 days, the treatment may be reapplied. Lindane offers no particular advantage over other agents. The potential for toxicity is frequently mentioned; however, the short exposure time required in the treatment of pediculosis minimizes

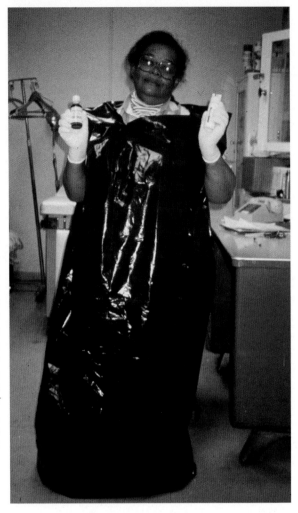

bacterial infections of skin should be treated with antibiotics as indicated. Lindane (Kwell™) has potential neurotoxicity and should not be used in the following situations: immediately following a warm bath; in individuals with extensive dermatitis; in infants and young children; in pregnant or lactating women; or in persons with seizure disorders or other neurologic disorders. Most cases of lindane neurotoxicity have occurred when this medication was applied improperly or used repeatedly.

Resistance to lindane (Kwell™) and permethrin (Elimite™) has been reported. Ivermectin (Stromectol™) 200 ug/kg as a single oral dose can be used for head lice treatment failures (does not affect viability of nits). Ivermectin should not be used with children who weigh less than 15 kg.

Body Lice

The initial treatment of body lice is somewhat controversial. Because most body lice live on clothing, many clinicians do not treat infested individuals with medication, while others choose Elimite cream or Kwell lotion. Either of these can be applied for 8-12 hours, and may eradicate any lice or nits that linger on the body hair. In either case, clothing and bed linens must be discarded or decontaminated by laundering in the hot cycle for 15-30 minutes, dry cleaning, dusting clothing with 1% malathion powder or 10% DDT powder, or by storing clothes for two weeks at 75-85°F.

Pubic Lice

Individuals with pubic lice may be treated with either permethrin (Elimite™, Acticin™, Nix™) or pyrethrin (A200™, RID™). Lindane is no longer recommended for pubic lice. The preparation should be applied to infested and adjacent hairy areas (especially the pubic mons and perianal regions) as well as the thighs, torso, and axillary regions in hairy individuals. Neglecting to treat these areas is a common cause of treatment failures. Infested eyelashes can be treated with petrolatum 2-5 times a day for 8-10 days (followed by removal of nits), 1% yellow oxide of mercury ointment four times a day for two weeks, or 0.25% physostigmine ophthalmic ointment two times a day for three days. Clothing, bed linens, and other fomites should be laundered at a high temperature or dry-cleaned. Sexual contacts should be treated simultaneously. Notably, individuals with HIV/AIDS tend to have more severe infestations and to be unresponsive to conventional treatment.

the amount of systemic absorption and essentially eliminates this possibility.

Nit removal can be facilitated by dipping the fine-toothed comb in a solution of equal proportions of vinegar and water. After use, all combs and brushes should be soaked in pediculocide or boiled in water for up to one hour.

Household members should be treated at the same time. Clothing, bed linens, towels, and headgear should be machine-washed and dried (hot cycle) or dry-cleaned. Items that cannot be washed can be stored in plastic bags in a warm room (75-85°F/23.8-29.4°C) for two weeks (eggs hatch and nymphs starve). Brushes and combs may be discarded or washed in hot water (130°F/54.4°C) for 10-20 minutes or coated with pediculocide for 15 minutes and then cleaned in hot soapy water. Floors and furniture should be vacuumed to remove any hairs that may have been shed containing viable nits.

Pruritis may persist for weeks. Persistent pruritis may be treated with antihistamines such as hydroxyzine (Atarax™). Use of medium to high potency topical corticosteroids is controversial. Secondary

Prevention and Control

Infestations of head lice may be prevented by addressing overcrowded living conditions, by avoiding the sharing of hats, combs and brushes, and by periodic screening (e.g. of students).

Body lice infestations may be prevented with improved personal hygiene, including the frequent changing of clothes.

Infestations of pubic lice may be prevented if sexual or close body contact with an infested individual is avoided.

Summary

Lice are wingless, obligate, blood-leeching ecto-parasites of which only two species infest humans: *Pediculus humanus*, which is subdivided into head lice and body lice, and *Phthirus pubis*, or pubic lice. Lice are transmitted by close personal contact with an infected individual or by the sharing of fomites (e.g. clothing) used by an infested individual. Treatment includes the use of prescription and over the counter medications (head lice and pubic lice) and the cleaning or disposal of fomites (all types). Prevention and control measures include avoidance of sharing of grooming instruments (head lice), improving personal hygiene including regular changing and washing of clothing, avoidance of close personal contact with infected individuals, and regular screening of high-risk individuals.

Bartonella: A Complication of Lice

Bartonella is an aerobic, fastidious, gram-negative bacillus that causes a wide range of diseases, including bacillary angiomatosis and trench fever. *Bartonella quintana*, as opposed to the other species of Bartonella, is associated with exposure to body lice, homelessness, and low socioeconomic status. Several recent studies have demonstrated significant numbers of homeless individuals with positive serologic testing for *B. quintana* in this country and in others. One study done in downtown Paris examined homeless individuals with cutaneous parasitic infestations and found that increasing age of the individual and number of years of homelessness were both independently associated with a positive *B. quintana* serology. *B. quintana* causes bacillary angiomatosis, asymptomatic bacteremia, trench fever, and endocarditis. Each will be discussed briefly in this section.

The only known vector of *B. quintana* is the human body louse. It is unclear whether there are additional modes of transmission. There are several reported cases of *B. quintana* endocarditis in which the patient contacted cats or cat fleas but was not homeless and had no contact with lice.

Bacillary Angiomatosis
Prevalence and Distribution

Bacillary angiomatosis (BA) is usually a disease of immunocompromised individuals and is caused by both *B. henselae* and *B. quintana*. BA caused by *B. henselae* is associated with exposure to cats and their fleas and can cause disease of the liver and spleen and involve the lymph nodes. BA due to *B. quintana* is strongly associated with homelessness and the presence of lice and manifests itself more commonly as subcutaneous infection and bony invasion.

Symptoms and Diagnosis

The skin findings of bacillary angiomatosis (also known as epithelioid angiomatosis) are reddish or purple vascular papules or nodules that may be found anywhere on the skin or mucosa. These are often tender, bleed easily, and can range in size from very small lesions, much like cherry angiomas, to much larger pedunculated masses with a scaly collarette that measure several centimeters. Ulcerations may occur in the lesions. Peripheral satellite lesions may be present, as well as invasion and destruction of the underlying bone. The subcutaneous nodules are often tender and range in appearance from well-demarcated nodules to diffuse subcutaneous swellings that may be indurated.

Diagnosis is generally based on tissue histology or by culture.

Treatment and Complications

Several different antibiotics have been effective in treating bacillary angiomatosis. Treatments with macrolides, tetracyclines, or antituberculous agents have been used. A prolonged course of up to 2 months of treatment may be necessary. The skin lesions may not resolve with treatment.

Bartonella. This 1995 issue of The New England Journal of Medicine had two articles and an editorial about bartonella in homeless persons in Seattle and Paris.

Trench Fever

Trench fever was originally described in soldiers fighting in the trenches in World War I. This febrile illness causes significant morbidity, although it is rarely fatal. The causative agents are *B. henselae* and *B. quintana*.

Prevalence and Distribution

Trench fever has reemerged in the USA, primarily among homeless individuals (*B. quintana*) and among some individuals with tick bites (*B. henselae*).

Symptoms and Diagnosis

The clinical presentation of trench fever is quite variable and may include headache of sudden onset, paroxysmal and often very high fever, weight loss, malaise, severe musculoskeletal discomfort, and aseptic meningitis. Bacteremia may be chronic and accompanied by few clinical findings in homeless patients.

The diagnosis of trench fever is made by finding bacteremia, which can persist for weeks. *B. quintana* and *B. henselae* are slow growing organisms and can require 45 days of incubation.

Treatment and Complications

The most effective treatments are azithromycin (Zithromax™), with dosage of 500 mg per day, or erythromycin (Eryc™, E-mycin™) 2 gms per day. A course of 4 weeks may be necessary for treatment.

Bartonella Endocarditis

Four Bartonella species have been established as causing what had previously been classified as "culture negative" endocarditis. The most frequently isolated species is *B. quintana*, though other species including *B. henselae* have also been found to be causative agents of this serious infection of the heart valves.

Prevalence and Distribution

Homelessness, alcoholism, and contact with body lice are all independently and significantly associated with *B. quintana* endocarditis. These patients are also significantly less likely than other endocarditis patients to have underlying valvular disease. Other species of Bartonella have not shown similar associations.

Symptoms and Diagnosis

Diagnosis is confirmed by blood culture.

Treatment

No clear antibiotic regimen has been demonstrated to be the standard of care in the treatment of Bartonella endocarditis. A 4-6 week course of antibiotics is appropriate for the treatment of uncomplicated *B. quintana* bacteremia. Erythromycin (Eryc™, E-mycin™), azithromycin (Zithromax™), and doxycycline (Vibramycin™) are recommended. Treatment with doxycycline and gentamicin (Garamycin™) has been found to be effective in preventing relapses. Treatment of *B. quintana* endocarditis, in the absence of valve surgery, should continue for 4-6 months, with a bactericidal agent (for example an aminoglycoside or 3rd generation cephalosporin) added during the first 2-3 weeks of treatment.

Prevention and Control

No clear regimen that has been recommended to prevent Bartonellosis. Presumably the most important interventions would be those described in the section on body lice.

Summary

Bartonella causes a variety of illnesses, some of which occur more frequently in the homeless population. The primary vector appears to be the body louse. Several treatment regimens have been used for each of these illnesses, and there is very little at this point that can be reported as standard of care. ▦

The authors of this chapter gratefully acknowledge the invaluable contribution of Barry Bock, RN, who authored this chapter in the original Manual.

Lice Medication List

Generic	Brand	Cost
lindane	Kwell	$
permethrin	Elimite, Nix	$$
pyrethrins with piperonyl butoxide	A-200, RID	$
hydroxyzine	Atarax	$
ivermectin	Stromectol	$

Bartonella Medication List

Generic	Brand	Cost
erythromycin	E-Mycin, Eryc	$
azithromycin	Zithromax	$$
doxycycline	Vibramycin	$
gentamicin	Garamycin	$$

References

Fauci AS, Braunwald E, Isselbacher K, et al., eds. *Harrison's Principles of Internal Medicine.* 14th ed. New York: McGraw Hill, Inc.; 1998:2549.

Behrman RE, Kliegman RM, Jenson HB, eds. *Nelson Textbook of Pediatrics.* Philadelphia, PA: W.B. Saunders Company; 2000:2046-2047.

Mandell GL, Bennett JE, Dolin R, eds. *Principles and Practice of Infectious Diseases.* Philadelphia, PA: Churchill Livingstone; 2000:2971-2974.

Brouqui P, Lascola B, Roux V, Raoult D. Chronic Bartonella quintana bacteremia in homeless patients. *New England Journal of Medicine* 1995;340(3):184-189.

Comer JA, Flynn C, Regnery RL, et al. Antibodies to Bartonella species in inner-city intravenous drug users in Baltimore, Md. *Archives of Internal Medicine* 1996;156(21):2491-2495.

Foucault C, Barrau K, Brouqui P, Raoult D. Bartonella quintana bacteremia among homeless people. *Clinical Infectious Diseases* 2002; 35(6):684-689.

Fournier PE, Lelievre H, Eykyn SJ, et. al. Epidemiologic and clinical characteristics of Bartonella quintana and Bartonella henselae endocarditis: a study of 48 patients. *Medicine* 2001;80(4):245-251.

Gilbert DN, Moellering RC, Sande MA. *The Sanford Guide to Antimicrobial Therapy.* Hyde Park, VT: Antimicrobial Therapy, Inc.; 2001.

Guibal F, de La Salmoniere P, Rybojad M, et al. High seroprevalence to Bartonella quintana in homeless patients with cutaneous parasitic infestations in downtown Paris. *Journal of the American Academy of Dermatology* 2001;44(2): 219-223.

Jackson L, Spach D, Kippen D, al. E. Bartonella (Rochalimaea) quintana endocarditis in three homeless men. *New England Journal of Medicine* 1995;(332):419-423.

Ohl ME, Spach DH. Bartonella quintana and urban trench fever. *Clinical Infectious Diseases* 2000;31(1):131-135.

Raoult D, Ndihokubwayo JB, Tissot-Dupont H, et al. Outbreak of epidemic typhus associated with trench fever in Burundi. *Lancet* 1998;352(9125):353-358.

Schwartz GR. David K. Wagner PS, ed. *Principles and Practice of Emergency Medicine.* Baltimore: WIlliams and Wilkins; 1999.

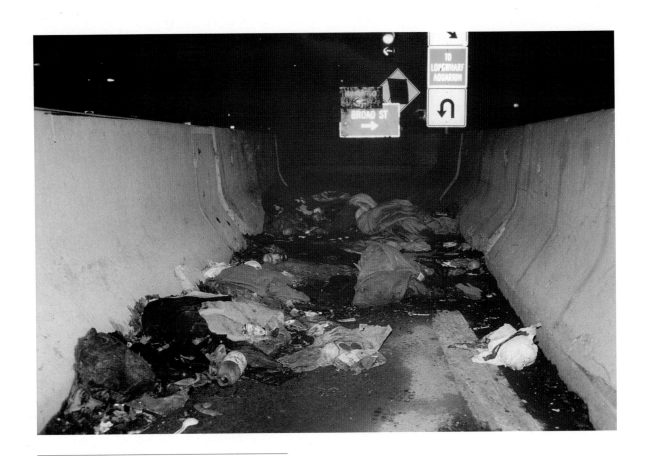

*Boston's Big Dig lasted for over a decade and changed
the city's landscape. These temporary Jersey barriers
divided a main street along the harborfront and became a
safe haven for many homeless rough sleepers.
Photo by James O'Connell MD*

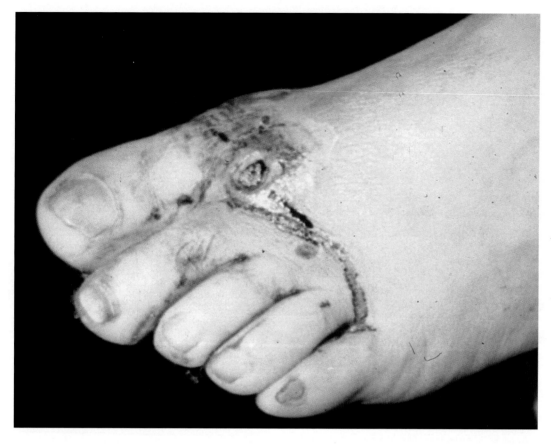

Maggots
(Myiasis)

Alison May, MD

Myiasis refers to the infestation of living vertebrates by maggots. Many different species of fly cause cutaneous disease, and several different syndromes have been described. The type most commonly seen in homeless persons is myiasis of wounds and body cavities, as seen above.

Flies are attracted to the blood and pus found in open wounds and body cavities. The flies lay eggs, and the larvae enter diseased skin or wounds soon after hatching. Many of these species remain confined to the necrotic tissue and keep the wound clean. Some species are able to invade viable tissues, and this can cause significant local destruction.

Treatment consists primarily of manual removal of the larvae and debridement (cleaning) of the affected tissue. We have had good success with the application of ether (or 15% chloroform in cooking oil) to the area prior to extraction. The larvae are immobilized and much easier to remove. ▓

Maggots.
This gentleman was seen in the Pine Street Inn with an open sore of his foot caused by pressure from his boot. Maggots invaded the wound and removed the necrotic tissue, keeping the area clean.
Photo by James O'Connell MD

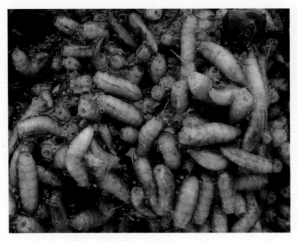 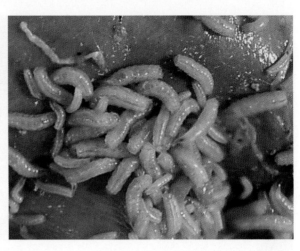

(left)
Maggots.
Flies are attracted
to open wounds and
lay eggs. The larvae
hatch and live on the
necrotic skin, keeping
the wounds clean.

(right)
Maggots.
Maggots can
sometimes invade the
viable tissue around
wounds and
body cavities.
Photos courtesy of
Richard Major
Australian Museum

References

Maguire J, Spielman A. Ectoparasite infestations, arthropod bites and stings. In: Braunwald E, Fauci AS, Kasper DL, et al., eds. *Harrison's Principles of Internal Medicine.* 15th ed. New York: McGraw-Hill; 2001:2622-2624.

Mathieu ME, Wilson BB. Myiasis. In: Mandell GL, Bennett JE, Dolin R, eds. *Mandell, Douglas, and Bennett's Principles and Practice of Infectious Diseases.* 5th ed. Philadelphia: Churchill Livingstone; 2000:2976-2979.

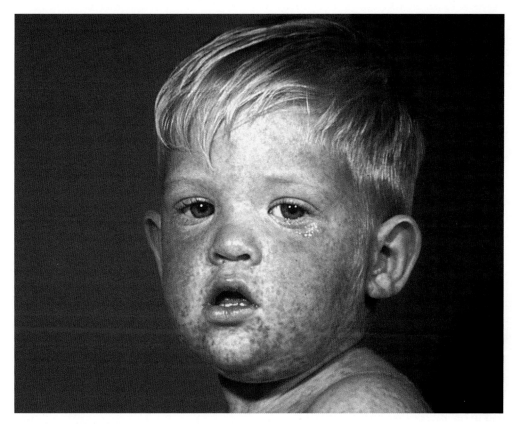

Measles

M. Anita Barry, MD, MPH

Measles is an acute, highly contagious disease caused by the measles (rubeola) virus and is a major cause of illness and death worldwide. Typical symptoms of the disease include fever, cough, runny nose (coryza), a blotchy red rash, and reddened watery eyes (conjunctivitis). The rash usually begins on the face and then progresses to involve the entire body. After 5 to 6 days, the rash usually fades in the same order of appearance, from face to extremities. Koplik spots, tiny blue-white bumps resembling grains of sand, may arise on the mucous membranes of the mouth. Their presence is strongly suggestive of a diagnosis of measles.

Complications of measles include middle ear infections (otitis media), diarrhea, pneumonia, and inflammation of the brain (encephalitis). Measles during pregnancy increases the probability of spontaneous abortion, premature labor, and low birth-weight infants. In rare circumstances, measles results in a degenerative neurologic illness (subacute sclerosing panencephalitis).

In the USA, 1 to 3 of every 1000 measles cases results in death. Children less than 5 years of age, those with severe malnutrition, and those who are immunocompromised (due to HIV/AIDS or other conditions) are at higher risk.

Prevalence and Distribution

Measles vaccine became available in the USA in 1963. Prior to the introduction of an effective vaccine, about half a million measles cases were reported nationwide each year. Since widespread vaccination against measles has been in place, the number of cases has declined by 99%. Currently fewer than 200 measles cases are reported in the USA each year, most of which are related to importation of the virus from other countries.

An increase in measles cases occurred from 1989 to 1991, primarily in large urban areas among racial and ethnic minority children younger than 5 years of age who had not been immunized in accordance with national standards. Intensive campaigns to vaccinate pre-school-aged children led to a rapid decline in cases. Outbreaks among school- and college-aged children, related to waning immunity

*Measles.
Typical facial rash of measles. This child has a fever, cough, runny nose, red and watery eyes, and this blotchy rash that began on his face and then spread to his entire body. Photo courtesy of the CDC*

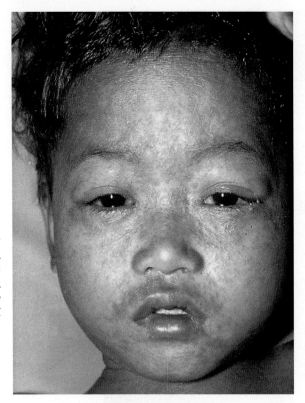

The likelihood of measles increases if an individual is not born in the USA, if there have been other measles cases in the area, or if the patient has traveled to other countries or other areas in the USA where a large number of measles cases have been reported.

A blood test (serology) to measure measles IgM antibody is typically used to diagnose measles. This test may not become positive until the rash has been present for 3 days and remains positive for about 1 month. A person who has an illness compatible with measles but has a negative initial IgM test obtained early after the onset of the rash should have the test repeated. In addition, a rubella (German measles) serology should be checked since symptoms of the two infections can appear similar. Other tests used to confirm a diagnosis of measles include viral culture of urine, blood, or nasopharyngeal secretions, and paired tests on blood specimens drawn about 2 weeks apart to look for rising IgG antibody titers.

Treatment and Prevention

Treatment for measles is supportive; no specific medication is used to eradicate the measles virus. Children with measles who are severely malnourished may require vitamin A supplementation. Because there is no effective treatment once the

or failure to respond to the measles vaccine (primary vaccine failure), have become uncommon since the introduction of a routine two-dose measles vaccination schedule. Prior infection with measles seems to provide lifelong protection against later exposures to the disease.

Transmission

Measles spreads when a person in the infectious stage of the disease disperses droplets carrying the virus into the air by coughing, sneezing, or talking. These droplets land on mucous membranes of other people or are inhaled from the air. Measles virus can last in the air of an enclosed area for up to 2 hours after an infectious person has left the room. The air ventilation system in a building can also disperse the virus from room to room. Measles typically occurs in late winter or spring.

The incubation period for measles is usually 8-12 days after exposure. Rash usually appears 14 days after exposure but can range from 7-18 days. Individuals are infectious from 3-5 days before until 4 days after the rash appears.

Diagnosis

Measles should be suspected in anyone who has the following signs or symptoms:
- a generalized rash;
- fever;
- cough, coryza, or conjunctivitis.

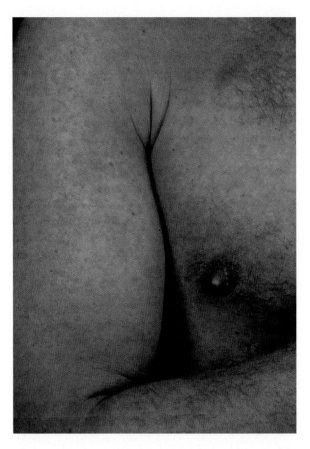

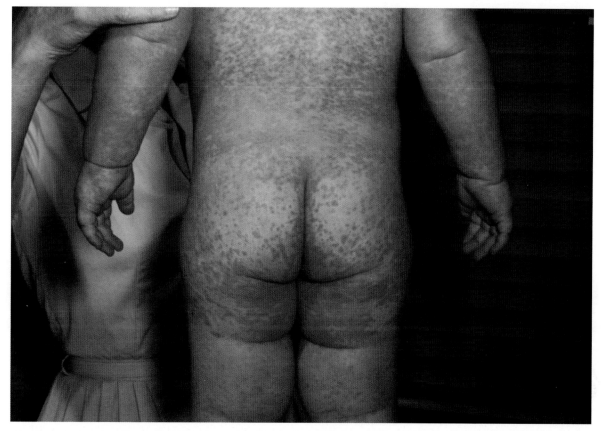

Child with Measles. This child with measles has the characteristic red blotchy rash on his buttocks and back during the third day of the illness. Photo courtesy of the CDC

disease occurs, prevention is crucial.

The routine childhood immunization schedule in the USA calls for children to receive two doses of MMR (measles, mumps, rubella) vaccine, with the first dose given at 12-15 months of age and the second given at 4-6 years of age. However, the second dose can be administered any time > 4 weeks after the first dose. Any child > 12 months of age whose immunization history is unknown should be offered two doses of MMR vaccine no less than four weeks apart.

Measles was so widespread in the USA until the mid-1950s that adults born prior to 1957 are likely to be immune to measles by virtue of prior infection. However, persons born in 1957 or later should have an assessment to determine if they are immune to measles. Adequate proof of immunity to measles includes written documentation of any one of the following:

- receipt of at least two doses of a measles containing vaccine given after 1/1/68, at least 4 weeks apart and when the individual was at least 12 months of age;
- a history of physician-diagnosed measles;
- laboratory evidence of immunity to measles based on serology (a blood test).

Individuals born after 1956 without documented immunity to measles should be offered two doses of MMR vaccine. Because of the particular

risk for transmission of measles once it occurs in a health care or shelter setting, workers in these settings, regardless of age, should have either documented immunity to measles as above or be offered two doses of MMR vaccine.

Measles vaccine should not be given to the following groups of people due to an increased risk of side effects from the vaccine:

- persons with current severe, febrile illness;
- people who had an immediate, severe allergic reaction to a previous dose of MMR vaccine;
- individuals with a history of anaphylaxis to neomycin or gelatin (vaccine components);
- persons with very low platelet counts;
- immunocompromised individuals as a result of disease (including HIV) or medication (e.g., steroids);
- pregnant women.

Women should be advised to avoid pregnancy for 4 weeks following the receipt of MMR vaccine. MMR is recommended for persons with asymptomatic HIV infection as well as those not severely immunocompromised by HIV. Because of potential interference with response to MMR vaccine, vaccination must be delayed following the receipt of blood or blood products such as immune globulin. The duration of the interval depends on the particular product administered.

Measles immunization can temporarily suppress the response to tuberculin skin testing, and if both TB testing and measles immunization are needed, they should be performed on the same day. If this is not possible, TB testing should be delayed until 4 to 6 weeks after vaccine administration. In general, MMR vaccine is not given to infants less than one year old because adequate antibody responses are not reliably produced.

Control

Suspected or confirmed measles cases should be reported immediately to the local health department. Public health officials can conduct an overall assessment of the risk to others within a shelter or other setting. To reduce the possibility of transmission of infection, people with confirmed or suspected measles who reside in larger shelters should be separated from guests and staff who may not be immune to the disease. If housing with an immune friend or relative is not an option, admission to an acute care facility may have to be considered. Shelters that admit persons for time periods of several weeks or longer should review any available immunization records for those being admitted. Providing MMR vaccine to those without a history of prior adequate vaccination may help to prevent outbreaks that could easily spread within a crowded environment. Those working in a shelter setting should ensure that they are immune to measles.

Post-Exposure Immunization

Susceptible persons exposed to measles may benefit from post-exposure prophylaxis. Two types of preventive treatment are available:

1. a single dose of MMR vaccine, if given within 72 hours of exposure, may prevent disease;
2. immune globulin (IG), given within 6 days of exposure, may prevent or modify the course of disease. IG is usually given to susceptible close contacts of measles cases who are at high risk for complications from measles. These include infants < 1 year of age, pregnant women, and immunocompromised persons. IG is recommended only for those at high risk and not as a general measure for outbreak control. If indicated, IG should be given as soon as possible after exposure to ensure maximum protection.

Summary

Measles is a serious disease caused by the rubeola virus. The most common signs and symptoms are a fever, a rash covering the entire body, red watery eyes (conjunctivitis), cough, and runny nose (coryza). Tiny blue-white bumps resembling grains of sand may be seen inside the mouth.

Measles is highly contagious. It spreads when a person with the disease talks, sneezes, or coughs, releasing infected droplets into the air. The droplets are then inhaled by others and can infect a person through the lining of the mouth, nose, or throat.

Measles can lead to serious complications, including middle ear infections, pneumonia, diarrhea, and inflammation of the brain (encephalitis). Pregnant women infected with measles have a higher risk of spontaneous abortion, premature labor, and low birth-weight infants.

An effective vaccine to protect against measles is available. Unless specifically contraindicated, susceptible persons and those with an unknown vaccine history should receive two doses of vaccine given at least 4 weeks apart.

If a suspected measles case is referred to a health care facility, that facility should be alerted to the possible diagnosis so that appropriate infection control measures can be in place to minimize the risk of spread to others.

Suspected measles cases should be reported immediately to the local health department. Control measures to minimize the spread of disease need to be implemented quickly to be effective.

Measles can spread easily and rapidly within crowded environments, and therefore all shelter staff should ensure that they are immune to measles. ∎

References

Centers for Disease Control and Prevention. Measles, mumps and rubella - vaccine use and strategies for elimination of measles, rubella,and congenital rubella syndrome and control of measles: Recommendation of the Advisory Committee on Immunization Practices (ACIP). *MMWR* 1998;47(RR 8):1-58.

Pickering LK, Peter G, Baker CJ, et al., eds. *The Red Book 2003: Report of the Committee on Infectious Diseases.* Elk Grove Village, IL: American Academy of Pediatrics; 2003:419-429.

Chin J, Ascher MS, eds. *Control of Communicable Diseases Manual.* Washington, DC: American Public Health Association; 2000.

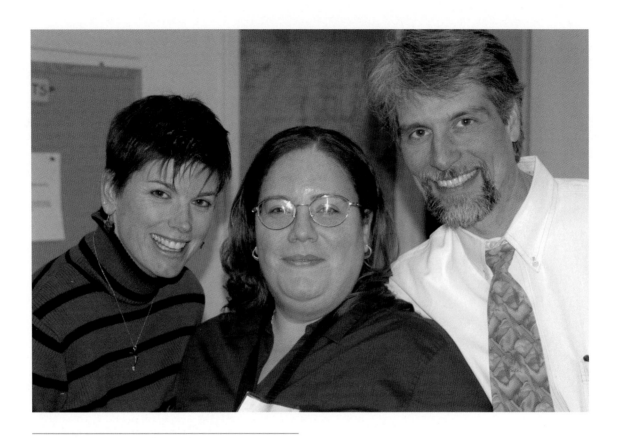

*Marisol Velazquez (center) celebrates the 10th anniversary
of McInnis House as well as her decade of service to BHCHP.
She is flanked by Kelly Keveaney RN and John Romano MD.
Photo by James O'Connell MD*

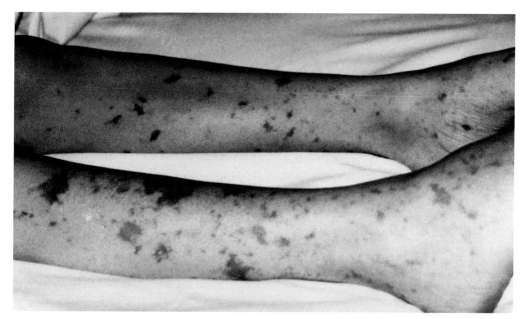

Meningococcal Disease

Janet Groth, MS, CFNP

Meningococcal disease is a very serious infection caused by the bacterium *Neisseria meningitidis*. Meningococcus is now the second most common cause of bacterial meningitis among children and the third leading cause among adults. Despite advances in antibiotics, the overall mortality in the USA is 13%.

Meningococcus has a particular affinity for the bloodstream and the lining around the brain, called the meninges. The severity of infection ranges from a transient fever with bacteremia to severe life-threatening illness. Infrequently, meningococcal infection causes pneumonia or conjunctivitis.

The clinical syndrome of meningococcal infection is similar to other types of meningitis. Symptoms may first appear as a respiratory tract illness, often followed by the abrupt onset of fever, headache, stiff neck, and vomiting. Changes in mental status may ensue, including confusion, drowsiness, stupor, and even coma. Infants may have fever with irritability, poor feeding, vomiting, or a high-pitched cry.

A specific feature in the presentation of meningococcal disease is the appearance of tiny hemorrhages, called petechiae. These are usually found on the trunk and lower extremities. Petechiae are present in 75% of patients with meningococcal infection.

Meningococcal infection is associated with high rates of morbidity and mortality. Even with optimal medical care and appropriate treatment, almost one in ten patients die from this disease, while as many as 20% are left with hearing loss, neurological impairment, or loss of a limb. In rare cases, meningococcal infection follows a fulminant course, known as Waterhouse-Friedrichsen Syndrome. This rapidly progressive disease, marked by hemorrhages into the skin, joints, and internal organs, can lead to septic shock and death even when appropriate antibiotics are started immediately.

A positive outcome of meningococcal disease depends on prompt diagnosis, early referral, and rapid treatment with antibiotics.

Prevalence and Distribution

Endemic disease is most common in children under the age of 5, particularly within the 6-12 month age group. Outbreaks are common among school age children and young adults in group settings, such as day care centers, military camps, and colleges. Freshman college students living in dormitories are at particular risk. This infection appears to be seasonal, with the majority of cases occurring in winter and early spring.

Transmission

Neisseria meningitidis spreads when carriers cough or sneeze infected secretions into the air that others inhale. The disease also spreads through infected nose and throat secretions that come into contact with the mucous membranes of others.

Waterhouse-Friedrichsen Syndrome. This rapidly progressive form of meningococcal disease is marked by hemorrhages into the skin and joints. Septic shock and death can result, even with appropriate antibiotics. Photo courtesy of the Meningitis Trust

The onset of disease usually occurs within 10 days (commonly 3-4 days), although longer intervals are possible.

Meningococcus inhabits the upper respiratory tract of a significant proportion of individuals without causing illness. It is not known why some who carry invasive strains of the bacteria become ill while others do not. Some speculate that a concurrent viral infection or exposure to passive or active cigarette smoke may diminish a person's resistance to *Neisseria meningitidis* that has colonized a person's upper respiratory tract, thus allowing illness to develop in someone who has been carrying the organism. Persons with certain immune deficiencies and persons without a spleen may be at increased risk for infection.

Diagnosis

Anyone suspected of meningococcal disease should have blood cultures and a lumbar puncture without delay. The organism may also be cultured from synovial, pleural, or pericardial fluid.

Treatment

Meningococcal Disease

Persons suspected of having meningococcal disease require intravenous antibiotic therapy and close supervision in a hospital setting. The disease calls for strict respiratory isolation for at least 24 hours after the beginning of antibiotic therapy. A third generation cephalosporin such as ceftriaxone (Rocephin™) in high doses is usually used initially to treat the infection. High doses of penicillin G or chloramphenicol for 1 to 2 weeks have also successfully treated this infection.

Colonization

Antibiotics other than ceftriaxone usually used to treat meningococcal infection do not reliably reach high enough concentrations in upper respira-

tory tract fluids to destroy the organism at the site of colonization in the nasopharynx. To eradicate the organism completely, patients treated with these antibiotics should also be treated with an antibiotic that is known to clear the nasopharynx of organisms, namely ciprofloxacin, ceftriaxone, or rifampin. Ciprofloxacin (Cipro™) 500 mg in a single oral dose can be given to adults but is not recommended for children under age 18 unless there is no alternative therapy. It is not recommended for pregnant or lactating women.

Ceftriaxone (Rocephin™) in a one-time dose at 125 mg for children less than age 15 and 250 mg for those ages 15 and above is an alternative course of therapy.

Rifampin (Rimactane™, Rifadin™) is a drug that has long been used to eradicate meningococcal colonization. Dosing is 5 mg/kg every 12 hours for 2 days in infants less than 1 month old, 10 mg/kg of body weight with a maximum of 600 mg every 12 hours for two days in all persons older than one month. For infants, the liquid form of rifampin is easier to administer. If liquid rifampin is unavailable, the contents of the capsules can be mixed with applesauce. Rifampin cannot be given to pregnant women or those with active liver disease.

Urine, stool, sweat, tears, and semen may turn orange-red when taking rifampin. Soft contact lenses can be permanently stained, so glasses should be worn while taking the medication. Rifampin may also diminish the effects of methadone and the effectiveness of birth control pills. Patients should use a barrier form of contraception (condoms, diaphragm) for the duration of the entire birth control pill cycle in which rifampin therapy occurs.

Prevention and Control

All persons who have been in close contact with a person with meningococcal disease should receive antibiotic prophylaxis with ciprofloxacin, rifampin, or ceftriaxone. The risk of developing disease from such contact varies with the duration and closeness of exposure. In general, persons with less than 20 hours of contact in the week prior to illness are likely to be at less risk than those with a longer duration of contact. However, persons with direct mucous membrane exposure to secretions from an infected person's nose or throat are at higher risk. Such types of exposure include:

- mouth-to-mouth resuscitation;
- kissing;
- mouthing toys;
- sharing food, glasses, bottles, or cigarettes.

Rash from Meningococcus. A characteristic feature is the appearance of tiny hemorrhages on the skin, called petechiae. When glass is pressed against the skin, the petechiae do not blanche or lose their color. Photo courtesy of the Meningitis Trust

Identified close contacts should be evaluated for rifampin, ciprofloxacin, or ceftriaxone prophylaxis within 24 hours of exposure. Refer to the treatment section above for dosages. If antibiotics cannot be initiated within 10 days of exposure, the efficacy is diminished.

Due to the emergence of resistant strains of *Neisseria meningitidis* and possible non-adherence with recommended antibiotic prophylaxis, caregivers should monitor all close contacts for at least 2 weeks following the diagnosis of the initial case. We recommend that smaller shelters, where families or adults live for weeks or months, hold any new admissions until all identified persons at risk within the shelter have received prophylaxis with ciprofloxacin, rifampin, or ceftriaxone. If compliance with therapy cannot be assured, then admissions should further be held until 2 weeks following the diagnosis of the last case of meningococcal disease. Any close contact who develops a febrile illness should go to an acute care facility immediately for evaluation. Staff or caregivers should notify the facility ahead of time to ensure that precautions are taken to lessen the risk of exposure to others.

A vaccine is available for certain strains of *Neisseria meningitidis* (namely A, C, Y, and W-135) but is not routinely given to the general population. The vaccine is recommended solely for control of outbreaks involving certain serogroups. The vaccine is not effective in children under the age of 2 years.

Massachusetts and most other states require that confirmed cases of meningococcal illness be reported to the local board of health immediately.

Summary

Meningococcal disease is a serious bacterial infection that most commonly causes varying degrees of infection in the blood or meninges (the linings covering the brain). This illness can be life threatening and occurs most commonly in infants and young adults.

Initial symptoms can be similar to an upper respiratory tract illness, followed by the abrupt onset of fever, headaches, stiff neck, vomiting, and occasionally a change in behavior. Infants may have a fever, appear irritable, have a high-pitched cry, and feed poorly. Petechiae, or tiny hemorrhages into the skin, may appear on the trunk or legs in both adults and children.

The spread of meningococcal disease occurs when infected individuals cough or sneeze into air that is then inhaled by others. Direct exposure to an infected person's saliva will also spread this infection.

Those suspected of having meningococcal disease must be evaluated as soon as possible in an acute care setting. Respiratory isolation, antibiotic therapy, and close monitoring are required.

Persons likely to be at greatest risk from exposure include those who have spent 20 or more hours with the infected person in the week preceding the illness, and those who have contact with the infected person's nose and throat secretions through activities such as sharing toys, food, glasses, or bottles. These "close contacts" should be evaluated as soon as possible for antibiotic therapy (ciprofloxacin, rifampin, or ceftriaxone) to prevent this illness.

If a suspected or confirmed case of meningococcal disease occurs in a shelter, the local board of health must be notified immediately. This agency can help the shelter in identifying people at risk and instituting measures to control the spread of this potentially fatal disease. ▟

Meningococcal Disease Medication List		
Generic	**Brand Name**	**Cost**
ceftriaxone	Rocephin	$$$$$
chloramphenicol	Chloromycetin	$$$$$
ciprofloxacin	Cipro	$$$
penicillin G		$$$
rifampin	Rifadin, Rimactane	$$$

References

Centers for Disease Control and Prevention. Control and prevention of meningococcal disease. Recommendations of the Advisory Committee on Immunization Practices (ACIP). *MMWR* 1997;46(RR-5):1-9.

Centers for Disease Control and Prevention. Control and prevention of serogroup C meningococcal disease. Evaluation and management of suspected outbreaks. Recommendations of the Advisory Committee on Immunization Practices (ACIP). *MMWR* 1997;46(RR-5):13-21.

Rosenstein NE, Perkins BA, Stephens DS, et al. Meningococcal disease. *The New England Journal of Medicine* 2001;344(18):1378-1386.

Rosenstein NE, Perkins BA, Stephens DS, Lefkowitz L, et al. The changing epidemiology of meningococcal disease in the United States, 1992-1996. *The Journal of Infectious Diseases* 1999;180(6):1894-1901.

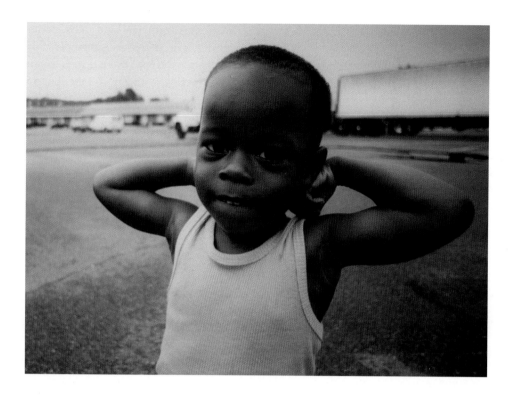

Pertussis (Whooping Cough)

Johnye Ballenger, MD, FAAP

P ertussis, commonly known as whooping cough, is a highly infectious disease of the respiratory tract caused by the bacterium *Bordetella pertussis*. In a young child it can be very serious and may cause pneumonia, apnea, seizures, cerebral hemorrhage, and even death. Newborns and infants not yet immunized are at the highest risk for serious infection and complications. Other people at risk include young adults who were not immunized as children or whose immunity from the vaccine routinely given in childhood has waned.

Three Stages of Pertussis

The course of pertussis involves three stages. Each stage lasts an average of 2 weeks. The usual incubation period is 7 to 10 days.

Catarrhal stage

Stage I is the catarrhal or "cold-like" stage. This usually begins with mild cold symptoms: sneezing, runny nose, tearing, and mild conjunctival infection. Later in this phase, a mild cough develops and soon becomes worse. The pertussis bacteria is most easily spread from one person to another during the first stage.

Paroxysmal stage

Stage II is the paroxysmal or "coughing" stage. During this stage, the cough becomes harsh, dry, and irritating. Spasms of sudden coughing happen in clusters or repetitive bursts, lasting 10 to 20 seconds. These episodes often end with a deep breath that causes the characteristic "whooping" sound. Vomiting, cyanosis, and exhaustion often follow these bursts of coughing.

Paroxysmal coughing is more common at night but can happen several times a day to several times an hour. External stimuli (cold air and smoke) and internal stimuli (stress) can trigger the episodes. The paroxysmal stage usually lasts 1 to 2 weeks but may last 4 weeks or longer.

Convalescent stage

Stage III is the convalescent or "recovery" stage, normally lasting several weeks. The cough becomes milder and less frequent during this phase. If a person develops an upper respiratory infection such as bronchitis during the third stage, the paroxysms will increase. Despite the cough, people are usually not infectious at this point in the course of the disease.

In older children and adults, the disease may be somewhat milder or atypical, sometimes with only a cough that lingers for several weeks.

This exuberant boy is flexing his muscles for our photographer in the parking lot of the motel where he lived with his mother and two brothers for one year.
Photo by Stephen Savoia

Transmission

Pertussis spreads by direct contact with secretions from the nose or throat of an infected person, or by breathing the droplets dispersed in the air when an infected person coughs.

Pertussis most easily passes between people in the initial catarrhal stage of illness, often before diagnosis. While the organism can spread throughout the course of illness, the degree of infectivity decreases with time and depends on environmental conditions, such as crowding and ventilation.

Diagnosis

Diagnosis of pertussis depends on a patient's history and a physical examination. Caregivers should suspect pertussis in anyone with:
- a new cough lasting 14 days or more; or
- a cough followed by vomiting that lasts 7 days or more.

A confirmed diagnosis depends on culturing secretions from the nose and throat in the early stages of the disease. Culturing must be done on media that specifically supports the growth of *Bordetella pertussis* organisms. The local or state health departments can provide information about obtaining these kits. People on antibiotic therapy and those who have been ill for several weeks are less likely to have positive cultures.

In addition, a blood test to detect antibodies to pertussis is available on a limited basis and can be used for diagnosis.

Treatment

A person diagnosed with pertussis needs strict respiratory isolation for 5 days from the initiation of antibiotic treatment. Staff should not admit infected children to a shelter until they have completed 7 days of medication. If antibiotic treatment is impossible, the patient should remain isolated until 3 weeks after the onset of paroxysms.

Young children need careful management because the paroxysms may make feeding and breathing difficult. Also, thick mucous in the nose and throat can block the airways. Some children may need frequent suctioning to remove the mucous. In cases with severe complications, such as respiratory distress or dehydration, hospitalization may be required.

For children and adults, the antibiotic of choice is erythromycin (E-mycin™, Eryc™). However, for those individuals unable to tolerate erythromycin, newer macrolides, such as clarithromycin (Biaxin™) and azithromycin (Zithromax™), may be as effective as erythromycin and have fewer adverse side effects and better compliance. The course of the illness may be less severe if the patient receives antibiotic treatment during the incubation period or early in the catarrhal stage (stage I). Treatment begun after the paroxysmal stage (stage II) does not change the course of the illness. However, antibiotic treatment after stage II will prevent further spread of the disease by killing the remaining bacteria in the body.

The dose of erythromycin estolate is 40-50 mg/kg/day, orally, divided into 4 daily doses for 14 days. The maximum daily dose is 2 grams. The dose of clarithromycin is 15-20 mg/kg/day, orally, divided into 2 daily doses for 7 days. The maximum daily dose is 1 gram. The dose of azithromycin is 10-12 mg/kg/day, orally, as 1 dose daily for 5 days. The maximum daily dose is 500 mg.

Prevention

Immunization with pertussis vaccine is the most important measure to prevent the spread of the organism. Immunization is particularly important for young children in whom the disease is likely to be most severe.

The pertussis vaccine is a combination of diphtheria and tetanus toxoids and acellular pertussis in a single shot called DTaP. The recommended immunization series consists of 5 doses. Infants usually receive the first dose between the ages of 6 and 8 weeks. Additional doses are given at 4 months and 6 months of age. The fourth dose comes at 18 months of age, completing the primary series. Children receive the fifth dose between the ages of 4 and 6 years. This schedule may need modification for children who have not followed a normal immunization schedule. (For more information, refer to the immunization schedules in Part 5.) Pertussis vaccine is not usually recommended for those over 7 years of age.

The rates of local reactions (erythema and induration at the injection site), fever, and other common systemic symptoms (drowsiness, fretfulness, and anorexia) are substantially lower with acellular pertussis vaccines than with the whole-cell pertussis vaccines. Rare, potentially more serious adverse events associated with the older DPT, such as seizures, have been found to occur less frequently after DTaP. The decision to give pertussis vaccine to infants and children with underlying neurologic disorder is difficult and must be made on an individual basis, after careful consideration of the risks and benefits. Deferral of pertussis immunization should be considered in infants and children known to have, or suspected of having, an unstable or evolving neurological disorder that may predispose the child to seizures or neurological deterioration. The Red Book outlines the different categories of neurologic disorders and relevant recommendations.

Control

Caregivers should report suspected and confirmed cases of pertussis to the local health department, which can provide information about control measures.

When there has been an outbreak of pertussis in a community or shelter, the health department or consulting pediatrician may decide to begin DTaP vaccine schedule as early as 2 weeks of age with subsequent doses given as often as every 4 weeks. Generally, 3 doses will provide protection from the disease in 80% of children.

Close contacts under 7 years of age who have had at least 4 doses of vaccine should receive a booster dose unless they received a dose in the past 3 years. Children under 7 years of age with no history of DTaP vaccine or with less than 4 doses of DTaP should begin the vaccination schedule or continue on schedule.

In addition, appropriate antibiotic treatment in the dosages described above is recommended for all household contacts and other close contacts. This is because vaccine-induced immunity does not prevent disease in all cases. Also, older children and adults may develop a very mild case of pertussis that may still be transmitted to others.

All contacts to a case of pertussis should be watched closely for respiratory symptoms (sneezing, runny nose, tearing, conjunctivitis, and later, a mild cough) for 2 incubations periods (28 days) after the last exposure. New suspected cases should be promptly referred to a health provider for evaluation.

Special Considerations for Homeless Populations
Family shelters

Pertussis can create considerable problems in a family shelter, because children under 12 months are at greatest risk of infection and complications.

Anyone exposed to an infected person for more than one hour in a close setting (play group, dining area, etc.) is a close contact. These people will need antibiotic prophylaxis, as discussed above, to prevent them from developing pertussis.

The recommended course of treatment for pertussis is 14 days. After the first 7 days of antibiotic therapy, infected people (including close contact with symptoms after exposure to an active case) no longer pose a risk to other guests or staff. Close contacts who do not show symptoms are not considered infectious.

This 7-day period of infectivity during treatment presents a special problem for group settings. The average time from exposure to the onset of disease is only 7 to 10 days. Usually an exposed person will not have had time to complete 7 days of antibiotics before beginning to show symptoms. This person may then be able to spread infection to others, creating another group of close contacts.

One solution is the provision of separate accommodations for all identified close contacts during the first 7 days of preventive treatment. This is often impractical. Therefore, staff and guests who will spend more than one hour with any close contact during the first 7 days of prophylaxis will also need to take antibiotics.

A shelter should not discharge a close contact to another shelter or group setting until completion of at least 7 of the 14 days of prophylactic therapy.

Adult shelters

In larger adult shelters, prophylaxis of all guests is clearly an impractical solution. Targets for prophylaxis should include adults and children who have shared indoor airspace with a confirmed case for at least 10 hours per week or more while the person was considered contagious. Caregivers should also consider treatment for close contacts who interact with children of any age. Prophylaxis is especially important for anyone who has contact with children under 12 months and those who have not had at least 3 doses of pertussis vaccine.

Summary

Pertussis or whooping cough is a serious infection that primarily affects the upper respiratory areas. It is spread by direct contact with infected secretions from the nose or throat or by breathing infected droplets in the air where an infected person has coughed.

Generally, pertussis begins with symptoms like a cold. The illness progresses with a cough that becomes dry and harsh and occurs in bursts especially at night. The person may turn blue while coughing. The episode may end with a large intake of air that sounds like a whoop. Vomiting and exhaustion can follow these events. Older people infected with pertussis may have a less serious illness.

Complications are greatest in children under one year and include serious problems with the lungs or brain.

Treatment of pertussis requires antibiotics and supportive care. Strict respiratory isolation is necessary for the infected person until 5 days after antibiotics have been started.

Pertussis can be prevented through the routine vaccination of children.

People of any age who have been exposed to an infected person should also see a health provider for preventive therapy with antibiotics.

The local board of health or appropriate health agency must be informed of any person who has been diagnosed with pertussis as soon as possible. The agency can also provide information about the risk to the rest of the shelter guests and staff and can help with instituting control measures. ⬛

Pertussis Medication List

Generic	Brand Name	Cost
erythromycin	E-mycin, Eryc	$
clarithromycin	Biaxin	$$$
azithromycin	Zithromax	$$

References

Pickering LK, Peter G, Baker CJ, et al., eds. *The Red Book 2003: Report of the Committee on Infectious Diseases.* Elk Grove Village, IL: American Academy of Pediatrics; 2003:472.

Centers for Disease Control and Prevention. Guidelines for the Control of Pertussis Outbreaks. Centers for Disease Control and Prevention; Atlanta, GA, 2000. http://cdc.gov/nip/publications/pertussis/guide.htm

Centers for Disease Control and Prevention. Pertussis---United States, 1997-2002. *MMWR* 2002;51(4):73-76.

Guris D, Strebel P, Bardenheier B, et al. Changing epidemiology of pertussis in the United States: increasing reported incidence among adolescents and adults, 1990-1996. *Clinical Infectious Diseases* 1999;28(6):1230-1237.

Yih W, Lett S, des Vignes F, et al. The increasing incidence of pertussis in Massachusetts adolescents and adults, 1989-1998. *Journal of Infectious Diseases* 2002;182(5):1409-1416.

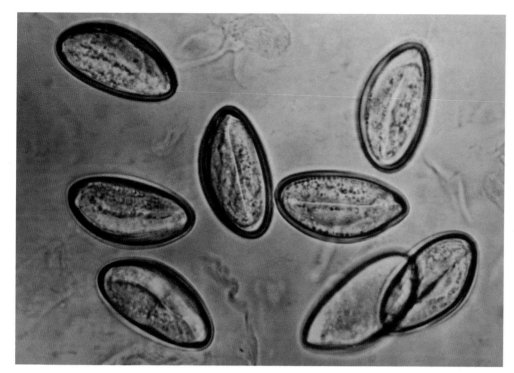

Pinworm

Maya Mundkur Greer, MSN, APRN, BC

The pinworm, or *Enterobius vermicularis*, is a parasite that commonly infects the intestines of humans. The male is 2 to 5 millimeters long and lives in the lower gastrointestinal tract. Females can be twice as long as males. Eggs take 1 to 2 months to mature in the gastrointestinal tract and become large enough to migrate. Pregnant females typically migrate to the rectal area to lay eggs, often during the night. Pinworms may also deposit their eggs along the perineum and even in the vagina. The females usually die after depositing their eggs.

Humans are the only known natural hosts; pinworms do not live in dogs and cats.

Clinical Course

Pinworm infection can cause intense itchiness in the perianal region. Persistent scratching can produce an excoriated rash. The discomfort from pinworms usually results in restless sleep. Thankfully, the infection is self-limited, and serious complications are rare.

Prevalence

Pinworm infection occurs worldwide and is very common. Prevalence rates are higher among pre-school and school-aged children. Up to 50 percent of institutionalized persons may be infected. While infection in adults is far less common, children with pinworms often infect parents and other household members.

Variables that increase risk of infection include: age (5–10 years old); presence of other children in the living area or living in an institution; sharing beds; and living in a warm, moist climate.

Transmission

Pinworm infection can be spread in several ways, most commonly by direct contact with the eggs. People can continually reinfect themselves by scratching the perianal area and touching their mouths or touching objects that are then eaten or placed in the mouth.

Pinworms also spread through indirect contact when someone touches clothes, underwear, or bedding that contain eggs. These eggs can then spread to food, toys, or other objects that often go into children's mouths. Eggs can also be dispersed around a room when contaminated articles are shaken, causing the eggs to settle into dust. In ideal conditions, the eggs can live up to 3 weeks on bedding, clothing, and dust; however, less than 1 out of 10 eggs will be alive after 2 days at room temperature.

Pinworm Eggs. These eggs of the human parasite Enterobius vermicularis, or "human pinworm", have been captured on cellulose tape. Photo courtesy of the CDC

A third mode of transmission is "retro-infection". This happens when the pinworms reinfect the host by hatching in the perianal region and then migrating back into the rectum.

Diagnosis

Perianal and perineal itching, especially at night, and a rash coupled with insomnia are the most common complaints of pinworm infection. However, many pinworm infections are entirely without symptoms.

The presence of pinworms can be confirmed in one of two ways. The first is direct observation of the adult worms around the anus, perineum, or entrance to the vagina. The optimum time to see the worms is 1 to 2 hours after a child has gone to bed or on awakening in the morning. A flashlight will help with the search. A second test is to observe the eggs, which are about the size of the head of a pin, under a microscope. A 2-inch strip of scotch tape can be applied to the child's perianal area in the morning before the child awakens. The tape may then be transferred to a glass slide for examination.

Pinworms can be identified about 50% of the time after a single attempt at one of these tests. These tests should be repeated over 3 to 5 consecutive mornings before accepting a negative result. Pinworm infection usually runs in families, and a diagnosis in one person calls for the examination of all family and household members.

Treatment

Most people in single family households will get rid of pinworms without treatment. Unfortunately, larger group settings such as shelters and day care centers facilitate transmission and persistent infection. Breaking the cycle of reinfection through direct and indirect contact can be very difficult. Early treatment and thorough examination of family members and close friends will increase the chances of eradication. If children in different families are diagnosed with pinworms within a short time, the entire shelter or day care facility may require treatment.

Pyrantel pamoate (Antiminth™) kills pinworms at dosages of 11 mg/kg to a maximum dose of 1 gram. Antiminth™ can be used in people of all ages and is not contraindicated in pregnant women. Some people develop headaches and stomach pains when taking the drug, but these side effects are uncommon. Antiminth™ is currently available without a prescription. Brand names include "Pin-X" and "Reese's Pinworm Medication".

Mebendozole (Vermox™) is an antihelminthic that comes in chewable tablets of 100 mg and has few side effects. Available by prescription, this medication is not recommended for pregnant women or children under two years of age.

Albendazole (Albenza™) is a pinworm medication available by prescription that is usually reserved for infections that are not cleared by the other preparations. A single 400 mg tablet is given by mouth. Once again, this medication is not recommended for pregnant women or children under the age of two.

Treatment with a second dose of medication (Vermox™, Antiminth™, or Albenza™) 14 days after the first dose has a cure rate of 90 percent. In rare circumstances 4 to 6 treatments may be necessary to get rid of the infection.

Vaseline™ and other over the counter creams or ointments can help relieve the itching caused by pinworms when applied to the perianal area.

Prevention and Control

The control of pinworms calls for personal and environmental hygiene. Staff must be particularly sensitive to an individual's feelings of guilt or embarrassment. Pinworms can infect the cleanest household. When discussing hygiene, staff should emphasize the ease of transmission and frequency of reinfection. Pinworms can spread easily to a whole family and throughout an entire family shelter unless the source is treated.

During treatment for pinworms, the linens, bedclothes, underwear, and toys of infected individuals should be washed in hot (131°F/55°C) soapy water. If washing is not possible, then the articles should be thoroughly vacuumed. Before cleaning, you can avoid dispersing the eggs into the air by handling every article with minimal shaking. Staff and guests should damp dust, damp mop, and/or vacuum the living space of infected guests and common rooms daily for several days after treatment to reduce the number of eggs that may reside in dust.

If the entire shelter needs treatment, all linens, bedclothes, and living space should be considered infected. Guests and staff should clean all articles and spaces as described above.

The following measures also help to reduce transmission:

- discourage scratching in the anal area;
- the use of gloves and close fitting bed clothes can be helpful;
- trim nails to minimize biting;

- wash hands with warm, soapy water before preparing, serving, or eating food and after using the toilet or changing diapers.
- avoid shaking or fanning the bedding.

Summary

Pinworms are tiny worms that live in a person's intestines. Female pinworms crawl to the rectal area at night to lay eggs, causing the infected person to itch and to sleep restlessly. While uncomfortable, pinworms rarely cause serious complications. However, they are easily spread among people who live or play closely together, particularly children. When a child scratches, the eggs of pinworms can get on the hands and under the fingernails. The child can then put his or her hands into the mouth or onto objects such as toys or food. The eggs are also easily spread around a room when infected linen or clothing is shaken.

When one person in a family is found to have pinworms, the entire family needs to be examined. When the infected person and close contacts are treated early, there is little risk to the rest of the shelter. If several cases happen in different families, the entire shelter may need treatment.

Pinworms reappear easily, but careful hygiene reduces the prospect of reinfection during treatment. You should consult the local board of health and caregivers for specific control measures regarding this infection. ∷

Pinworm Medication List		
Generic	**Brand Name**	**Cost**
albendazole	Albenza	$$$
mebendazole	Vermox	$
pyrantel pamoate	Antiminth (Pin-X, Reese's Pinworm Medication)	$

References

Pinworm infection. In: Pickering LK, et al., eds. *2000 Red Book: Report of the Committee on Infectious Disease.* Elk Grove Village, IL: American Academy of Pediatrics; 2000:449-451.

Bundy DAP, et al. Nematodes limited to the intestinal tract (Enterobius vermicularis, Trichuris trichuira, and Capillaria phillippinensis). In: Strickland GT, ed. *Hunter's Tropical Medicine and Emerging Infectious Diseases.* Philadelphia: WB Saunders; 2000:719-726.

Drugs for parasitic infection. *Medical Letter on Drugs and Therapeutics* 1998;40(1017):1-12.

Enterobiasis (Pinworm disease). In: Benenson AS, ed. *Control of Communicable Disease in Man.* Washington D.C.: American Public Health Association; 1990:157-159.

Hearns VL. Pinworms. In: Rakel RE, ed. *Saunders Manual of Medical Practice.* Philadelphia: W.B. Saunders; 2000.

Nelson JD, Bradley JS. *Nelson's Pocket Book of Pediatric Antimicrobial Treatment.* Lippincott Williams and Wilkins; 2000.

Pinworm infestation. In: Berkow R, ed. *The Merck Manual.* Rahway, New Jersey: Merck and Company; 2000: 2363-2364.

Owen RL. Parasitic diseases. In: Sleisenger MH, Fordtran JS, eds. *Gastrointestinal Disease: Pathophysiology, Diagnosis, and Management.* Philadelphia: W.B. Saunders Company; 1989.

Urbach AH. Pinworms. In: Burg FD, et al., eds. *Gellis and Kagan's Current Pediatric Therapy.* Philadelphia: WB Saunders Company; 1999.

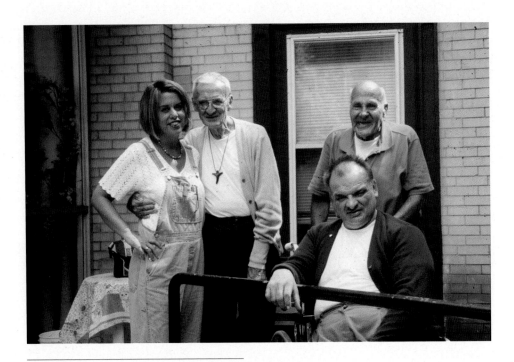

*BHCHP nurse practitioner Denise Petrella visits
several patients recuperating from major illnesses
at a nursing home. Each of these men had lived
for several decades on Boston's streets.
Photo by James O'Connell MD*

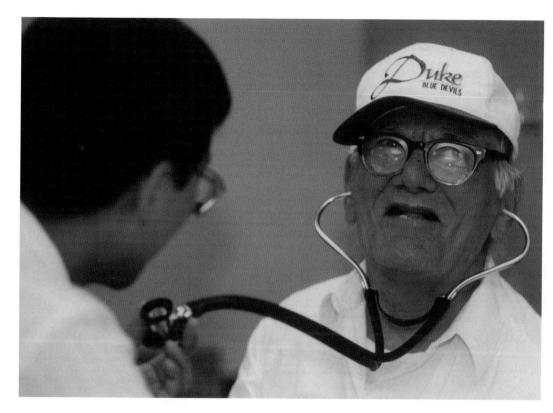

Community Acquired Pneumonia

Jill S. Roncarati, PA-C
John Bernardo, MD

The term community-acquired pneumonia (CAP) refers to a common lower respiratory infection diagnosed by a combination of some or all of the following: clinical signs and symptoms; an infiltrate seen on chest radiography; and abnormal laboratory values. CAP occurs outside of the hospital or within 48 hours after hospital admission in a patient who has not been recently hospitalized and is not living in a long-term care facility. Pneumonia acquired while hospitalized or while living in an inpatient setting is referred to as "nosocomial pneumonia".

Prevalence and Distribution

More than 4 million adults are diagnosed with community-acquired pneumonia in the USA each year, resulting in close to 1.5 million hospitalizations. According to the Infectious Disease Society of America (IDSA), pneumonia is the sixth leading cause of death in the USA, with greater than 14% mortality among hospitalized patients. Pneumonia affects men and women equally; however, those with predisposing conditions such as dysphagia, esophageal disease, or altered consciousness have a greater chance of succumbing to the illness. Higher risk groups include: homeless persons who are 35-55 years old; persons with co-morbid diseases such as asthma, COPD, tuberculosis, and a history of smoking; and individuals who abuse drugs and/or alcohol.

Mode of Transmission

CAP usually occurs when bacteria from the upper respiratory system or undigested material in the stomach are aspirated into the lung. Infection can also occur by the inhalation of aerosolized material or by the seeding of microorganisms in the lungs through hematogenous spread, the least common route. Persons suffering from the co-morbid diseases described above usually are more likely to have contracted CAP through aspiration.

Symptoms and Diagnosis

The most common signs and symptoms are cough (with or without sputum production), fever, chills, tachypnea (rapid breathing), tachycardia (a rapid heart rate), pleuritic chest pain (chest pain that worsens or "catches" with inhalation), dyspnea

Dr. Stephen Hwang of BHCHP finds a creative approach to speaking with this deaf man during a clinic visit at St. Francis House Day Shelter. Photo by Stephen Savoia

Table 1:

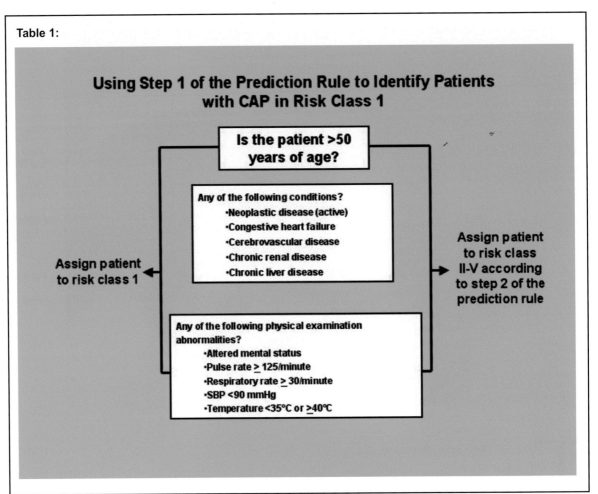

Using Step 1 of the Prediction Rule to Identify Patients with CAP in Risk Class 1

Is the patient >50 years of age?

Any of the following conditions?
- Neoplastic disease (active)
- Congestive heart failure
- Cerebrovascular disease
- Chronic renal disease
- Chronic liver disease

Any of the following physical examination abnormalities?
- Altered mental status
- Pulse rate ≥ 125/minute
- Respiratory rate ≥ 30/minute
- SBP <90 mmHg
- Temperature <35°C or ≥40°C

Assign patient to risk class 1

Assign patient to risk class II-V according to step 2 of the prediction rule

PORT Pneumonia Severity Index, Step 1. Prediction rule to identify those patients with CAP in Risk Class 1. Courtesy of UpToDate. www.uptodate.com

(sensation of difficult breathing), altered mental status, dehydration, and hemoptysis (coughing up blood). Clinical findings include a temperature greater than 100°F (>37.8°C), heart rate over 100, respiratory rate greater than 25, room air oxygen saturation <90%, and an exam showing rhonchi or focal rales on auscultation of the lungs, decreased breath sounds, and bronchophony.

If pneumonia is suspected, the IDSA recommends a chest x-ray along with several laboratory tests: complete blood count with a differential, serum creatinine, blood urea nitrogen, glucose, electrolytes, and liver function tests. Vital signs along with oxygen saturation by oximetry or by blood gas analysis should always be assessed. Two blood cultures and Gram's staining of sputum, with a culture and sensitivity evaluation, also should be ordered before antibiotics are given. Other tests to be considered may include HIV screening, PPD skin testing for tuberculosis, and Legionella or influenza (viral) cultures. Since tuberculosis can also present like community-acquired pneumonia in those who are at-risk for TB, the PPD status of the patient should be verified. If past results are either unknown or negative, a PPD should be planted in

persons at-risk for TB. If the PPD has been positive in the past, the chest x-ray and sputum samples should be evaluated for active TB. Sputum should be tested for acid fast bacilli (AFB) by smear and culture on three separate sputum samples, taken at least 8 hours apart, to help rule out tuberculosis.

Although the chest x-ray is accepted as the "gold standard," the sensitivity and specificity have not been well-studied. For example, in a patient with dehydration or early in the disease process, an infiltrate (i.e. pneumonia) may not be recognized by the chest radiograph. Thus, an alternative standard, based on a combination of clinical symptoms and findings, chest radiography results, laboratory data, and clinical response to anti-microbial treatment, may be better. However, chest radiography usually is useful to help assess severity of the disease process and the response to therapy over time.

Gram's stain of the sputum, usually available within hours, can contribute useful information. The Gram's stain should be inspected for the presence of neutrophils and for the identification of the predominant bacteria. A large number of squamous epithelial cells (>25/hpf) suggests the sample is saliva rather than sputum and should be discarded. According to a study of homeless persons in Boston in 2001 conducted by the authors of this chapter, the three most common microorganisms that cause community-acquired pneumonia in adults are *Streptococcus pneumoniae*, *Haemophilus influenza*, and *Staphylococcus aureus*. With aspiration pneumonia, the responsible microorganism is often an anaerobe or a combination of anaerobes and the above aerobic organisms. The primary anaerobes found to cause aspiration pneumonia in adults are Peptostreptococcus, *Fusobacterium nucleatum*, Prevotella, and Bacteroides species. If an anaerobic infection is suspected, a transtracheal aspiration from the lower airways may be obtained for culture and sensitivity studies. This will avoid contamination of the sample by anaerobes that inhabit the oral cavity.

The decision to hospitalize a patient with pneumonia can be difficult. To help clinicians with this dilemma, a Pneumonia Severity Index (PSI) has been derived by the Pneumonia Patient Outcome Research Team (PORT) after a very lengthy prospective cohort study involving almost 15,000 adults who presented to emergency rooms with radiographic evidence of pneumonia. Based on the risk of death within 30 days of presenting to the emergency room, the PSI is a 2-step process that stratifies patients into 5 risk classes. The PSI is a very useful clinical tool that utilizes the decision-making processes that clinicians typically use during a clinic visit.

The first step is to identify patients with pneumonia on chest x-ray who are at very low risk (Class1): under the age of 50 and without any of 11 demographic variables, co-morbid conditions, physical findings, or laboratory results. These persons can be treated as outpatients with close follow-up, but do not usually require hospitalization. Please see Table 1.

The second step in the PSI assigns the remaining patients to classes 2 through 5, based upon a total point score. This score involves adding the age in years (age minus 10 points for females) to the points for each risk factor that is present. The risk factors and points are detailed in Table 2, which is adapted from the IDSA. The point assignments for Classes 2-5 are depicted in Table 3.

Patients in Class 1 and 2 do not usually require hospitalization and can be followed as outpatients. Those in Class 3 require a brief hospital stay, while those in Class 4 and 5 almost always require hospitalization, and sometimes even admission to an Intensive Care Unit.

Table 2: Risk Factors and Assigned Points

Risk Factors	Points
Demographic factors	
Age for men	Age (years)
Age for women	Age (years) – 10
Nursing home resident	+10
Coexisting illnesses	
Neoplastic disease (active)	+30
Chronic liver disease	+20
Congestive heart failure	+10
Cerebrovascular disease	+10
Chronic renal disease	+10
Physical examination findings	
Altered mental status	+20
Respiratory rate ≥ 30/minute	+20
Systolic blood pressure < 90 mmHg	+20
Temperature < 35°C or ≥40°C	+15
Pulse ≥ 125 beats/minute	+10
Laboratory and radiographic findings	
Arterial pH <7.35	+30
Blood urea nitrogen ≥ 30 mg/dL (11 mmol/L)	+20
Sodium < 130 mmol/L	+20
Glucose ≥ 250 mg/dL	+10
Hematocrit <30 percent	+10
Partial pressure of arterial oxygen < 60 mmHg*	+10
Pleural effusion	+10

*or an oxygen saturation of <90 percent on pulse oximetry

PORT Pneumonia Severity Index, Step 2. The risk factors with assigned points used to determine the total score for Risk Classes 2 to 5.

Treatment and Complications

Treatment consists of oral or intravenous antibiotics, hydration, and over-the counter-analgesics such as acetaminophen (Tylenol™) for minor arthralgias, myalgias, and fever. Antibiotics are ideally prescribed according to which microorganism is causing the infection. Efforts should be made to determine the type of microorganism in order to decrease antibiotic resistance, avoid unnecessary exposure to medication side effects, and

Table 3

CLASS	POINT ASSIGNMENT
Class 2	≤70
Class 3	71-90
Class 4	91-130
Class 5	>130

PSI Risk Classes.

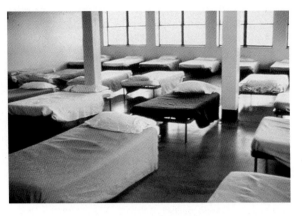

prevent worsening of disease by using an antibiotic not active against the infecting bacteria.

The initial choice of antibiotic is made empirically. After 24-48 hours, when microbiology laboratory tests are complete (such as sputum Gram's staining and culture results), an antibiotic sensitive to the bacteria causing CAP should be confirmed and prescribed. Performing such laboratory tests is often impossible or the test results are equivical; in such cases, empirical treatment is continued. According to the IDSA, certain conditions can predict certain pathogens. The most pertinent correlations can be found in Table 4 from the IDSA.

The IDSA also recommends the following classes of antibiotics agents, in no particular order, for the empirical treatment of outpatients: a macrolide, doxycycline (Vibramycin™), or a fluoroquinolone, as these classes of medications have the greatest activity against *Streptococcus pneumoniae, Mycoplasma pneumoniae,* and *Chlamydia pnuemoniae.* Please refer to the Medication List at the end of this chapter for the most commonly used medications in these classes of antibiotics. Special consideration should be taken to different regional sensitivity to these medications. For elderly patients

or those who will have difficulty with medications that are dosed several times per day, a once-a-day fluoroquinolone or macrolide may be a good option. However, a fluoroquinolone should not be used in individuals at-risk for tuberculosis. While this class of drugs has excellent activity against the *M. tuberculosis* bacteria, their use as a single agent may lead to fluoroquinolone drug resistance if the person actually has tuberculosis pneumonia (see chapter on Tuberculosis). Furthermore, these drugs may cause clinical improvement in TB patients and mask the underlying disease. In this situation, the TB remains incompletely treated, and the patient is permitted to remain in the community or shelter and become a public health risk for TB transmission.

Prevention and Control

A *Streptococcus pneumoniae* vaccine active against the 23 most prevalent types is available and should be administered to all people over 65 years of age, those over 2 years of age with chronic pulmonary disease, those at risk for aspiration pneumonia (such as chronic alcohol and drug abusers), and those with HIV. This vaccine needs to be administered every 5 years. Influenza vaccine should also be given yearly to those at risk for pneumonia. Drug and alcohol treatment programs should always be encouraged to provide vaccinations to their clients.

Special Considerations for Homeless Populations

In homeless persons with pneumonia, aspiration should be suspected in those who use drugs or alcohol as well as those with known upper gastrointestinal conditions. An antibiotic effective against anaerobes should be used, such as penicillin V (Pen-Vee K™), metronidazole (Flagyl™), or clindamycin (Cleocin™). Treatment regimens can

Table 4	
Medical Condition	**Most Common Pathogen**
Chronic obstructive pulmonary disease (COPD) or smoking	*Streptococcus pneumoniae, Haemophilus influenzae, Moraxella catarrhalis,* and Legionella species
Alcoholism	*Streptococcus pneumoniae* and anaerobes
Poor dental hygiene	Anaerobes
HIV infection in the early stages.	*Streptococcus pneumoniae, Haemophilus influenzae,* and *Mycobacterium tuberculosis*
HIV infection in the later stages	All pathogens from the early stages as well as *P. carinii,* Cryptococcus, and Histoplasma species
Influenza in community	Influenza, *Streptococcus pneumoniae, Staphylococcus aureus, Streptococcus pyogenes,* and *Haemophilus influenzae*
Aspiration or airway obstruction	Anaerobes, *Streptococcus pneumoniae, Haemophilus influenzae,* and *Staphylococcus aureus*
Intravenous drug abuse	*Staphylococcus aureus,* anaerobes, *Mycobacterium tuberculosis,* and *Streptococcus pneumoniae*

be difficult to complete for homeless persons, especially with complicated drug regimens that require dosing every 4 or 6 hours or when there is no safe place to store medicines. Medications taken once a day, such as fluroquinolones or macrolides, may encourage successful completion of an antibiotic course. In some cases, the cost of prescribed antibiotics and accessibility to medications for persons without health insurance should be considered.

The availability of a safe place to convalesce can be as important as taking medications as prescribed. Homeless persons with pneumonia often are not ill enough to be admitted to the hospital but are much too sick and vulnerable for the shelter system or the streets. Shelters often close their doors during the daytime, sending guests to the streets until the doors re-open again in the late afternoon or evening. If a homeless person is ill, navigating this system can prolong or worsen the illness. Requesting or advocating for a homeless patient with pneumonia to be admitted to the hospital is thus worthwhile. An alternative to hospitalization is a day care unit or a medical respite unit, such as the Barbara McInnis House, a 92-bed facility in Boston, Massachusetts. These facilities may provide nursing care and other resources to help patients adhere to treatment plans and recover in a safe environment.

Summary

A constellation of clinical signs and symptoms should lead the clinician to a diagnosis of pneumonia in the appropriate setting. Clinical findings may be noted even before changes appear on chest x-ray. An effort to perform diagnostic microbiologic laboratory studies should be made as soon as the diagnosis is suspected. Antibiotics are usually started empirically at the outset based on the clinical presentation and then changed if necessary when the diagnostic tests become available. If the patient is homeless, ease of administration of treatment regimes (such as once a day dosing), cost of medications, health insurance status, and having a place to convalesce should be considered. Immunizations such as the influenza vaccination and Pneumovax should be considered as a prevention measure. Where TB is a risk, the PPD status should be verified. If the patient is not connected with a primary care provider or already has primary care, follow up care should be arranged. ▪

Community Acquired Pneumonia Medication List		
Generic	**Name Brand**	**Cost**
acetaminophen	Tylenol	$
clindamycin	Cleocin	$$
doxycycline	Adoxa, Doryx, Monodox, Vibramycin	$
Fluroquinolones		
ciprofloxacin	Cipro, Cipro XR	$$$
levofloxacin	Levaquin	$$$
Macrolides		
azithromycin	Zithromax	$$
clarithromycin	Biaxin	$$$$
erythromycin	Eryc, E-mycin	$
metronidazole	Flagyl, Florazole ER	$
penicillin V	Pen-Vee K, Veetids	$

References

Bartlett JG, et al. Practice guidelines for the management of community-acquired pneumonia in adults. *Clinical Infectious Disease* 2000;31:347-382.

Metlay JP, Fine MJ. Testing strategies in the initial management of patients with community-acquired pneumonia. *Annals of Internal Medicine* 2003;138(2):109-118.

Moser RL. *Primary Care for Physician Assistants.* New York: McGraw-Hill; 1998.

Auble TE, Yearly DM, Fine MJ. Community-acquired pnemonia: risk stratification and the decision to admit. UpToDate, 2002. http://www.uptodate.com

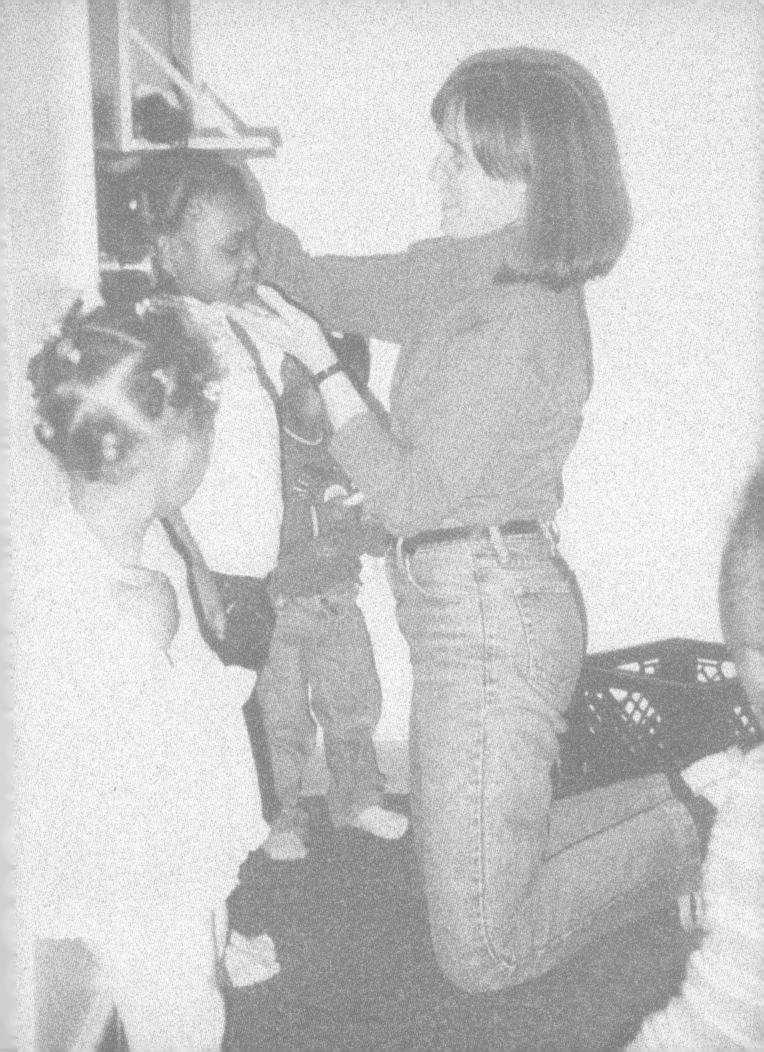

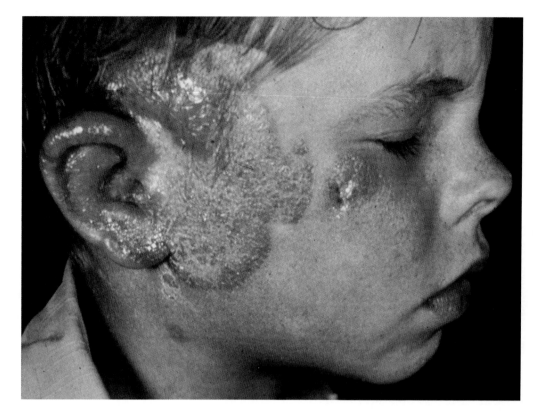

Ringworm

Sarah McSweeney-Ryan, MD
Megan Sandel, MD

Ringworm refers to infections caused by several fungi, commonly called tinea, that can grow on skin, hair, or nails. The descriptive name "ringworm" comes from the characteristic rash that grows outward in the shape of a ring, with worm-like borders and normal skin in the middle.

Each of these fungal infections is named for the part of the body infected. The most common sites are:

- tinea capitis, on the scalp;
- tinea corporis, on the body, excluding the groin, feet, hands, beard region, and scalp;
- tinea pedis ("athlete's foot") and manus, on the feet and hands;
- tinea unguium, under the nails;
- tinea cruris ("jock itch"), on the groin area.

Infection of the scalp is especially troublesome, as it may cause permanent hair loss when untreated. Ringworm infection of the nails can be difficult to eradicate and can cause severe damage to the fingernails and toenails.

Tinea pedis is very common among homeless persons living in shelters and on the streets. A separate chapter has been devoted to this particular form of ringworm. For more information please see the Tinea Pedis chapter.

Prevalence and Distribution

In the USA fungal infections are the second most commonly reported skin disorder. Acne is the most common. Approximately one out of every five people will eventually develop a tinea infection.

The site of tinea fungal infections varies widely among different age groups:

- fungal infections of the scalp and skin (tinea capitis or tinea corporis) are common in young children, while infections of the feet and toes are not. Approximately 3-8% of children in the USA are infected with tinea capitis. Some people are "carriers" of tinea capitis but are themselves not symptomatic. These "carriers" often unknowingly infect and reinfect other people in their homes and therefore pose a challenge to treatment;
- fungal infection under the nails (tinea unguium) is more common in adult and elderly populations;
- "athlete's foot" (tinea pedis) is common in adolescents and adults and spreads easily within families and institutions;

Tinea Corporis. This young boy has an itchy ring-like rash involving the face and ear. The borders are clearly marked, the central area is clear, and there is prominent scaling of the skin. Photo courtesy of the CDC

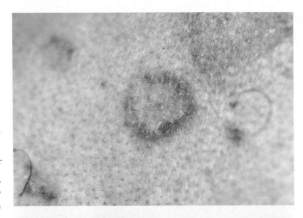

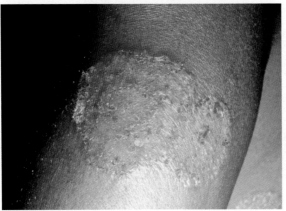

- sharing clothes and contact with infected pets, including dogs, cats, and guinea pigs, are additional ways that fungi can be spread to the skin.

Some types of fungal infections can spread from one part of the body to another. Most people who have tinea cruris also have tinea pedis. Fungal infection of the toes can spread to the toenails, resulting in tinea unguium.

Persons with ringworm are infectious for as long as the cultures of the lesions show the presence of fungi or as long as the skin lesions persist.

Diagnosis
Clinical

The term ringworm describes the appearance of ring-shaped lesions with raised (worm-like) edges. Ringworm typically refers to tinea corporis, the skin lesions. The raised borders are red, often with clear or normal appearing skin in the center of the "ring". The rash is often mildly itchy.

Scalp infection (tinea capitis) can be inflammatory or non-inflammatory. Sore, boggy pustules and hair loss characterize inflammatory infections. Inflammation of the hair follicles causes the hair to break off and the scalp to become scaled and red. The infection may spread locally, creating a larger circle of lost hair, or may be diffuse over the entire scalp. Non-inflammatory tinea capitis produces little scaling, redness, or pustules. The hair shaft can break at the scalp causing a "black dot" appearance.

Fungal infection of the hands and feet (tinea manus and pedis) frequently involves the webbed area between the fingers and the toes, where the skin may become red, cracked, and eroded. Dryness and fine white scaling on the palms of the hands or bottom of the feet can also be evidence of fungal infection. Due to the breakdown of the skin barrier, secondary bacterial infections of the feet may occur. This often leads to pain and swelling of the feet.

Nails infected with fungus (tinea unguium) will generally thicken, become brittle, ridged, and finally split. Caseation produced by the infection causes a tan to brown discoloration of the nail plate. The infection may make the nail very difficult to cut.

"Jock itch" (tinea cruris) is characterized by the scaling of skin and itchy, red irritation of the groin and inner thighs that extends symmetrically to the front of the thighs. The rash usually spares the penis and scrotum. The appearance of the rash can be confused with candida (yeast) infections, which typically have small "satellite" lesions outside the border of the rash.

- fungal infection of the groin (tinea cruris), commonly called "jock itch", typically occurs in young adult men, especially those who wear athletic equipment.

The prevalence of fungal infections has racial variations as well. Fungal infection on the scalp and head (tinea capitis) is more common in African-American children than in Caucasian children.

Fungal infections are more common in people with weak immune systems. Since fungal infections can promote the growth of other bacteria on the skin, clinicians should closely monitor the progress of fungal infections in those who are immunocompromised.

Transmission

Ringworm infection occurs most often through direct contact with an infected person, animal, or surface. Broken or irritated skin promotes transmission, as does warmth and humidity for some fungi. Damp places such as bathroom floors, shower stalls, and rugs often provide ideal opportunities for transmission of the fungi that cause ringworm:

- walking barefoot on an infected surface can result in fungal infection of the feet and toes;
- combs, hats, and barber's instruments can spread ringworm to the scalp and skin;

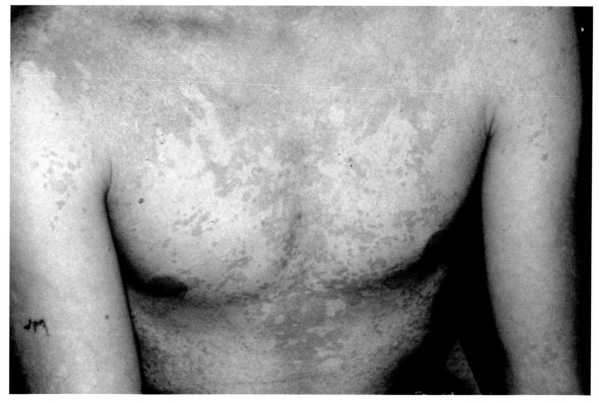

*Tinea Versicolor.
This chronic,
asymptomatic fungal
infection of the skin
is marked by areas
of hypopigmentation
which become
especially prominent
during exposure to
sunlight.
Photo by
Howard Koh MD*

Laboratory

To confirm the diagnosis, a piece of hair, nail, or skin from an active border of the rash may be scraped or clipped off and examined under a microscope. The specimen should first be dissolved in potassium hydroxide preparation (KOH). Since microscopic exams are often negative, a culture using a special medium (Sabouraud's agar) may be necessary. Fungi grow slowly so these results may take weeks.

Examination of the scalp with a Wood's light to demonstrate fungal infection is of limited use. Some fungi will appear bright green under such a light. However, the fungus which most commonly causes tinea capitis in the USA does not fluoresce under this light.

Treatment

Fungal infections are treated by two primary routes: topical or systemic medications. Topical antifungal medication is appropriate initial treatment for skin infections (tinea corporis, pedis, manus, and cruris), unless the infection involves an extensive area. Oral or systemic treatment with antifungal medications is required for all infections involving the scalp or nails (tinea capitis and unguium) and for fungal skin infections that do not respond to topical treatment.

Topical treatment is typically with an antifungal cream, such as clotrimazole (Lotrimin™ 1% cream or lotion), terbinafine (Lamisil™), ketoconazole (Nizoral™), or one of many others. These lotions or creams should be applied once or twice a day to the entire rash and at least 2 centimeters beyond the borders of the rash for a minimum of four weeks. Treatment should generally be continued for one week after resolution of rash.

Systemic antifungal therapy for tinea capitis or other skin infection resistant to topical treatment is typically with griseofulvin, once a day for 4-8 weeks or until 2 weeks after resolution of symptoms. In adults, tinea capitis may be treated with oral terbinafine as a first line medication. There is some evidence that oral terbinafine is a better first line medication for children as well, though current recommendations are for the use of griseofulvin.

Griseofulvin may cause headaches and gastrointestinal disturbances and should always be taken with fatty foods. Griseofulvin can also temporarily interfere with normal liver enzymes, necessitating frequent tests to monitor liver function, especially when treating refractory cases for prolonged periods or using doses of 20 mg/kg or higher.

Nail infections (tinea unguium) are very difficult to treat and are frequently resistant to treatment with oral griseofulvin. Improved cure rates have been seen with the use of oral terbinafine and itraconazole for the treatment of fungal nail infection. Treatment with terbinafine is for a minimum of 6 weeks, and treatment with itraconazole (Sporanox™) is for a minimum of 3 months. These medications may have side effects on the gastrointestinal system, especially the liver. In resistant fungal nail infections, removal of the nail bed may be necessary.

An anti-dandruff shampoo containing selenium sulfide, such as Selsun™ (1% available over the counter or 2.5% by prescription), can eliminate some of the spores in the scalp and can also be applied to the body to help prevent spread of the infection to others. Infected people do not need to wear a cap during treatment.

Prevention and Control

Persons who have had close contact with an individual infected with ringworm should be informed of the signs of this fungal infection and instructed to see a health care provider should any of these appear on the skin, scalp, feet, hands, or nails.

When a case of ringworm occurs in a shelter, staff and guests should be reminded of the need for contact precautions. Guests should avoid walking barefoot and also avoid sharing clothes, hats, hair combs, or brushes. After showering, guests with tinea pedis should dry the body first and the feet last in an attempt to prevent spread of the fungus to the groin or body.

Most fungal infections thrive in warm, damp environments. Clean and dry cotton clothes should be worn, and tight fitting shoes and clothing should be avoided. The prevention and control of ringworm depends upon appropriate treatment and follow-up.

Summary

"Ringworm" refers to several diseases caused by fungi that can invade the skin, scalp, and nails. Depending on the location of the infection, mild to moderate inflammation can occur. Complications include loss of hair and damage to the toenails and fingernails. While seldom life threatening, fungal infections may lead to local bacterial infections of the skin, especially in people with poor immune systems.

Ringworm spreads by direct contact with infected areas on the skin, scalp, or nails. Ringworm may be spread by contact with contaminated bathroom floors, shower stalls, tubs, benches, combs, and brushes. Treatment generally involves either antifungal pills or antifungal cream, depending on the area infected and the severity of the infection. ■

The authors of this chapter gratefully acknowledge the invaluable contribution of Ben Siegel, MD, who authored this chapter in the original Manual.

Ringworm Medication List

Generic	Brand Name	Cost
clotrimazole	Lotrimin	$
griseofulvin	Fulvicin-u/f, Grifulvin-V, Grisactin 500	$$
ketoconazole	Nizoral	$
selenum sulfide	Selsun	$
terbinafine	Lamisil	$$$
Itraconazole	Sporanox	$$$$$

References

Pickering LK, Peter G, Baker CJ, et al., eds. *The 2000 Red Book: Report of the Committee on Infectious Diseases*. Elk Grove Village, Illinois: American Academy of Pediatrics; 2000:569-574, 673.

Elewski BE. Tinea capitis: a current perspective. *Journal of the American Academy of Dermatology* 2000;42(1):1-20.

Friedlander SF, Aly R, Krafchik B, et al. Terbinafine in the treatment of Trichophyton tinea capitis: a randomnized, double-blind, parallel-group, duration-finding study. *Pediatrics* 2002;109(4):602-607.

Weinstein A, Berman B. Topical treatment of common superficial tinea infections. *American Family Physician* 2002;65(10):2095-2102.

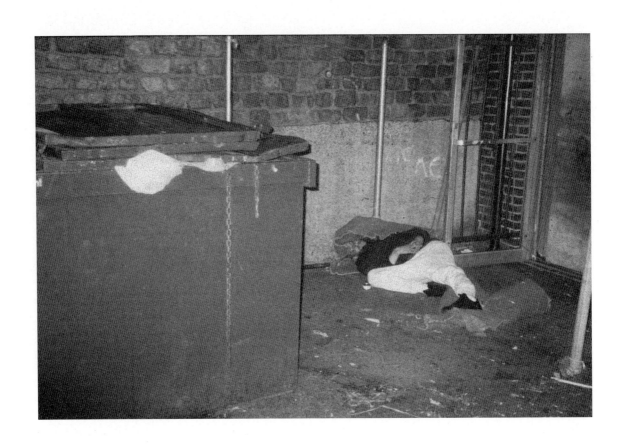

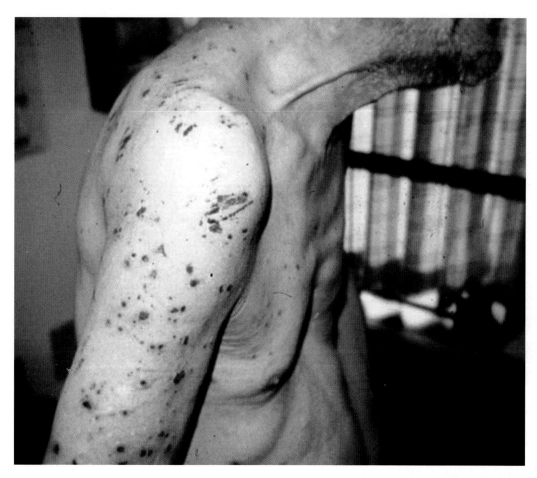

Scabies

Alison May, MD

S cabies is caused by *Sarcoptes scabiei, var. hominus*, the microscopic mite that burrows into a human host to obtain nutrients. Scabies is an extremely contagious infestation that causes an intensely itchy or pruritic rash anywhere on the body, but especially on the trunk, folds of the skin, and on the extremities. Similar to lice, scabies has afflicted humankind for thousands of years and spreads efficiently in crowded living situations such as shelters. Scabies is found worldwide, infesting approximately 300 million people annually and occurring in all climates, socio-economic classes, and races.

Transmission

Fertilized female mites burrow into human skin to the base of the epidermal stratum corneum. They lay 2-3 eggs a day in these burrows. The eggs hatch as nymphs, which mature in these burrows and return to the skin surface as adults about 2 weeks later. Mating then occurs, and the cycle is repeated as the gravid (pregnant) female mites burrow into the skin of the same or a different host. Full-grown female mites are rounded and about 0.35 mm long with 4 pairs of legs. Scabies is generally transmitted by intimate contact, but transmission also occurs by fomites (often in clothing or bedding).

Symptoms and Diagnosis

The extent of disease is variable and depends on the personal hygiene and immune status of the infected individual, as well as the duration and degree of infestation. More severe disease usually occurs in individuals who are less attentive to personal care or whose sensation is impaired in some way. Scabies cause extreme pruritis, or itchiness, due to the immunologic reaction to the burden of mites, their eggs, and their excreta. Initial infection can remain asymptomatic for up to 6 weeks, whereas reinfection causes an immediate hypersensitivity reaction. Symptoms are generally worse at night or after showering.

Scabies.
This man came to our clinic complaining of a cough and was diagnosed with a trilobar pneumonia. He had an incidental scabies infestation. Note the linear burrows of the mite. Photo by James O'Connell MD

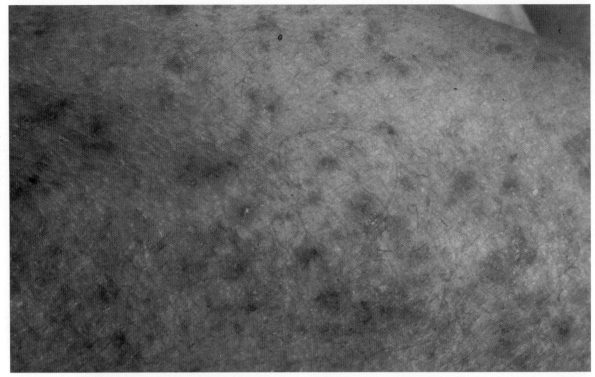

*Scabies Rash.
A popular eruption of the skin, with faint linear or wavy ridges where the mites have burrowed under the skin. This rash is intensely itchy.
Photo by Irwin Freedberg MD*

The dermatological findings of scabies are generally erythematous papules and excoriations, most commonly affecting the interdigital web spaces, wrists, elbows, anterior axillary folds, periumbilical area , buttocks, and the penis. Dark, slightly elevated linear epidermal burrows, generally up to 15 mm long, can also be found, usually in the interdigital web spaces or wrists. A vesicular dot at one end of the burrow can indicate the location of the mite. Scabies can also cause reddish-brown nodules, which are most frequently found in the groin and male genitalia or in the axillae. Less commonly, scabies can present as a more bullous or vesicular eruption. The head, neck, palms, and soles are usually spared, except in infants and young children, in whom these areas are frequently involved.

Norwegian (or crusted) scabies is a severe variant that most commonly occurs in institutionalized, debilitated, or immunosuppressed individuals. The load of parasite is much higher (generally thousands of mites as opposed to 5-10 mites in more classic scabies), and the disease is therefore much more contagious. This variant of the disease has a different appearance, with diffuse crusting of plaques and nodules. The nails can also become thickened with subungual debris. In some patients with Norwegian scabies, the lesions may be more hyperkeratotic and psoriaform, with little or no pruritis, all features which may delay diagnosis.

Another variant of scabies, *S. scabiei var canis*, causes dog mange and can infest humans who have contact with the animal. The mite cannot reproduce on the human host, and therefore no burrows are seen in this variant. Treatment of the infested animal results in resolution of the human symptoms as well.

Definitive diagnosis of scabies can be made microscopically by visualization of the mites, eggs, or a fecal pellet. Mineral oil should be dropped onto a burrow or unexcoriated papule, which should then be unroofed by scraping with a sterile #15 scalpel blade. The material obtained should be examined under microscopic low power.

Treatment and Complications

Until recently, topical lindane 1% lotion (Kwell™) was the standard treatment for scabies. Generalized seizures have been reported after repeated applications of lindane, and clinicians must exercise caution when using this medication. The risk seems to be greater in small children (because of their high surface area-to-mass ratio), in people with neurological disease, or when lindane is applied after a warm bath (vasodilation increases absorption). This toxicity, as well as concerns about possible resistance to lindane, have resulted in the use of permethrin 5% cream (Elimite™) as the treatment of choice for scabies. A single application of permethrin is usually sufficient when applied to a clean and dry body after a tepid bath or shower. The entire skin surface should be covered from chin to toes with a thin layer of the agent, including the

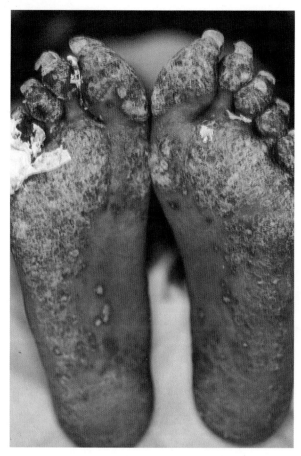

area behind the ears, between the fingers and toes, the groin, between the buttocks, and under finger and toenails. The medicine should be left on for 8-10 hours and then washed off. The patient should then put on clean clothes. The treatment may be repeated in 1 week if necessary. Permethrin is safe for children over 2 months of age.

Though less desirable for the reasons already discussed, lindane 1% lotion (Kwell™) may be used and should be applied in the same way as permethrin. Lindane should not be used in pregnant or nursing women or in young children.

Another alternative treatment is 6% precipitated sulfur in petrolatum which is safe in pregnancy, lactation, and for children younger than 2 months old. This medication is applied nightly for 3 consecutive nights and washed off completely 24 hours after the final application. This agent is messy, stains, and has an odor, but it is quite effective.

One oral regimen is available. A single dose of ivermectin 200 mcg/kg (Stromectol™) has been found to be effective in healthy patients as well as in many patients with HIV infection and crusted scabies. Patients with severe disease may require a second or third treatment or may require concomitant treatment with a topical scabicidal agent. Experience with ivermectin in the treatment

of scabies is limited, and its use should therefore be considered experimental. Ivermectin should not be used in pregnancy or in children who weigh less than 15 kg.

After treatment is completed, clothing and bed linens used during the 3 days preceding treatment should be discarded or machine washed in hot, soapy water and then dried in the hot setting

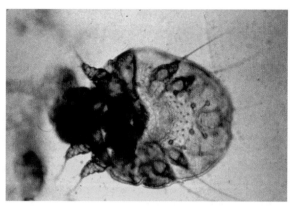

of a household dryer. The treatment of intimate contacts is recommended, even when they are asymptomatic.

In Norwegian scabies, topical agents should be applied to the scalp, under the nails, and to the face excluding the areas surrounding the eyes, nose, and mouth. Multiple sequential regimens may be required. In addition, treatment with a keratolytic agent such as 6% salicylic acid may be necessary in order to assure adequate penetration of the scabicidal agents. Because of the extremely infectious nature of this variant, isolation of the index case is extremely important, and treatment of the environment as well as of exposed contacts is indicated.

Pruritis may persist for several weeks after treatment for scabies, even though effectively treated patients are no longer infectious after one day. Antihistamines and calamine lotion are effective for relief of these symptoms. Topical steroids or glucocorticoids can be helpful in the relief of pruritis after successful treatment is completed.

In addition to scabicidal agents, all patients should trim their fingernails. Permethrin should be reapplied to the hands whenever they are washed during treatment.

Repeated treatment with any scabicidal agent may cause an allergic contact dermatitis. Other complications of scabies include secondary eczema or impetigo that are generally caused by *Staphylococcus aureus*. Oral antibiotics may be necessary to treat secondary bacterial infections. Some strains of streptococci have also been found to cause a

(far left)
Norwegian Scabies. This man with HIV/AIDS has Norwegian scabies of his feet with marked hyperkeratosis. Intense nocturnal pruritis is highly characteristic of these often polymorphic lesions. Photo by Jon Fuller MD

(near left)
Sarcoptes scabiei. This mite causes scabies and is seen here under the microscope. Photo by Howard Koh MD

superinfection that can lead to glomerulonephritis.

Prevention and Control

Prevention and control are largely described in the preceding sections. Mites can generally survive for around one day away from the human host, so surfaces that cannot be washed should be vacuumed. Close contacts of patients with scabies should be treated at the same time as the index case.

Summary

Scabies is an intensely pruritic eruption caused by a mite that burrows under the skin. It is highly contagious and is spread by close personal contact or by the sharing of clothing or linens. Scabies can be effectively treated by the application of topical agents. Prevention of spread of the disease is dependent on the appropriate laundering of clothing and linens, as well as treatment of close contacts of anyone who has scabies. ▪

The author of this chapter gratefully acknowledges the invaluable contribution of Barry Bock, RN, who authored this chapter in the original Manual.

Scabies Medication List

Generic	Brand Name	Cost
1% lindane lotion	Kwell	$
permethrin 5% cream	Elimite	$$
ivermectin 200 mcg/kg	Stromectol	$

References

Maguire J, Spielman A. Ectoparasite infestations, arthropod bites and stings. In: Braunwald E, Fauci AS, Kasper DL, et al., eds. *Harrison's Principles of Internal Medicine.* 15th ed. New York: McGraw-Hill; 2001:2622-2624.

Meinking TL, Taplin D, Hermida JL, et al. The treatment of scabies with ivermectin. *New England Journal of Medicine* 333(1):26-30.

Mathison GE. Of mites and men: lessons in scabies for the infectious diseases clinician *Clinical Infectious Disease* 1998;27(3):646-648.

Orkin M, Maibach HI. Scabies and Pediculosis. In: Wonsiewicz M, Englis MR, Bauer L, eds. *Fitzpatrick's Dermatology in General Medcine.* 5th ed. New York: McGraw-Hill; 1999:2677-2680.

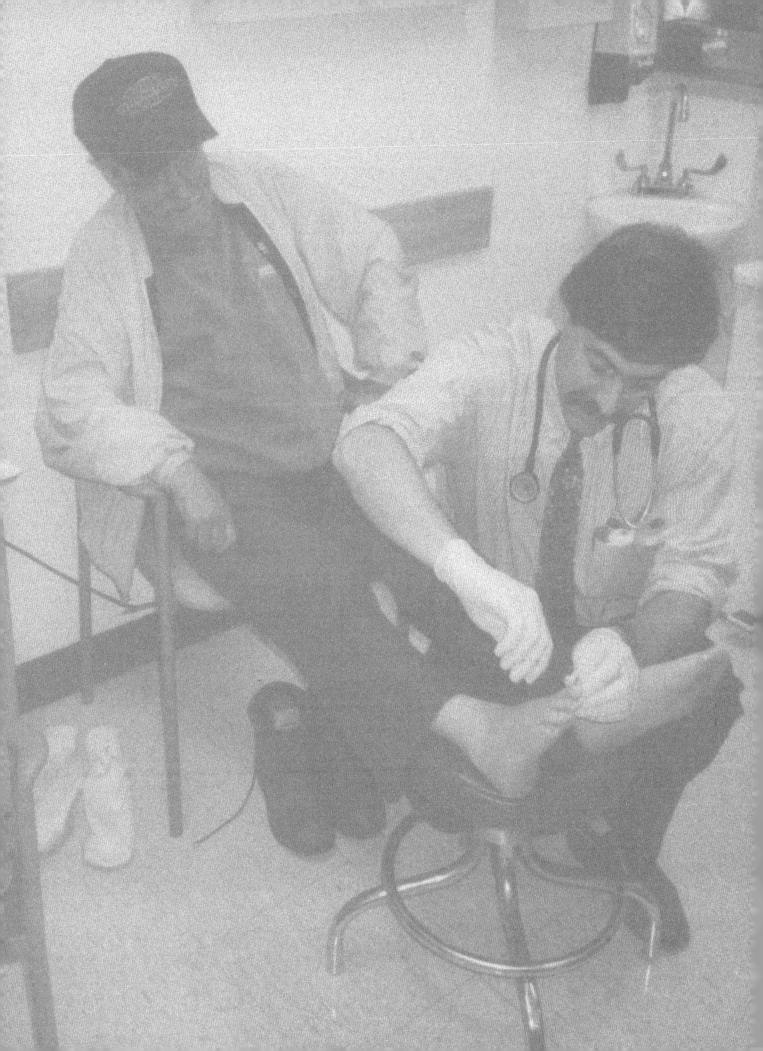

Sexually transmitted diseases (STDs) are discussed in the following two chapters. We have chosen a different approach for this important public health topic because of the complexity, breadth, and multiple dimensions of these diseases. Persons may have one or more STDs. Some may be without symptoms, while others can present with an array of overlapping syndromes. The diagnosis is rarely made solely on a clinical basis, but usually requires laboratory and microbiological studies.

With such diversity and so much overlap, Dr. Noreen Hynes of Johns Hopkins University Schools of Medicine and Public Health has graciously divided STDs into two broad clinical categories. Part I discusses the causes of genital "sores" while Part II focuses on the inflammatory STDs that cause "drips" or discharges. Rather than chapters on each specific disease, an anatomic approach has been taken that focuses on the specific site of the clinical findings. For each physical sign or symptom, such as a vaginal discharge or urethritis, the differential diagnosis is offered and discussed. We hope that this will be practical for clinicians in the field caring for homeless persons, and will help give a framework for approaching this increasingly complex topic.

The following outlines are offered as a guide to the diseases discussed in the next two chapters.

STDs, Part I: Genital Sores

I. Ulcers (Genital Ulcer Disease)
   Herpes Simplex Virus
   Primary Syphilis
   Chancroid

II. Non-Ulcerative Genital Lesions
   Genital Warts
   Pubic Lice
   Scabies
   Secondary Syphilis
   Molluscum Contagiosum
   Genital Candida Dermatitis

STDs, Part II: Drips and Discharges

I. Acute Inflammatory STDs in Women
   A. Lower Genital Tract STDs
      1. Vaginitis
         Bacterial Vaginitis (BV)
         Trichomoniasis
         Vulvovaginal Candidiasis (VVC)
      2. Mucopurulent Cervicitis (MPC)
         Gonorrhea
         Chlamydia
         Herpes Simplex Virus
   B. Upper Genital Tract STDs
      (Pelvic Inflammatory Disease)
         Gonorrhea
         Chlamydia

II. Acute Inflammatory STDs in Men
   A. Urethritis
      Gonococcal Urethritis
      Non-Gonococcal Urethritis
   B. Epididymitis
      Gonorrhea
      Chlamydia

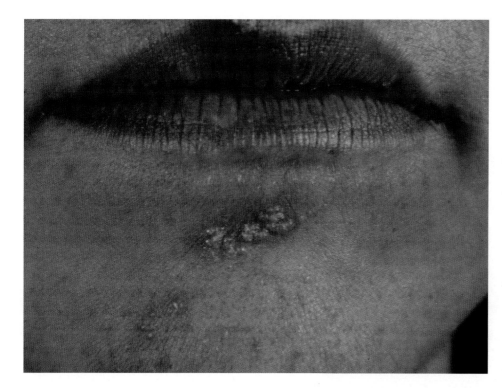

Sexually Transmitted Diseases, Part I : Genital Sores

Noreen A. Hynes, MD, MPH

S exually transmitted diseases (STDs) can be caused by numerous pathogens including viruses, bacteria, parasites, fungi, and ectoparasites. These infections cause a spectrum of disease from asymptomatic infection to an array of often overlapping syndromes that make clinical diagnosis alone inadequate for predicting the cause of the infection. Untreated or inadequately treated STDs can have long-term adverse consequences, particularly for women and their fetuses and newborn infants. STDs presenting as either genital sores, either ulcers or non-ulcerative lesions, have been shown to enhance the acquisition and transmission of human immunodeficiency virus (HIV). Early detection, treatment, partner notification services, and education targeting behavior modification are all critical components of interrupting the transmission of STDs. These prevention and control elements have to be more rigorously and creatively pursued among certain at-risk groups, including guests in homeless shelters, to help interrupt the ever-expanding "hidden epidemic" of STDs. When possible, diagnostic testing should be available at the point of patient care and directly observed single-dose therapy offered whenever the efficacy of this approach has been demonstrated for a particular STD.

Oral Herpes Simplex. Small clear blisters are grouped on a reddish base and are frequently painful. This lesion lasts about 7-10 days, and recurred twice each year in this patient. Photo by Irwin Freedberg MD

A General Approach to the STDs

Every sexually active individual not in a long-term mutually monogamous relationship who is seen in the clinic should be considered at risk for newly incident STDs, both asymptomatic and symptomatic. A routine STD screening history and physical examination should be obtained on all at-risk patients, regardless of the presenting complaint. Contacts of patients treated for bacterial STDs or trichomoniasis should be treated and also offered screening for HIV infection, if indicated. Contacts of persons with viral STDs should be tested for the presence of infection and offered screening for HIV, if indicated. Sexually active persons, with or without symptoms, should undergo diagnostic testing for treatable STDs and be offered HIV counseling and testing. Those with symptoms should have further evaluations based upon the clinical

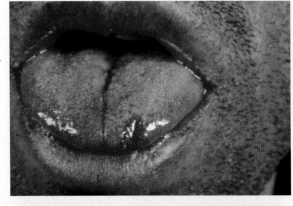

(top)
Oral Herpes Simplex.
This painful
inflammation of
the tongue can be
accompanied by a
low-grade fever and
swollen neck glands.
The symptoms
usually resolve in
about two weeks.
Photo by
Irwin Freedberg MD

(bottom)
Genital Herpes
Simplex.
This HSV infection of
the anus and rectum
is very painful.
Photo by
Howard Koh MD

syndrome noted at presentation. Most of the STD clinical syndromes fall into two general categories: "sores" and "drips/discharges". The approach to these general syndrome categories is discussed in this and the following chapter.

I. Genital Ulcer Disease (GUD)

Sexually transmitted genital sores can be subdivided into two groups - genital ulcers and other genital sores. Although certain "classic" presentations of genital sores may suggest a particular diagnosis, clinical diagnosis alone is neither sensitive nor specific enough as the only diagnostic modality.

Causes of Genital Ulcer Disease

Although there are numerous causes of genital ulcer disease (GUD), the three most common in the USA are:

- herpes simplex virus (HSV), the most common GUD;
- primary syphilis, a cause of GUD that is increasing in many areas; and
- chancroid, a very infrequently diagnosed GUD.

Other much less commonly seen GUDs include lymphogranuloma venereum (LGV) and granuloma inguinale, both of which are bacterial STDs rarely diagnosed in the USA.

Signs and Symptoms

The physical characteristics of the lesion, the temporal evolution of the lesion, lymph nodes draining the area, and the presence or absence of pain or itching may provide clues to the diagnosis.

HSV classically begins with a pruritic macule that rapidly develops into one or more vesicles that upon rupture cause painful, shallow ulcers with a scant amount of associated fluid. On average, the lesions appear within 6 days following a primary exposure to an asymptomatic viral shedder. Tender bilateral lymphadenopathy is most likely to be seen with primary HSV GUD, whereas non-tender unilateral lymphadenopathy may be seen in recurrent disease. However, a broad spectrum of associated signs and symptoms can be seen, particularly with recurrent ulcerative disease and in immunocompromised persons. Except in severely immunocompromised persons the symptoms will resolve without treatment, but all symptomatic persons are treated to decrease their risk for HIV acquisition or transmission. The infection is life-long, and recurrences of clinical symptoms are not uncommon, although the severity and duration are usually less impressive than that noted with primary disease.

Primary Syphilis causes a temporal spectrum of acute and chronic manifestations. The chancre is the classically painless ulcer of primary syphilis. The chancre occurs 10 to 90 days after exposure. It begins as a macule, evolves to a papule, and then a painless indurated ulcer with a sharply demarcated border on a smooth red base. Single ulcers are the rule, but multiple lesions are not uncommon. The chancre occurs at the point of contact; hence, oral and rectal chancres can be seen. Non-tender, firm, enlarged regional lymph nodes are seen at this stage of infection. The chancre will resolve without treatment, but the infection will not.

Chancroid is a very uncommon cause of GUD that intermittently is identified in outbreak settings. A small papule evolves into a classically painful and deep ulcer with a purplish border and "dirty" yellow to gray exudate with enlarging, tender lymph nodes that often suppurate over the course of 2 to 3 weeks.

Complications of GUDs

Some GUDs can cause complications related to local extension of the lesions (HSV, chancroid) or spread of the infectious organism to extragenital sites (HSV, syphilis).

HSV. Genital HSV can result in local or systemic complications that are seen more frequently with primary infection and in women. Local extension of disease is most commonly seen in immunocompromised persons. The ulcers may coalesce and continue to spread. Secondary bacterial infection is uncommon and is seen more frequently in immunocompromised persons. Neurological complications include aseptic meningitis (particularly common in primary infection), transverse myelitis, urinary retention, and constipation. Transmission to the newborn can occur during parturition, particularly when lesions are present.

Primary Syphilis. The chancre of syphilis represents the first stage of early infection. Untreated syphilis is a systemic disease that can lead to neurologic, ophthalmologic, cardiovascular, skeletal, or gastrointestinal complications. Pregnant women with untreated syphilis remain potentially infectious for the fetus for 4 years following initial infection.

Chancroid. This cause of GUD is rarely is associated with ulcer superinfection. In uncircumcised men, cicatrix formation with phimosis is a late complication and may require circumcision to cure.

Prevalence

HSV. Approximately 45 million Americans are estimated to be infected with genitally-acquired HSV. By the age of 35 years, approximately 25% of adults are infected. Most have asymptomatic infection although they continue to intermittently shed the virus. About one million new infections with this persistent pathogen are genitally acquired each year.

Primary Syphilis. The chancre of syphilis is a short-lived lesion and thus the incidence and prevalence are essentially the same. Statistics are only available for combined primary and secondary syphilis (the most infectious forms of syphilis). Over 6000 cases were reported in 2002. After a significant decline, cases are increasing. Risk groups include residents in urban and rural indigent areas, men who have sex with men, and commercial sex workers and their contacts.

Chancroid. The prevalence and incidence of chancroid is less than 300 cases per year nationwide.

Diagnosis

HSV. The diagnostic gold standard is culture. A Tzanck smear is positive in only 50% of cases and may be useful in the outpatient setting with classic-appearing lesions. PCR remains a research tool. Serology is only useful if negative for both

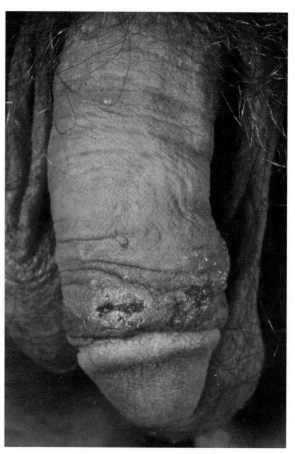

Genital Herpes Simplex.
Several small blisters on the shaft of the penis in addition to areas of erosion. The differential diagnosis of these latter lesions would include chancres due to syphilis.
Photo by Irwin Freedberg MD

HSV-1 and HSV-2 to rule out HSV as the cause of the ulcer.

Primary Syphilis. Darkfield microscopy is the gold standard for the diagnosis of primary syphilis. Antibody to cardiolipin, as measured by the rapid plasma reagin (RPR) test, will yield a low antibody titer in 80% at the time of presentation. If the RPR is positive, a treponemal antibody test, such as the MHA-T and the FTA-Abs, is necessary to confirm the diagnosis. These treponemal antibody-specific tests cannot be used alone for diagnosis because they remain positive for life. Hence a positive test does not mean the infection is new or untreated.

Chancroid. Culture is the diagnostic test of choice. However, the sample must be carefully collected and transported using a cotton or calcium alginate in special transport media. Most state health department laboratories can provide diagnostic laboratory assistance.

Treatment

The treatment of genital ulcer disease due to syphilis or chancroid should utilize directly observed, single dose therapy at the time of diagnosis. Genital herpes requires different regimens for primary and recurrent lesions.

HSV. Acyclovir (ACV), valacyclovir (VACV),

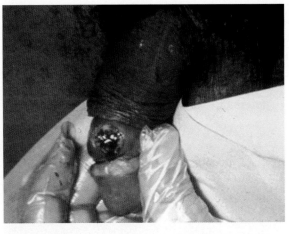

and famciclovir (FCV) are all effective against herpes simplex virus.

First clinical episode of genital HSV:
- ACV 400 mg orally three times a day for 7-10 days, or;
- ACV 200 mg orally five times a day for 7-10 days, or;
- VACV 1 gm orally twice a day for 7-10 days, or;
- FCV 250 mg orally twice a day for 7-10 days.

Recurrent genital HSV:
- ACV 200 mg orally five times a day for 5 days, or;
- ACV 800 mg orally twice a day for 5 days, or;
- VACV 500 mg orally twice a day for 3-5 days, or;
- VACV 1 gm orally once a day for 5 days, or;
- FCV 125 mg orally twice a day for 5 days.

Suppressive therapy (for persons with > 5 recurrences per year):
- ACV 400 orally twice a day, or;
- VACV 500 mg orally once a day, or;
- VACV 1 gm orally one a day, or;
- FCV 250 mg orally one a day.

Primary Syphilis. The treatment of choice for all stages of syphilis is parenteral penicillin. Treatment of primary and secondary syphilis is benzathine penicillin G 2.4 million units intramuscularly in a single dose. Some public health experts recommend a second dose one week after the first dose, particularly in HIV-infected persons and pregnant women. Patients with penicillin allergy who are pregnant or whose compliance with alternative therapy cannot be ensured must be desensitized and treated with benzathine penicillin G. In non-pregnant patients with penicillin allergy, doxycycline

100 mg orally twice a day for 14 days can be used. Preliminary data suggests that a single 2-gram dose of azithromycin may be effective. However, many patients experience moderate to severe gastrointestinal upset at this dose of azithromycin.

Chancroid. Recommended single-dose regimens include azithromycin 1 gm or ceftriaxone 250 mg intramuscularly. Up to 10 percent of patients with chancroid are co-infected with syphilis and some public health experts recommend concomitant treatment for primary syphilis. Multi-day regimens include ciprofloxacin 500 mg orally twice a day for three days, or erythromycin base 500 mg orally three times a day for 7 days.

Follow-up

Patients with syphilis and chancroid require follow-up to ensure adequacy of treatment.

Syphilis. Treatment failure can occur with any regimen. Therefore, reassessment is needed. Patients whose signs or symptoms persist or recur or who, after 6 months, have a sustained fourfold rise in nontreponemal antibody titers compared with the maximum or baseline titer measured on the day of treatment have probably failed treatment or have been reinfected. A lumbar puncture with a CSF analysis is needed in such cases to rule out neurosyphilis.

Chancroid. Patients should be re-examined 3 to 7 days after initiation of treatment to determine if treatment is successful, i.e. significant improvement in symptoms in 3 days and objective improvement in ulcers by 7 days. Failure to improve requires consideration of an alternative diagnosis or the need for treatment longer than 2 weeks.

Prevention and Control

Syphilis, chancroid, and the genital form of HSV are spread only by sexual contact and can be prevented by abstaining from sexual activity or engaging in a long-term mutually-monogamous relationship in which both partners are uninfected at the outset. Condoms do not cover all potentially exposed areas and are less effective in preventing STDs transmitted by direct skin-to-skin contact, including syphilis, chancroid, and genital HSV, than STDs transmitted by secretions, such as gonorrhea, Chlamydia, and trichomoniasis.

Syphilis and chancroid cases are reportable by law to the local or state health department, who will undertake further investigation and partner notification activities that focus on interrupting transmission of these diseases. Many persons benefit from partner notification services, and shelter guests with diagnosed STDs should be encouraged to make their partners aware of potential STD risk and urge them to seek diagnosis and treatment.

All sexually active shelter guests, particularly women in the childbearing years, HIV-infected persons, and those with a history of a previous STD, should receive a syphilis test every year as part of routine primary care. Pregnant women should have a cardiolipin-based syphilis screening test at the time of the initial prenatal visit, during the third trimester of pregnancy, and again at the time of delivery. Guests diagnosed with any STD, particularly GUD, should be encouraged to receive HIV counseling and testing services.

II. Non-Ulcerative Genital Lesions

Five common STDs and one sexually-associated disease can manifest as non-ulcerative genital skin lesions:

- genital warts
- pubic lice (phthriasis)
- scabies
- secondary syphilis
- molluscum contagiosum
- genital Candida dermatitis.

While considered STDs, both scabies and molluscum contagiousum can frequently be transmitted non-sexually. Candida is not considered an STD, but is commonly seen in sexually active persons, particularly women.

Signs and Symptoms

The signs and symptoms associated with each of the non-ulcerative STD genital skin lesions may be helpful in suggesting a diagnosis. The appearance of these STDs can be very similar to other dermatolgoical conditions, and a definitive diagnosis cannot be made clinically without supportive tests.

Genital Warts. These lesions are caused by several human papillomavirus (HPV) strains. Genital warts can have variable appearances, ranging from flat to verrucous-appearing (condylomata acuminata), and can be confused with other genital lesions. They can be single or multiple in number. Although HPV has been causally linked to cervical cancer and probably other ano-genital squamous cell cancers, visible genital warts have a lower oncogenic potential than asymptomatic infections. In men, warts are commonly seen around the glans penis and the distal penis. Intraurethral warts are not

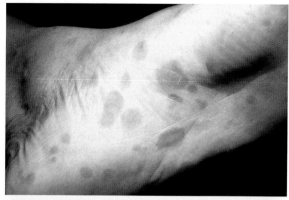

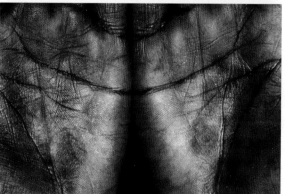

(top)
Secondary Syphilis. This itchy rash of the soles of the feet was accompanied by muscle aches and generalized lymphadenopathy. Note the "copper coin" lesions. Photo by Howard Koh MD

(bottom)
Secondary Syphilis. This man presented with a rash of the palms of his hands, the soles of his feet, and the roof of his mouth. He complained of fatigue and a loss of appetite, and did not recall a chancre in the past. Photo by Irwin Freedberg MD

uncommon. In women, visible warts are common at the introitus and on the vagina. Cervical warts may be noted at the time of a speculum examination in women. Perirectal warts can be seen in both sexes, with a greater frequency in persons who engage in anal receptive intercourse. Patients with genital warts may complain of itching.

Pubic Lice. Pubic lice appear as adult lice or nits on the pubic hair and may be difficult to see. Erythematous skin is often seen beneath the hair shaft containing the nit. Pruritis is a hallmark of this ectoparasitic infestation. If the person has not been previously infested with pubic lice, redness or itching may not be present for the first 5-7 days. Itching occurs within 24 hours in persons who have had a previous infestation. Please see chapter on Lice.

Scabies. Scabies can be identified by the findings of linear, red, excoriated areas between the fingers, at the belt line, the external genitalia, abdomen, and buttocks. In addition to the classic mite burrow of scabies, the lesions can be urticarial, eczematous, nodular, papular, or pustular. Pruritis may be severe, often worse at night or in a warm environment. Immunocompromised persons may develop severe infestations of disease with diffuse, large crusted lesions. This form of disease is known as crusted or Norwegian scabies and is associated with the presence of a very large number of ectoparasites. Please see chapter on Scabies.

Table 1: Differential Diagnostic Features of Sexually Transmitted Genital Ulcer Diseases

FEATURE	PRIMARY HSV	RECURRENT HSV	SYPHILIS	CHANCROID	LGV	GRANULOMA INGUINALE
Incubation period	2-14 days	Recurrence usually within 6-9 months of primary HSV	10-90 days	1-14 days	3-21 days	Unknown; likely 1 to 16 weeks
Initial lesion	Papule→ vesicles→ ulcer	Papule→ vesicles→ ulcer	Papule→ ulcer	Papule→ ulcer	Papule→ pustule→ ulcer	Papule or nodule→ ulcer
Ulcer border	"Punched out", erythematous	"Punched out", erythematous	Sharp, demarcated	Purplish, undermined	Variable, may be missed	Beefy red, rolled up edges
Ulcer base	Red, smooth	Red, smooth	Red, smooth	"Dirty" yellow to gray exudate	Variable	Beefy red
Ulcer depth	Superficial	Superficial	Superficial	Deep, evacuated	Variable	Variable with granulomatous tissue
Ulcer discharge	Serous, scant	Serous, scant	Serous, scant	Purulent to hemorrhagic	Variable	Variable
Number of ulcers	Multiple, may coalesce	Multiple, may coalesce	Usually one	Usually 1 to 3	Usually one	Usually one
Ulcer induration	None	None	Firm (consistency of an Oxford shirt collar buttonhole)	Rare, usually soft	Variable	Moderate firmness
Pain	Common, may be severe	Common, usually less severe	Rare	Usually, can be severe	Uncommon	Rare
Pruritis	Common	Common	Rare	Rare	Rare	Rare
Lymph node enlargement	Bilateral, firm, tender, inguinal area	Uncommon, unilateral, non-tender, inguinal area	Non-tender, firm, inguinal area	Very tender, enlarged and may suppurate	Tender, inguinal and femoral nodes, may suppurate	Uncommon

Secondary Syphilis. The classic genital lesions of secondary syphilis are condylomata lata. These are red, moist, raised, glistening, wheal-like lesions that are often mistaken for the condylomata acuminata caused by HPV infection. Other common lesions include mucous patches (reddish, ulcer-like lesions with a purplish border that can be seen on the penis, scrotum, vagina, vulva, perirectal area, or the mouth), macular-papular eruptions that can be found on the genitalia or other skin surface, and classic "copper coin" lesions most notable on the palms and soles. The lesions of secondary syphilis appear weeks to months after exposure to syphilis and may occur after the disappearance of the chancre of primary syphilis, while the chancre is still present, or in the absence of a history of a chancre having been present. Little or no itching is associated with these lesions. This stage of syphilis is a systemic disease and non-dermatologic findings may be present, including sore throat, headache, fever, malaise, weight loss, general lymphadenopathy, and hepatitis. Circular lesions may be seen on the facial skin of darker pigmented persons.

Molluscum Contagiosum. The lesions caused by molluscum contagiosum virus can appear anywhere on the genitalia and on the skin of the hands and face. They appear as papular, smooth, pearly-white, centrally umbilicated, non- or minimally pruritic lesions, usually 3-5 mm in size. Caseous material can be expressed from the central umbilicated area. Normal hosts may have 10-20 lesions, whereas immunocompromised persons may develop hundreds of lesions.

Genital Candida Dermatitis. This infection is not sexually-transmitted but is commonly considered to be sexually-associated, i.e. found more commonly in persons with STDs than in those without STDs. In women, the dermatitis covers a spectrum from non-specific pruritic patches of erythema to severe erythema and peeling of the hair-bearing part of the labia majora. The affected area may be bounded by a rim of scaling and superficial pustules (satellites). In men, Candida produces red papules or plaques on the glans of the uncircumcised penis. Lesions are rarely seen on the shaft of the penis or the scrotum. Moderate to severe pruritis is seen.

Complications

Genital Warts. More than 30 types of HPV can infect the genital tract. Visible warts are associated with the minority of these infections. HPV infection can be associated with cancer; the association is lowest for visible warts when compared with asymptomatic infection. In women, HPV can cause cancer of the cervix, vulva, vagina, and anus. Heterosexual men have a very small risk of penile cancer. Men who have sex with men have an increased risk of anal cancer. Certain groups are at increased risk for developing very large genital warts, including persons with decreased cell-mediated immunity due to HIV, Hodgkin's disease, immunosuppressive drugs, or pregnancy. These large warts can become locally destructive.

Pubic Lice and Scabies. Persons with pubic lice or scabies, on rare occasion, may develop local bacterial cellulitis in excoriated areas.

Secondary Syphilis. Certain complications seen in secondary syphilis are related to high levels of circulating immune complexes, including patchy alopecia, iritis, anterior uveitis, glomerulonephritis, or nephrotic syndrome. In addition, acute neurosyphilis can occur during this stage, manifested as meningoencephalitis, meningitis, or hearing loss. All cases of neurosyphilis require treatment with parenteral penicillin for 10-14 days. Untreated syphilis may result in long term complications of the skeletal, cardiovascular, or central nervous systems.

Molluscum Contagiosum. The most frequent complication of infection is an eczematous reaction 3-10 cm in diameter around individual lesions. This reaction occurs 1-15 months after the onset of the lesion and disappears when the lesion resolves. Lesions neither worsen during pregnancy nor appear to affect the outcome of pregnancy.

Genital Candida Dermatitis. Persistent or recurrent infection may be noted in immunocompromised persons. Longer course therapy may be needed in such cases.

Prevalence

No reliable prevalence estimates are available for pubic lice, scabies, molluscum contagiosum, or genital Candida dermatitis.

Genital Warts. HPV is the most common viral STD in the USA; about one percent of the sexually active population has genital warts. Peak prevalence is in persons 17-33 years of age.

Secondary Syphilis. The lesions of secondary syphilis are short lived and resolve without treatment, although the person is still infected and at risk for long-term complications from infection. In an untreated person, the lesions of secondary syphilis can recur. Statistics are only available for combined primary and secondary syphilis. Together these two stages are the most infectious stages of syphilis. Over 6000 cases were reported in 2002. After a significant decline, cases are increasing. Risk groups include residents in urban and rural indigent areas, men who have sex with men, and commercial sex workers and their contacts.

Diagnosis

All sexually active shelter guests with atypical genital warts, undiagnosed genital rash, or genital lesions should have a screening test for syphilis.

Genital Warts. The diagnosis of genital warts begins with a thorough clinical examination using a bright light and a lens to evaluate small lesions. All persons with genital warts should have a screening test for syphilis because genital warts and lesions of secondary syphilis are often confused. A negative rapid plasmin reagin (RPR) test essentially rules out secondary syphilis. Because cervical and vaginal lesions often accompany lesions of the external genitalia in women, a speculum examination should also be performed. Cytologic examination of cervical (Pap smear) and anal specimens are also an integral part of the examination, particularly in women and in men who have sex with men. Some experts recommend anoscopy when perianal or perineal warts are seen or the person has a history of anal receptive intercourse. Although visible warts are much less commonly associated with cancer, co-infection with several virus types is not uncommon, including oncogenic strains. Detection of HPV DNA by molecular-based assays, although not currently in routine clinical use, is an area of active development and may soon be integrated into primary care practice.

Pubic Lice. The diagnosis begins with a careful history followed by a thorough physical examination. The louse and the nits should be visible with the naked eye, although a hand lens and bright light are very useful. The eyelashes and axillary hair may also be infested.

Scabies. The appearance of the lesions cannot be relied upon to make a definitive diagnosis of scabies. A hand lens and bright light should be used to examine burrows. To make the burrows more visible, rub fountain pen ink on the suspect area and then wipe the area with isopropyl alcohol. The burrow will then be visible. The area is then scraped with a #15 scalpel blade to disrupt the top of the

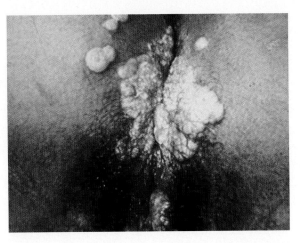

burrow. This scraping is placed on a microscope slide with a coverslip and examined with the oil immersion microscope lens for the presence of mites, eggs, or fecal pellets.

Secondary Syphilis. The diagnosis of secondary syphilis is made in the presence of any lesion consistent with secondary syphilis on an individual with a history of unprotected sexual contact who has a positive RPR and a positive confirmatory treponemal antibody test.

Molluscum Contagiosum. Diagnosis can be made clinically in the setting of classic pearly lesions with central umbilication. Histology or electron microscopy of a biopsy specimen will identify the virus in atypical lesions.

Genital Candida Dermatitis. The diagnosis is made with a 10% potassium hydroxide slide preparation from a swab specimen collected from a moist area of the lesion. The slide will show budding yeasts and pseudohyphae.

Treatment

Genital Warts. The primary goal is to remove symptomatic warts. In most cases wart removal results in a wart-free period. Notably, if left untreated, visible warts may resolve on their own, remain unchanged, or increase in number or size. Removal of visible warts may decrease infectivity. Persons with fewer than 11 visible warts or a total visible wart area of less than 1 cm by 1 cm can receive either point of care treatment by the clinic health care provider or be given a patient-applied treatment. More complicated warts, including those on mucosal surfaces, should be referred for management. Those who do not respond to one treatment type should be retreated with another modality. Recommended regimens for external genital warts include:

- clinic provider administered treatment;
- cryotherapy with liquid nitrogen or cryoprobe. Repeat application every 1-2 weeks. This is the only recommended therapy for use during pregnancy;
- podophyllin resin, 10% to 25% in a compound tincture of benzoin. Apply a small amount to each wart and allow to air dry. Limit application to an area <10 cm^2 or <0.6 mL per session. Some experts recommend thorough washing of the area in 1-4 hours after the application. Repeat treatment every week, as needed;
- trichloroacetic acid (TCA) or bichloro-acetic acid (BCA) 80% to 90%. Apply a small amount only to the warts and allow to dry, indicated by "frosting" of the lesions. If too much acid is applied, cover the area with baking soda or liquid soap to remove the excess acid. Repeat weekly, if needed;
- surgical removal by tangential scissors excision, tangential shave excision, curettage, or electrosurgery;
- patient-applied treatments;
- imiquimod 5% cream, applied three times weekly.

Pubic lice. Agents used to treat pubic lice should NOT be applied to the eyes or eyelashes. Eyelash infestation is managed by applying occlusive ophthalmic ointment to the eyelid margins twice a day for 10 days.

Bedding and clothing should be decontaminated by machine washing, machine drying using the heat cycle, dry-cleaning, or removing from the body for 72 hours. There is no need to fumigate living quarters. All persons with pubic lice should be evaluated for other STDs. The recommended treatments include:

- permethrin 1% cream rinse applied to affected areas and washed off within 10 minutes. Some public health experts prefer this treatment to lindane because it has less potential for toxicity;
- lindane 1% shampoo applied for 4 minutes to the affected area and then thoroughly washed off. DO NOT USE in pregnant women or children < 2 years;
- pyrethrins with piperonyl butoxide applied to the affected area and washed off after 10 minutes.

Scabies. The recommended regimen for the treatment of scabies is 5% permethrin cream applied to the entire body from the neck down and washed off after 8 to 14 hours. Clothing and bedding should be decontaminated by either dry cleaning or machine washing followed by drying using the hot cycle. Alternatively, the clothing and bedding can be removed from all bodily contact for 72 hours. Fumigation is not needed. Some public health experts recommend the use of ivermectin 200 μg/kg orally that is repeated 14 days after the initial treatment rather than permethrin cream for immunocompromised persons and other special groups, including guests in homeless shelters. Lindane has increasingly fallen into disfavor by many clinicians due to associated adverse effects, and it cannot be used in pregnancy.

Secondary Syphilis. Recommended treatment regimens for primary and secondary are the same. The treatment of choice for all stages of syphilis is parenteral penicillin. Treatment of primary and secondary syphilis is benzathine penicillin G 2.4 million units intramuscularly in a single dose. Some public health experts recommend a second dose one week after the first dose, particularly in HIV-infected persons. Patients with penicillin allergy who are pregnant or whose compliance with alternative therapy cannot be ensured must be desensitized and treated with benzathine penicillin G. In non-pregnant patients with penicillin allergy, doxycycline 100 mg orally twice a day for 14 days can be used.

Molluscum Contagiosum. The goal of treatment is to hasten the resolution of individual lesions in an effort to decrease autoinoculation (particularly among immunocompromised persons) and to decrease transmission to others (particularly to immunocompromised persons). It is important to note that no treatment is very effective in immunocompromised persons who have a high likelihood of recurrence:

- direct destruction;
- cryotherapy with liquid nitrogen may be useful for small lesions when fewer than 10 are present;
- expression of the lesion core by direct pressure may be useful if fewer than 5 lesions are present. Care must be taken to avoid reinoculation;
- excisional curettage followed by application of a chemical irritant, such as silver nitrate or iodine, to the area.

Genital Candida Dermatitis. Visible genital, perineal, and perianal lesions can be treated by a single dose of fluconazole 150 mg orally. Immunocompromised persons may require re-treatment.

Some experts recommend several days of treatment for this group. Alternatively, an over-the-counter topical antifungal cream can be applied for 3-7 days. The area should be cleansed with mild soap and tepid water and be blotted dry each day until the lesions have resolved. In those using cream therapy, cleansing should precede cream application. In males, the foreskin should be retracted during the cleansing, drying, and cream application process.

Follow-up

Genital Warts. In most patients there is usually no need for further follow-up after warts have cleared. However, in immunocompromised persons for whom recurrences are common, repeated evaluations may be helpful in detecting early recurrence and initiating re-treatment. Annual cervical cytological evaluation is recommended for all women with or without genital warts. Some experts recommend follow-up anoscopy for patients with previously diagnosed anal warts.

Pubic lice. Patients should be evaluated after 1 week if symptoms persist. Re-treatment may be needed if lice are found or nits are observed at the hair-skin interface. Re-treatment should utilize a different regimen than that used initially.

Scabies. At the time of initial treatment, patients should be informed that itching and rash might last as long as 2 weeks after treatment. Patients with crusted scabies should be re-evaluated 1 week after therapy, particularly if a topical agent was utilized for initial treatment. Some experts recommend re-treatment after 1-2 weeks if the patients are symptomatic, whether or not live mites are seen.

Secondary Syphilis. Treatment failure can occur with any regimen. Therefore, re-assessment is necessary. Persons whose signs or symptoms persist or recur, as well as those individuals who, after 6 months, have a sustained fourfold rise in non-treponemal antibody titers compared with the maximum or baseline titer measured on the day of treatment, have probably failed treatment or have been reinfected. A lumbar puncture with a CSF analysis is needed in such cases to rule out neurosyphilis.

Molluscum Contagiosum. Follow-up after treated lesions have resolved is not necessary in most cases. In HIV-infected persons, periodic follow-up and early treatment of recurrent lesions may be useful.

Genital Candida Dermatitis. There is no need for follow-up after treated lesions have resolved. Immunocompromised individuals with recurrent disease should have follow-up one week after treatment.

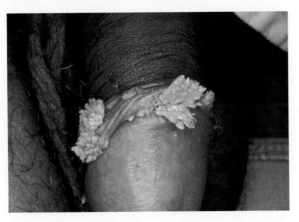

Condyloma Accuminata. These genital warts are caused by human papillomavirus (HPV). In men, these warts are commonly seen around the glans penis and the distal penis, as depicted here. Photo by Irwin Freedberg MD

Prevention and Control

Among the 6 non-GUD genital lesions discussed in this chapter only genital warts, secondary syphilis, and pubic lice are exclusively transmitted in adults by the sexual route; scabies and molluscum contagiosum are transmitted by sexual and non-sexual routes; genital Candida dermatitis is not sexually transmitted. All of the STDs listed here are transmitted by lesion-to-skin contact. The sexual transmission of these conditions can be prevented by abstaining from sexual activity or by engaging in a long-term and mutually monagamous relationship in which both partners are uninfected at the outset. Condoms do not cover all potentially exposed areas during sexual activity, and are therefore less likely to be effective for the STDs discussed in this chapter than for those transmitted by contact with genital secretions, such as gonorrhea, Chlamydia, and trichomoniasis.

All forms of syphilis, including secondary syphilis, are reportable by law to the local or state health department who will undertake further investigation and partner notification activities that focus on interrupting syphilis transmission. For pregnant women, syphilis screening should be undertaken at the time of the initial prenatal visit, during the third trimester of pregnancy, and again at the time of delivery.

Many persons benefit from partner notification services. Shelter guests with diagnosed STDs should be encouraged to make their partners aware of potential STD risk and urge them to seek diagnosis and treatment.

All sexually active shelter guests, particularly women in the childbearing years, HIV-infected persons, and those with a history of a previous STD, should be offered syphilis screening every year as part of routine primary care. Guests diagnosed with any STD should be encouraged to receive HIV counseling and testing services.

Summary

Ulcers or non-ulcerative lesions of the genitalia due to STDs are often present when shelter guests come to the clinic for other health-related problems. It is critically important to include a sexual history and focused physical examination for all sexually active patients to provide treatment and interrupt further transmission when possible. Key concepts to keep in mind when caring for shelter guests with STDs include:

- single dose, directly observed therapy is the preferred form of therapy when such a regimen is proven to be efficacious;
- persons with genital ulcer disease are at increased risk for HIV acquisition and transmission (if HIV infected);
- the presence of one STD increases the risk for a second STD and also is a marker for possible exposure to HIV. Therefore, all patients diagnosed with an STD should receive HIV counseling and testing, as indicated;
- women and their unborn children bear the greatest burden of adverse outcomes from STDs;
- women are more likely to have asymptomatic STDs than men;
- syphilis and chancroid are reportable diseases, and local or state health departments must be notified. ▪

STDs Part I: Genital Sores Medication List

Generic	Brand Name	Cost
acyclovir (oral)	Zovirax	$
acyclovir (ointment/cream)	Zovirax	$$$
azithromycin	Zithromax	$$
benzathine penicillin G	Bicillin L-A	$
ceftriaxone	Rocephin	$$$$$
ciprofloxacin	Cipro	$$$
doxycycline	Vibramycin	$$
famciclovir	Famvir	$$$
fluconazole	Diflucan	$
ivermectin	Stromectol	$
lindane 1% shampoo	Kwell	$
permethrin 5% cream	Elimite	$$
permethrin 1% cream rinse	Nix	$$
pyrethrins with piperonyl butoxide	RID, A-200	$
valacyclovir	Valtrex	$$$$

References

Centers for Disease Control and Prevention. Sexually transmitted disease treatment guidelines. *MMWR* 2002;51(RR06;1).

Holmes KK, Sparling PF, Mardh P-A, et al., eds. *Sexually Transmitted Diseases.* 3rd ed. New York, New York: McGraw Hill; 1999.

Hynes NA. *Johns Hopkins POC-IT Antibiotic (ABX) Guide.* https://www.hopkins-abxguide.org/. Last updated 2003 with planned ongoing updates.

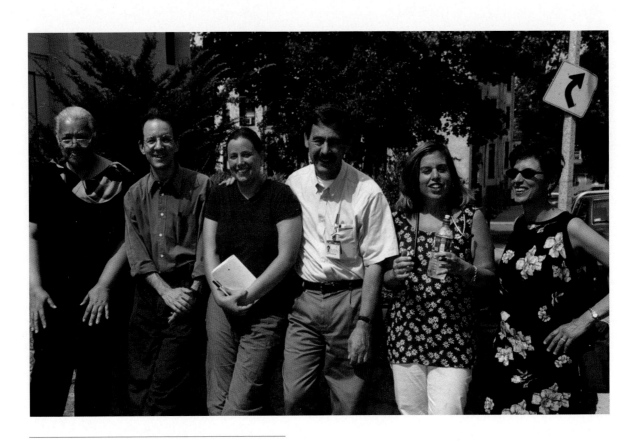

Ellen Dailey (left), Chair of the Consumer Advisory Board
and Vice Chair of the BHCHP Board of Directors, relaxes
after a meeting at McInnis House with Stefan Kertesz MD,
Carol Waldmann MD, Phil Pulaski MD, Denise Petrella NP,
and Claire Carlo MD.
Photo by James O'Connell MD

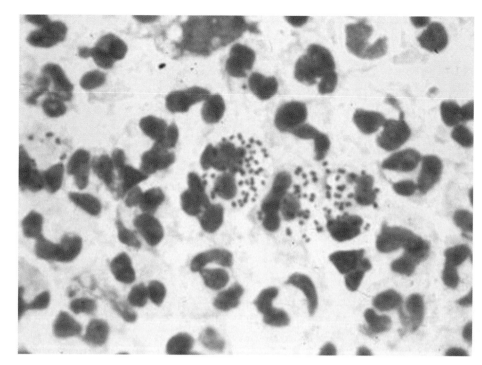

Sexually Transmitted Diseases, Part II: "Drips" & Discharges

Noreen A. Hynes, MD, MPH

exually transmitted diseases (STDs) associated with discharges or "drips" are usually caused by one of three types of pathogens - bacteria, viruses, or parasites. One non-STD fungal infection, candidiasis, is seen frequently among active persons and is considered in this group. Although inflammatory STDs are classically associated with discharges, these infections cause a spectrum of disease from asymptomatic infection to an array of often overlapping syndromes that make clinical diagnosis alone inadequate for predicting the cause of the infection. Untreated or inadequately treated STDs associated with discharges can have long-term adverse consequences, particularly for women and their fetuses and newborn infants. These inflammatory STDs enhance the acquisition and transmission of human immunodeficiency virus (HIV). Early detection, treatment, partner notification services, and education targeting behavior modification are critical components of interrupting the transmission of STDs. Prevention and control elements must be rigorously and creatively pursued among certain at-risk groups, including guests in homeless shelters, to interrupt the ever-expanding "hidden epidemic" of STDs.

Gonococcal Urethritis. Gram stain of the urethral discharge in this man shows many polymorphonuclear leukocytes with intracellular Gram negative diplococci. Photo courtesy of the CDC

General Approach to Patients at Risk for STDs

Every sexually active patient not in a long-term, mutually monogamous relationship who is seen in the clinic should be considered at risk for newly incident STDs, both asymptomatic and symptomatic. Whenever possible, a routine STD screening history and physical examination should be obtained on all at-risk patients, regardless of the presenting complaint. Contacts of patients treated for bacterial STDs or trichomoniasis should be

treated and offered screening for HIV infection, if indicated. Contacts of persons with viral STDs should be tested for the presence of infection and offered screening for HIV, if indicated. Sexually active persons, with or without symptoms, should undergo diagnostic testing for treatable STDs and be offered HIV counseling and testing. Those with symptoms of STDs should have further evaluations based upon the clinical syndrome noted at presentation. Single dose, directly-observed therapy should

Table 1: Vaginal Discharge and Vaginitis Features

Feature	Normal Female Vaginal Fluid	Bacterial vaginosis	Trichomoniasis	Candidia vulvovagintitis
Discharge Characteristics • Amount • Consistency • Color	Usually scant Flocculant, non-homogeneous White or clear	Moderate to heavy Homogeneous; coats vaginal walls Grey or white	Heavy Homogeneous; often frothy Yellow, green, white	Moderate to heavy "Cheesy", clumpy, adherant plaques on erythmatous base White
Classic symptoms	None	Increased discharge Odor often	Increased discharge Odor often External dysuria Pruritis	Increased discharge No odor Severe vulvar pruritis
Usual secretion pH	< 4.5	≥ 4.5	≥ 5.0	<4.5
Microscopic exam of secretions	Saline prep Epithelial cells: normal Organisms: Lactobacilli predominate	Saline prep Epithelial cells: Clue cells Organisms: No/few lactobacilli	Saline prep Organism: Motile trichomonads	10% KOH prep Epithelial cells: Lysed by KOH Organism: budding yeast/ pseudohyphae
"Whiff" test outcome	No odor	Fishy smell	Fishy smell at times	No odor

be used for treatment when an approved regimen exists.

Most of the STD clinical syndromes fall into two general categories: "sores" and "drips/discharges". The approach to genital "sores" was discussed in the previous chapter. This chapter will address STDs associated with discharges or "drips".

Inflammatory STDs Presenting as Discharges

Inflammatory STDs can cause diffuse manifestations, many of which are gender-specific rather than pathogen-specific. Therefore, the associated syndromes will be grouped by gender for discussion of the clinical presentations, prevalence, complications, diagnosis, and treatment, and follow-up. Prevention and control strategies will be discussed together after the clinical section of the chapter. The clinical syndromes for discussion include:

Acute Inflammatory STDs in Women
- lower genital tract inflammatory STDs in women (vaginitis, mucopurulent cervicitis)
- upper genital tract inflammatory STDs in women (pelvic inflammatory disease or PID)

Acute Inflammatory STDs in Men
- urethritis
- acute epididymitis

I. Acute Inflammatory STDs in Women:

A. Lower Genital Tract STDs

Vaginal discharge caused by a lower genital tract STD may be due to inflammation or infection of the vagina or the cervix, with vaginitis predominating. The presence of vaginal discharge should lead the practitioner to question the patient further about related signs and symptoms and should be followed by a directed physical examination that should include, at a minimum, inspection of the external genitalia and a bimanual examination. The pathogens associated with vaginal discharge include:
- *Neisseria gonorrhoeae,* the causative agent of gonorrhea;
- *Chlamydia trachomatis,* the causative agent of Chlamydia;
- *Trichomonas vaginalis,* the causative agent of trichomoniasis;
- bacterial vaginosis, a disruption of the

vaginal floral ecology;
- *Candida albicans,* the causative agent of vulvovaginal candidiasis;
- herpes simplex virus.

Vaginitis

Causes of vaginitis

Three common causes of inflammatory vaginitis are trichomoniasis, bacterial vaginosis, and candidiasis. Woman commonly present with a complaint of vaginal discharge or vulvar itching and irritation and may complain of the presence of a vaginal odor. Bacterial vaginosis (BV) is caused by a disruption of the normal acid-rich vaginal flora. BV has only been shown to be an STD in women who have sex with women. Otherwise, it is considered a high-risk marker for the presence of an STD.

Signs and symptoms

A detailed history to obtain a good description of the vaginal discharge in terms of amount, odor, and the presence or absence of pruritis is essential to the diagnosis of vaginitis. An examination of the external genitalia, vagina and cervix is very important:

- vulvovaginal candidiasis (VVC) is most likely to be associated with vulvar pruritis, erythema, and a "cheesy" discharge;
- trichomoniasis usually has vulvar pruritis and a frothy green-yellow discharge that is malodorous;
- BV often has a watery malodorous discharge.

Co-infection is common and signs and symptoms often overlap. Thus a laboratory diagnostic evaluation is necessary.

Diagnosis

Evaluation of a shelter guest with suspected vaginitis must rely on a good history, a physical examination, and the examination of the discharge. The amount, consistency, and location of the discharge should be noted. Two samples of the discharge should be collected from the vaginal wall with a swab. The specimen should not be contaminated with cervical mucous. The color of the discharge on the swabs should be noted in comparison to a fresh white cotton swab. Using pH indicator paper, roll the first swab directly onto the paper and note the pH of the secretions (normal vaginal fluid has a pH of 4.0 to 4.5). Mix the content of the second swab separately into a drop of saline on one slide and a drop of 10% potassium hydroxide (KOH) on

a second slide. Immediately smell the KOH slide to determine if there is a "fishy" odor. Then place cover slips on both the saline and KOH slides for microscopic examination.

Bacterial vaginosis:
- pH of vaginal fluid >4.5;
- fishy odor on KOH "whiff" test;
- "clue" cells on microscopic examination of the saline slide;

Trichomoniasis:
- pH of vaginal fluid >4.5;
- fishy odor on KOH "whiff" test (common);
- motile trichomonad parasites on microscopic examination of the saline slide.

Vulvovaginal candidiasis:
- pH of < 4.5;
- no fishy odor on KOH "whiff" test;
- yeast, budding yeast, and pseudohyphae on microscopic examination of the KOH slide.

Prevalence

- Bacterial vaginosis. BV is the most prevalent cause of vaginal symptoms among women of childbearing age. Data on the prevlance of BV varies widely because differing diagnostic criteria have been used and differences in the population sampled. In women attending STD clinics the prevalence is between 25 and 40 percent. Prevalence is essentially zero for women who are not sexually active.
- Trichomoniasis. Prevalence rates of trichomoniasis in women range from 5 to 10% in the general population to 50 to 60% in female prison inmates and commercial sex workers. In women who report vaginal complaints, the prevalence of trichomoniasis is 20 and 50%.
- Vulvovaginal candidiasis. VVC affects 70 to 75% of women at least once during their lives, of whom 40 to 50% will have at least one recurrence. Prevalence data are minimal at best, but some estimates suggest a prevalence of up to 200 per 100,000 women per year. Prevalence is highest among women who are pregnant, HIV-infected, or have diabetes mellitus.

Complications

- Bacterial vaginosis. BV during pregnancy is associated with adverse pregnancy out-

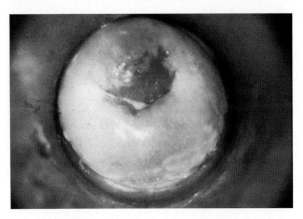

cator (5 gm) intravaginally at bedtime for 7 days.

- Trichomoniasis. The treatment is metronidazole 2 grams orally in a single dose.
- Vulvovaginal candidiasis. When possible, shelter guests should receive a single 150 mg oral tablet of fluconazole. Alternatively, there are 5 over-the-counter intravaginal preparations and 8 prescription formulations that can be used for varying numbers of days.

comes, including premature rupture of the membranes, premature labor, premature birth, and post-partum endometritis. Newer data strongly suggest that untreated symptomatic BV is also a risk factor for pelvic inflammatory disease (PID).

- Trichomoniasis. Potential complications of untreated trichomoniasis infection include pelvic inflammatory disease (PID) and rarely perinephric abscess or meningitis.
- Vulvovaginal candidiasis. Untreated, symptomatic VVC may result in secondary bacterial infection of excoriated areas.

Treatment

Any patient found to have motile trichomonads should be treated, whether or not associated with symptoms. BV and VVC should only be treated in symptomatic women with the exception of asymptomatic pregnant women with BV and a history of a previous preterm delivery.

- Bacterial vaginosis. The Centers for Disease Control and Prevention (CDC) provides general recommended and alternative regimens for the treatment of STDs. In the shelter setting, many experts prefer to designate single dose, directly observed therapy regimens as the recommended approach for treatment of STDs where such an approved treatment exists. This regimen uses metronidazole 2 grams orally as a single dose. This dose will concomitantly treat trichomoniasis, if present. Other CDC recommended regimens include:
1) metronidazole 500 mg orally twice a day for 7 days; or
2) metronidazole gel 0.75%, one full applicator (5 gm) intravaginally, once a day for 5 days; or
3) clindamycin cream 2%, one full appli-

Mucopurulent Cervicitis (MPC)
Causes of mucopurulent cervicitis

Vaginal discharge due to mucopurulent cervicitis can be associated with STDs as well as other non-infectious conditions. Sexually-transmitted causes of MPC include *C. trachomatis, N. gonorrhoeae,* and herpes simplex virus (HSV). Additionally, *T. vaginalis* and HSV can infect the cervix without producing cervical and vaginal discharge. However, evidence of inflammation is present when examining a gram stain of cervical secretions in the absence of visible mucopus.

Signs and symptoms

Women with MPC often complain of the recent onset of increasing amounts of yellow to green vaginal discharge. On speculum examination, mucopus is usually visible in the cervical os. Small amounts of mucopus may not be visible to the naked eye, but the tip of a cotton swab of sample secretions from the cervical os will be distinctly yellow when compared to the tip of a fresh swab (positive swab test). In the absence of mucopus, edema or easy bleeding of the region of cervical ectopy suggests cervicitis and some experts consider these to be the equivalent of MPC. Importantly, cervical infection with *N. gonorrheoae, C. trachomatis,* or HSV may be present without any clinical findings in more than 50% of cases. The importance of a laboratory diagnosis cannot be overemphasized due to the potential for severe adverse outcomes in women with untreated cervical infections.

Diagnosis

A sample of cervical secretions should be collected and tested for *N. gonorrhoeae, C. trachomatis,* and HSV. A Gram stain of cervical secretions is not a definitive diagnostic tool in women. Although the identification of Gram negative diplococci requires treatment for presumed gonorrhea, other non-gonococcal organisms can have this appearance in women. Additionally, Gram stain is negative in over 50% of infected women. Rectal cultures should also be collected because up to 50% of women with cervical gonococcal infection will have rectal colonization without a history of anal receptive intercourse. This may be the only site of infection in up to 10% of women. A throat culture for gonorrhea should also be collected, if history suggests possible exposure. This is occasionally the only site of infection and appears to be associated with a higher incidence of disseminated infection. Vaginal secretions should be collected and examined for evidence of vaginitis as previously described. Definitive diagnostic tests are key because as many as 40% of MPC cases are not associated with an isolated pathogen.

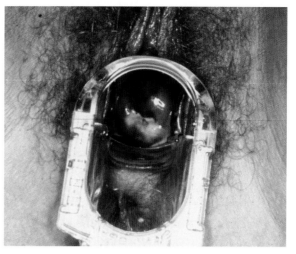

Gonorrhea of the Cervix. Gonorrhea often involves the cervix in women and may be asymptomatic. Pelvic inflammatory disease can be a complication. Photo by Nicholas Fiumara MD

Prevalence

Data on the prevalence of MPC is scant at best. Some estimates have indicated that 18% of women visiting STD clinics for the first time will have evidence of MPC on examination. The prevalence of the individual STD pathogens associated with MPC vary greatly and depend upon the population studied.

- Gonorrhea prevalence, although decreasing in recent years, has shown upward trends in some risk groups and some areas of the country. Asymptomatic, untreated infection among females is a critical factor in the persistence of this infection in a community.
- Chlamydia is the most common reported bacterial STD worldwide. Prevalence figures for all clinical forms of Chlamydia cervical infection range from 3 to 5% in asymptomatic sexually active women to 20% in women presenting to STD clinics.
- HSV can affect the cervix alone without involving the external genitalia. The prevalence of this site of infection is unknown, whether alone or in combination with external genitalia infection. HSV manifesting as MPC may be the result of a primary infection or reactivation of an existing infection. Among women with primary genital HSV infection, up to 90% may have HSV cervicitis. The prevalence of cervicitis with recurrent HSV is unknown.

Complications

The complications associated with MPC are related to the infecting pathogens.

- Gonorrhea can cause local and systemic complications, including pelvic inflammatory disease, disseminated gonococcal infection, endocarditis, and meningitis. Pregnant women can pass the infection to the newborn during parturition leading to ocular, respiratory, or disseminated infection.
- Chlamydia can cause both local and systemic complications, including pelvic inflammatory disease, perihepatitis, and (rarely) endocarditis. In immunocompromised persons, it can cause bronchitis and pneumonitis.
- HSV manifesting as MPC may be the result of a primary infection or reactivation of an existing infection. It is unknown whether solitary HSV infection of the cervix is associated with the same spectrum of complications as genital herpes, but it is assumed to be similar (See previous chapter).

Treatment

The results of sensitive tests for gonorrhea, Chlamydia, and HSV should be used to guide treatment for MPC unless there is a high likelihood that the woman has either a gonorrhea or Chlamydia infection. In such cases, empiric treatment should be considered if the prevalence of either or both of these infections is known to be high among the shelter guest population in your community. It is important to remember that MPC can persist despite repeated courses of antibiotics, and these women only rarely have gonorrhea or Chlamydia infection.

- Empiric MPC therapy. See the treatment for gonorrhea below.
- Chlamydia. Azithromycin 1 gram orally as

a single dose, directly observed therapy is the preferred form of treatment in shelter guests. This treatment appears to be safe and effective in pregnant women.

- Gonorrhea. Treatment depends on the amount of fluroquinolone-resistant *N. gonorrhoeae* in the shelter population. Shelters located in Hawaii and California have a high prevalence and fluroquinolones should not be used for treatment. Cephalosporin-resistant gonorrhea is also increasing, and practitioners should check with local or state health departments for information regarding resistance in your area. Cefixime, an oral cephalosporin used for single dose therapy, is no longer available. If Chlamydial infection has not been ruled out at the time of treatment for gonorrhea, concurrent treatment is the standard of care because Chlamydia accompanies 10 to 30% of gonococcal infections, and the cost of treatment is less than the cost of testing. Any of the following single dose, directly-observed treatments are effective in the treatment of cervical, rectal, or oropharyngeal gonococcal infection:
  - ciprofloxacin 500 mg orally in a single dose, or;
  - ofloxacin 400 mg orally in a single dose, or;
  - levofloxacin 250 mg orally in a single dose, or;
  - ceftriaxone 125 mg IM in a single dose. This treatment is suitable for pregnant women.
  - In penicillin-allergic pregnant women, spectinomycin 2 gm IM as a single dose can be given. Follow-up cultures are required if spectinomycin is used.

  If Chlamydia has not been ruled out, then a single oral dose of azithromycin 1 gram should be given at the time of treatment for gonorrhea.

B. Upper Genital Tract Infection (Pelvic Inflammatory Disease or PID)

Causes of Pelvic Inflammatory Disease

Approximately two-thirds of all PID cases are due to STDs, usually *C. trachomatis* or *N. gonorrhoeae*. The remaining cases of PID are due primarily to anaerobic Gram-positive cocci and *Escherichia coli*. Several other organisms appear to be associated with a small number of cases. Many cases of PID appear to be polymicrobial. All the organisms are believed to cause PID following ascension of the organisms to the upper genital tract via the endometrium. PID includes infection involving any of the structures of the upper genital tract, including the endometrium (endometritis), fallopian tubes (salpingitis), or pelvic peritoneum (peritonitis). Tubo-ovarian abscess is also included within the PID spectrum.

Signs, Symptoms, and Diagnosis

Acute PID has a wide spectrum of clinical presentations and is difficult to diagnose. Many asymptomatic or minimally symptomatic cases are known to carry a high burden of long-term adverse outcomes, including infertility, ectopic pregnancy, and chronic pelvic pain. Definitive diagnosis of PID is dependent upon the upper genital tract structure involved, requires a technically-demanding procedure (such as laparoscopy), and is expensive. As a result, the diagnosis and empiric treatment of PID are usually based upon clinical findings alone.

Empiric treatment for PID should be initiated in any sexually active woman at risk for STDs if either of the following criteria is present:
- uterine or adnexal tenderness;
- cervical motion tenderness.

Other symptoms that may suggest the presence of PID include:
- dysuria;
- monometrorrhagia;
- dyspareunia;
- new onset of pain with menses.

Additional physical findings that help to support the diagnosis of PID include the following:
- oral temperature >38.3°C (>101°F);
- abnormal cervical or vaginal mucopurulent discharge (MPC is common);
- laboratory documentation of *C. trachomatis* or *N. gonorrhoeae* cervical infection;
- elevated C-reactive protein;
- elevated erythrocyte sedimentation rate.

Prevalence

The prevalence of PID is unknown. However, approximately 60% of PID cases are asymptomatic, 36% associated with mild to moderate symptoms, and 4% classified as severe infection. Among women infected with *N. gonorrhoeae*, approximately 10 to 20% have PID. *C. trachomatis* is thought to be associated with the greatest number of "silent" PID cases, with up to 80% of Chlamydia cervical infections in women thought to be asymptomatic.

Treatment and Follow-up

The empirical regimens recommended for PID aim to cover the broad-spectrum of likely pathogens. Antibiotics are aimed at treating gonorrhea, Chlamydia, anaerobes, Gram negative facultative bacteria, and Streptococcus. For milder cases, oral therapy or mixed parenteral and oral therapy can be given. Ongoing parenteral therapy should be provided in the inpatient setting. All patients with PID should demonstrate clinical improvement within 72 hours of treatment initiation. Patients who do not improve should be reevaluated in the inpatient setting. Those failing inpatient therapy should be further evaluated for the need for surgical intervention. The criteria for hospitalization of women with suspected PID include:

- a surgical emergency, such as appendicitis, can not be ruled out;
- pregnancy (PID can occur in the first trimester);
- the presence of a tubo-ovarian abscess;
- a high fever, nausea and vomiting, or severe illness;
- inability to follow or tolerate an outpatient oral regimen; and
- failure to respond clinically within 48 to 72 hours to oral therapy.

The treatment of PID is divided into outpatient and inpatient regimens. Outpatient treatment, which should not be used in pregnant women, consists of either an oral or a mixed oral and parenteral regimen. The oral regimen is as follows:

- ofloxacin 400 mg twice a day for 14 days; or
- levofloxacin 500 mg once a day for 14 days;
- metronidazole 500 mg twice a day for 14 days is optional as a second drug. Some experts recommend that this be included in the oral regimen for vulnerable populations, including those represented among shelter guests.

The mixed oral and parenteral regimen is:

- ceftriaxone 250 mg IM as a single dose plus doxycycline 100 mg orally twice a day for 14 days;
- metronidazole 500 mg orally twice a day for 14 days is optional as a second drug, with the same recommendations as above.

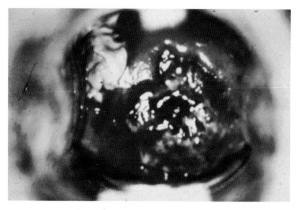

Two basic inpatient treatment regimens are utilized. One utilizes an IV cephalosporin with oral or IV doxycycline, while another uses IV clindamycin together with gentamicin.

II. Acute Inflammatory STDs in Men

Urethritis
Causes of Urethritis

A "drip" or urethral discharge is the most frequent STD syndrome seen in men. Drips are usually classified as gonococcal (GCU) or non-gonococcal urethritis (NGU). The primary causes of NGU include *C. trachomatis, Ureaplasma urealyticum, Mycoplasma genitalium, Trichomonas vaginalis,* and HSV.

Signs and symptoms of urethritis

Most men with GCU and NGU have dysuria or genital itching in conjunction with urethral discharge. Approximately 75% of men with GCU have purulent discharge, whereas NGU is more likely to manifest with mucoid or clear discharge. Notably, 5 to 15% of men with gonorrhea and up to 70% of men with Chlamydia infection may be asymptomatic.

Diagnosis

The diagnosis of urethritis in men begins with a history and directed physical examination, followed by a microscopic examination of the urethral discharge by Gram staining. The finding of >5 polymorphonuclear leukocytes (PMNs) per high power oil-immersion field (1000X) confirms the presence of urethritis. The presence of intracellular gram negative diplococci is considered confirmatory for *N. gonorrhea* infection in men (not in women), and no further confirmatory testing for this pathogen is needed. Men who have recently engaged in anal receptive intercourse should have a rectal swab collected for culture. In exposed persons, a throat culture should also be collected. Testing for *C. trachomatis* is strongly recommended for all men with urethritis. Diagnostic testing for other pathogens should only be undertaken in those patients who have recurrent or persistent urethritis following treatment.

Prevalence

The prevalence of urethritis in men is unknown.

- GCU. Because the majority of men with GCU have symptoms and the incubation period is short, the incidence provides an approximation for this reportable disease. The highest prevalence is among men age 15 to 29 years and is highest in the summer months. Urban and rural low socioeconomic groups have a higher incidence than other groups. Rates of infection are increasing in men who have sex with men.
- Chlamydia urethritis. Routine testing of men for this reportable STD is much less frequent than routine testing in women and prevalence estimates are variable. It is estimated that 3 to 5% of all men with symptomatic urethritis are infected with Chlamydia. Among STD clinic attendees, Chlamydia urethritis prevalence may be as high as 20%, whereas pharyngeal infection prevalence may be between 3 and 6%.

Complications

- GCU. Complications of GCU include epididymitis, seminal vesiculitis, acute prostatitis, disseminated gonoccocal infection, and very rarely endocarditis and meningitis.
- Chlamydia urethritis. Complications of Chlamydia urethritis in men include epididymitis, Reiter's syndrome (urethritis, conjunctivitis, arthritis, and characterisitc mucocutaneous lesions), and tenosynovitis.

Treatment

The treatment of either GCU or NGU is the same as for cervicitis and MPC in women (see above).

Epididymitis
Causes of Epididymitis

Like PID, epididymitis can be caused by STDs (two-thirds of cases) and by non-sexually transmitted

pathogens. Men under the age of 35 years are more likely to have STD-associated epididymitis. Gonorrhea and Chlamydia account for essentially all of the STD-associated disease. *E. coli* accounts for most of the non-sexually transmitted infection and a small portion of the STD-associated infection in men who engage in insertive anal intercourse.

Signs and Symptoms

The predominant presenting features in epididymitis are unilateral scrotal pain and swelling, usually with associated discharge. However, because this presentation is also consistent with a surgical emergency - testicular torsion - immediate referral for a radionuclide or Doppler flow study is needed if the patient has the following constellation: 1) sudden onset, 2) excruciating pain, 3) age < 20 years, and 4) testicular elevation. If after this evaluation testicular torsion is not strongly suspected, epididymitis should be considered.

Diagnosis

The evaluation of a man with suspected epididymitis includes: 1) a Gram stain of urethral discharge for evidence of urethritis (either NGU or GCU); 2) culture or nucleic acid appllification test of the discharge for *C. trachomatis* and *N. gonorrhoeae*, and; 3) examination of the first voided uncentrifuged urine for white cells if the Gram stain of the discharge is negative.

Prevalence

No reliable data are available regarding the prevalence of epididymitis.

Complications

The most serious complications seen with epididymitis are infarction of the testicle and testicular abscess. Infertility is a poorly documented long-term adverse outcome.

Treatment

Empiric treatment is always indicated prior to culture results. Therapy for epididymitis includes both antimicrobials and adjunctive therapy including bed rest, scrotal elevation, and analgesia until fever and local inflammation have decreased. All patients should be re-evaluated within 72 hours of commencing treatment to assess response to therapy. Failure to respond requires a comprehensive re-evaluation including consideration of alternative diagnoses.

Treatment of epididymitis due to gonococcal or

Chlamydia infections is as follows:

- ceftriaxone 250 mg IM in a single dose; and
- doxycycline 100 mg orally twice a day for 14 days.

Treatment of epididymitis likely due to enteric organisms or in persons allergic or intolerant of the regimen above include the following:

- ofloxacin 300 mg orally twice a day for 10 days; or
- levofloxacin 500 mg orally once daily for 10 days.

Prevention and Control of Acute Inflammatory STDs

All health care providers have critical roles in the prevention and control of STDs. Among the acute inflammatory STDs, gonorrhea and Chlamydia are reportable diseases throughout the USA. Diagnosed cases should be reported to the local or state health department. STD and HIV reports are kept strictly confidential by these authorities.

Prevention messages that providers offer to shelter guests should be tailored to each patient's risk profile. Male latex condoms are highly effective in preventing the transmission of Chlamydia, gonorrhea, trichomoniasis, and sexually transmitted HIV. Condoms are only somewhat effective in preventing HSV transmission. Laboratory studies suggest that the female condom is an effective barrier to HIV. Nonoxynol-9 vaginal spermicides should be avoided because they can induce local inflammation in some women which may increase the risk for transmission and acquisition of HIV.

Many individuals exposed to STDs benefit from partner notification services. Providers need to encourage shelter guests diagnosed with STDs to urge their partners to seek evaluation for detection of a possible HIV.

Women bear the disproportionate burden of the long-term adverse consequences of STDs as do their fetuses and newborn infants. All pregnant shelter guests should be offered HIV counseling and testing in addition to testing for the inflammatory STDs, syphilis, and hepatitis B. A Papinicolaou smear should also be obtained. All sexually active female shelter guests who are not in a long-term, mutually monogamous relationship should be routinely offered screening and testing for STDs every 6 months. Women known to be commercial sex workers or to exchange sex for drugs, money, or life essentials should be offered STD screening and treatment whenever they present for primary care services.

Summary

STDs associated with discharges or "drips" may be present when a shelter guest comes to the clinic for other health-related problems. A sexual history and focused physical examination should be included for all sexually active patients to provide treatment and interrupt further transmission when possible. Key concepts to keep in mind when caring for shelter guests with STDs include:

- single dose, directly observed therapy is the preferred form of therapy when such a regimen is proven to be efficacious;
- persons with inflammatory STDs are at increased risk for HIV acquisition and transmission (if HIV infected);
- the presence of one STD increases the risk for a second STD and also is a marker for possible exposure to HIV. Therefore, all patients diagnosed with an STD should receive HIV counseling and testing, as indicated;
- women and their unborn children bear the greatest burden of adverse outcomes from STDs; women are more likely to have asymptomatic STDs than men;
- Chlamydia and gonorrhea are reportable diseases and must be reported to the local or state health department. ▰

STDs Part II: "Drips" & Discharges Medication List

Generic	Brand	Cost
metronidazole	Flagyl	$
metronidazole gel 0.75%	MetroGel-Vaginal	$$$
clindamycin cream 2%	Cleocin	$$
fluconazole	Diflucan	$
azithromycin	Zithromax	$$
ciprofloxacin	Cipro, Cipro XR	$$$
ofloxacin	Floxin	$$$$
levofloxacin	Levaquin	$$$
ceftriaxone	Rocephin	$$$$$
doxycycline	Adoxa, Doryx, Monodox, Vibramycin, Vibra-Tabs	$
cefotetan	Cefotan	$$$$$
cefoxitin	Mefoxin	$$$$$
clindamycin	Cleocin	$$
gentamicin	Garamycin	$$

References

Centers for Disease Control and Prevention. Sexually transmitted disease treatment guidelines. *MMWR* 2002;51(RR06;1).

Holmes KK, Sparling PF, Mardh P-A, et al., eds. *Sexually Transmitted Diseases.* 3rd ed. New York, New York: McGraw Hill; 1999.

Hynes NA. *Johns Hopkins POC-IT Antibiotic (ABX) Guide.* https://www.hopkins-abxguide.org/ Last updated 2003 with planned ongoing updates.

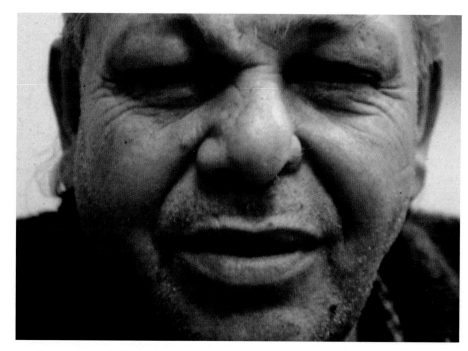

Sinusitis

Kathleen Fitch, MSN, APRN,BC, FNP
Gennine Zinner, RNC, ANP

S inusitis is ubiquitous among humans and one of the most common reasons health care office visits in the USA. In 1991 sinusitis accounted for more than 25 million visits to a primary care clinic and was the fifth most common diagnosis for which an antibiotic was prescribed. Expenditures for the treatment of sinusitis in the USA in 1996 were estimated at $5.8 billion, with 30% of this amount used for pediatric sinusitis.

Sinusitis develops from an interaction of environmental and host factors. The most common cause in all age groups is a viral upper respiratory infection (URI) that results in secondary bacterial overgrowth. Other causes of sinusitis include: allergic; fungal; mucosal or architectural abnormality; periodontal disease; immunologic factors; and environmental exposure to pollutants such as tobacco smoke. Clinicians must differentiate between acute viral sinusitis (common with colds and the flu) and bacterial sinusitis in order to prevent the over-prescription of antibiotics. (See chapter on The Proper Use of Antibiotics).

Prevalence and Distribution

Approximately one billion acute viral respiratory illnesses occur annually in the USA, with as many as 90% resulting in viral sinusitis. Fewer than 2% of viral URIs are complicated by secondary bacterial sinusitis. Children under 15 years of age and adults between 25 and 64 years of age are most frequently affected.

The most common cause of bacterial sinusitis is a viral URI. Seasonal trends in the incidence of bacterial sinusitis correlate with those of the common cold. However, bacterial sinusitis can occur throughout the year and is associated with allergy, swimming, and nasal obstruction due to polyps, foreign bodies, and tumors. The most common bacteria associated with acute sinusitis in adults include: *Streptococcus pneumoniae* (34%); *Haemophilus influenzae* (35%); and *Moraxella catarrhalis* (2%). In children, *M. catarrhalis* and *H. influenzae* are the most common pathogens isolated from acute sinusitis.

Viral sinusitis follows a well-established seasonal pattern, with annual epidemics in the fall, winter, and spring. Periods of inactivity are common during the summer months. Different virus families tend to have specific periods of high prevalence; rhinovirus is more common in early fall and late spring, whereas coronavirus, respiratory syncytial virus, and influenza virus are more common in winter and early spring.

Mode of Transmission

Sinusitis generally results from the following sequence of events. The virus is transmitted from

This man with a history of multiple allergies and a deviated septum had recurrent episodes of allergic sinusitis. Photo by James O'Connell MD

Figure 1

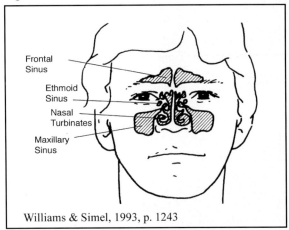

Frontal
Sinus

Ethmoid
Sinus

Nasal
Turbinates

Maxillary
Sinus

Williams & Simel, 1993, p. 1243

infected to susceptible persons, usually through coughing or sneezing, deposited into the nose, and transported to the posterior nasopharynx. Several inflammatory pathways are stimulated and result in engorgement of the nasal turbinates along with intercellular leakage of plasma into the nose and sinuses and discharge from seromucous glands and goblet cells.

The specific factors that determine whether bacterial invasion of the sinus will occur during a viral sinusitis are unknown. However, the nasal passages and nasopharynx are colonized with the same bacteria that commonly cause sinusitis and most likely serve as a reservoir for infection. Sneezing, coughing, and blowing the nose increase pressure differentials and may force bacteria-containing secretions to be deposited in the sinuses. Once deposited into the cavity of a swollen and obstructed sinus, the conditions are favorable for growth of the bacteria.

Prevention

Sinusitis may be prevented in several ways:

- prevention of the common cold by hand washing and covering the mouth when sneezing or coughing;
- protection against influenza by encouraging annual flu vaccines;
- use of prophylactic amantadine or rimandatine during periods of epidemic influenza;
- antihistamines can reduce swelling and prevent the entrance of both viruses and bacteria into the sinus cavities;
- fluids and the use of a humidifier or steam keep the mucous in the nasal passages from becoming thickened;
- cigarette smoke and adverse environmental

pollutants should be avoided whenever possible (but very difficult for persons living in shelters and on the streets); and

- educate individuals about viral URIs and how to manage initial symptoms, as well as when to seek evaluation from a doctor or health care provider.

Symptoms

Acute sinusitis is heralded by: nasal congestion; a purulent nasal discharge; a heightened sense of smell (hyposmia); facial pain that is often unilateral; pain in the upper teeth; eye pain; headache, often increasing in intensity when bending over; and a cough that is often worse at night. Fever, malaise, halitosis (bad breath), and a sore throat due to post-nasal drip can also occur. Acute sinusitis is usually preceded by a URI that worsens or does not resolve after 8-10 days. Most common colds and viral URIs resolve or are much improved by the end of one week.

Chronic sinusitis is more difficult to diagnose than acute sinusitis, and has a more subtle and indolent course. The symptoms are the same as those noted above but usually milder and persist for more than three months. This chronic infection is more common among immunocompromised persons, atopic individuals with allergies, and those with severe asthma. Different pathogens are involved in chronic sinusitis, requiring more broad-spectrum antibiotics and longer courses of treatment than required for acute sinusitis.

Diagnosis

Despite advances in technology, the diagnosis of sinusitis remains a challenge. The clinical diagnosis of acute bacterial sinusitis should be reserved for patients with symptoms lasting seven days or more and who have maxillary pain with tenderness in the face or upper teeth accompanied by purulent nasal secretions. Clinicians should be aware that most cases of acute sinusitis are viral and resolve without antibiotics. Bacterial sinusitis tends to be over-diagnosed and antibiotics prescribed too frequently. Because the symptoms are similar for acute viral and bacterial sinusitis, we recommend that antibiotics be held until symptoms have been present for at least seven days and reserved for those patients with the maxillary pain and purulent discharge noted above. Unfortunately, even the duration of symptoms is not always a reliable predictor of bacterial sinusitis, as many viral syndromes can last longer than a week. When symptoms have lasted longer than a week,

Table 1: Bacterial Etiology of Sinusitis

Organism	Percent of Adult Cases by Sinus Aspirate	
	Acute	Chronic
Streptococcus pneumoniae	40	7
Haemophilus influenzae	30	10
Moraxella catarrhalis	7	-
Anaerobic bacteria	8	50-100
Staphylococcus aureus	3	17
Streptococcus pyogenes	3	-
Streptococcus viridans	3	15
Gram-negative bacteria (including enteric gram-negative bacilli)	-	5

Table 2: Viral Etiology of Sinusitis

All viruses which cause upper respiratory tract infections may act as initiating triggers for sinusitis
Relatively mild tissue damage may result in a reduction of local mucosal immunity rendering the individual susceptible to secondary bacterial infection
The majority of bacterial sinusitis is probably initiated by a preceding viral infection

Adapted from Saccho, H. and Schoub, B., Lessons in Infectious Diseases, 4(12).

clinicians should investigate for allergic and fungal as well as bacterial causes of sinusitis.

The physical exam should include a fairly comprehensive head and neck exam together with examination of the lungs and cervical lymph nodes. Anterior rhinoscopy should be performed to check the appearance of inferior turbinates and nasal secretions, as well as for the presence of nasal polyps. Transillumination as a diagnostic tool is the subject of considerable controversy and is often limited by the skills and experience of the examiner. Cultures of nasal secretions are not generally useful, limited by lack of sensitivity for detecting sinusitis. Sinus puncture and aspiration of purulent secretions is the gold standard but not used much due to invasiveness and pain. This test is reserved for complicated cases and generally not performed in a primary care setting.

A CT scan is an excellent tool for diagnosis and has replaced sinus x-rays as the diagnostic image of choice for sinusitis. CT scans are not recommended for routine use, due to a lack of specificity and frequent abnormal findings in viral sinusitis. Clinicians may choose to reserve radiography with CT scans for antibiotic treatment failures.

Laboratory tests are not specific and thus not helpful in the diagnosis of bacterial sinusitis. Labo-

ratory investigation may be necessary in individuals with chronic or recurrent sinusitis in order to elucidate the underlying cause. Such testing may include HIV or other immunodeficiency testing, allergy testing, and even sweat chloride testing for cystic fibrosis (for children with recurrent symptoms).

Treatment

Most cases of sinusitis are viral and will generally resolve without antibiotic treatment. Once a bacterial etiology has been determined, the goal of treatment is twofold: relieve symptoms and cure the infection.

Symptomatic relief can be achieved with saline nasal spray, warm compresses, steam humidification, cough suppressants, and pain relievers. Nasal decongestants are useful but cause rebound congestion after three to five days; oral decongestants may be preferable. Nasal steroid sprays such as fluticasone (Flonase™) may help relieve swelling, especially in patients with allergic symptoms and polyps. However, both oral and topical steroids should not be used in non-allergic acute sinusitis but reserved for chronic cases and patients with a history of atopy. Antihistamines may also provide relief for rhinitis and various allergic symptoms.

Antibiotics are usually reserved for moderate to

severe cases. The emergence of drug-resistant strains of bacteria has created controversy in the treatment of acute bacterial sinusitis. Most consensus guideline committees still recommend the less expensive and narrow spectrum antibiotics as first-line therapy: amoxicillin (Amoxil™); doxycycline (Vibramycin™); and trimethoprim-sulfamethoxazole (Bactrim™, Septra™). The reasons for using these medications are the self-limited nature of sinusitis in most cases, the difficulty with the overuse of antibiotics in this common and often misdiagnosed infection, and the rare incidence of complications. Some clinicians argue that the high incidence of antibiotic resistance merits more aggressive use of broad-spectrum antibiotics as first-line therapy, specifically amoxicillin-clavulanate (Augmentin™), cefpodoxime (Vantin™), and levofloxacin (Levaquin™). However, we believe that the use of narrow-spectrum antibiotics is still the preferable treatment among homeless populations. The recommended course of treatment is 10 days for acute bacterial sinusitis and 3-8 weeks for chronic sinus infections.

Intravenous antibiotics are usually reserved for complicated infections or when intracranial or orbital extension is suspected. Fungal infections and those involving polyps are more complicated and may require surgery and different antibiotics. Referral to an otolaryngologist is necessary if symptoms worsen after 2-3 days of a broad-spectrum antibiotic or at any time that complications are suspected. Surgery may be necessary to clean and drain the sinuses, especially in the patient with recurrent episodes despite treatment. Consultation with an otolaryngologist is advised for these cases. Surgical repair of a deviated septum or nasal polyps may prevent recurrence.

With children, problems are often eliminated by removal of adenoids that block nasal and sinus passages. The most common type of surgery today is functional endoscopic sinus surgery, in which the natural openings from the sinuses are enlarged to allow adequate drainage.

Complications

Sinusitis very rarely can result in intracranial, orbital, and respiratory complications. Complications should be suspected whenever a patient reports a high fever, severe pain, extreme headache, visual changes, papillary or extraocular movement (EOM) abnormalities, or meningeal symptoms. Complications of sinusitis may include:

- chronic sinusitis;
- osteomyelitis (of facial bones);
- meningitis;
- orbital cellulitis or abscess (orbital complications more common in young children);
- abscess formation (brain) and subdural empyema;
- cavernous sinus thrombosis (and cortical vein thrombosis).

Bacterial resistance to certain common antibiotics may also occur, as well as exacerbation of asthma and bronchitis. Sinopulmonary disease is a generally recognized combination, especially when the condition has become chronic. Urgent referral to an otolaryngologist is in order if symptoms become markedly worse after 2-3 days of broad-spectrum antibiotics or if a provider notes possible signs of intracranial or orbital extension of infection.

Special Considerations for Homeless Populations

Homeless people are more likely to develop sinusitis than the general population due to both lifestyle and environmental risk factors. For example, smoking cigarettes is considered a risk factor for both acute and chronic sinusitis. Drinking alcohol causes nasal and sinus membranes to swell, which may inhibit the resolution of sinusitis and exacerbate symptoms. Drugs such as cocaine and heroin may have a deleterious effect on the nasal mucosa when "snorted" or ingested intranasally. Outside temperature fluctuations, poor hygiene, dehydration and poor nutrition, nasal trauma from falls or assaults, and constant exposure to environmental allergens and pollutants may all lead to frequent or complicated episodes of sinusitis.

Homeless people have a high incidence of upper respiratory illnesses and pulmonary disease when compared to the general population. These and various other co-morbid illnesses such diabetes, liver disease, and HIV/AIDS are associated with complicated and recurrent sinus infections.

Oral infections due to poor dental hygiene are endemic in homeless populations, further complicating the clinical presentation and successful treatment of sinusitis. Also, completing a full course of antibiotics may be difficult for the homeless patient and may lead to treatment failure or recurrence of symptoms. Various ancillary treatments, such as humidification with steam, are impractical for most shelter residents or people who sleep on the street and are thus likely neglected in the treatment of sinusitis.

Summary

Sinusitis is an extremely common infection, most likely with an even greater incidence in the homeless population. Viral sinusitis is far more common than bacterial, and the diagnostic challenge for clinicians is to distinguish between these two types of sinusitis. Judicious use of antibiotics is warranted, and antibiotics should only be prescribed when bacterial sinusitis is suspected or determined. The presence of typical symptoms for longer than one week, accompanied by purulent nasal discharge and facial pain over the maxillary area or upper teeth, are suggestive of a bacterial sinusitis. A careful examination of the head and neck, as well as the lungs and cervical lymph nodes, can help confirm a bacterial etiology. Offering adjunctive therapies such as sinus irrigation, antihistamines, decongestants, cough suppressants, and warm compresses are prudent for all cases of sinusitis, regardless of etiology. Avoiding unnecessary antibiotic use will help prevent drug resistance; overzealous use of antibiotics in the past has resulted in resistance among many strains of the common pathogens and changed the antibiotics of choice for this infection. Consultation with an otolaryngologist (ear, nose, and throat specialist) is recommended for patients with recurrent or resistant cases of sinusitis or when complications arise. ▉

Sinusitis Medication List

Generic	Brand Name	Cost
amoxicillin-clavulanate	Augmentin	$$$
cefpodoxime	Vantin	$$$
cefuroxime	Ceftin	$$$
fluticasone nasal spray 0.05%	Flonase	$$$
levofloxacin	Levaquin	$$$

References

Gwaltney JM. Acute community-acquired sinusitis. *Clinical Infectious Diseases* 1996;23(6):1209-1225.

Gwaltney JM. Acute sinusitis (rhinosinusitis). UpToDate; 2002. http://www.uptodate.com

Hickner JM, Bartlett JG, Bessner RE, et al. Principles of appropriate antibiotic use for acute rhinosinusitis in adults: background. *Annals of Internal Medicine* 2001;134(6):498-505.

Kaliner M. Medical management of sinusitis. *The American Journal of the Medical Sciences* 1998;318(1):21-28.

National Library of Allergy and Infectious Diseases. Fact sheet: Sinusitis. National Institutes of Health, 2002. http://www.niaid.nih.gov/factsheets/sinusitis.htm

Osguthorpe JD, Hadley JA. Rhinosinusitis: current concepts in evaluation and management. *Medical Clinics of North America* 1999;83(1):27-41.

Snow V, Mottur-Pilson C, Hickner JM. Principles of appropriate antibiotic use for acute sinusitis in adults. *Annals of Internal Medicine* 2001;134(6):495-497.

Switz KL. Determining the cause and relieving the discomfort of rhinosinusitis. *Journal of the American Association of Physician Assistants* 2000;13(3):25-8, 35-6, 39-42.

Williams JW, Simel DL. Diagnosing acute sinusitis by history and physical examination. *Journal of the American Medical Association* 1993;270(10):1242-1246.

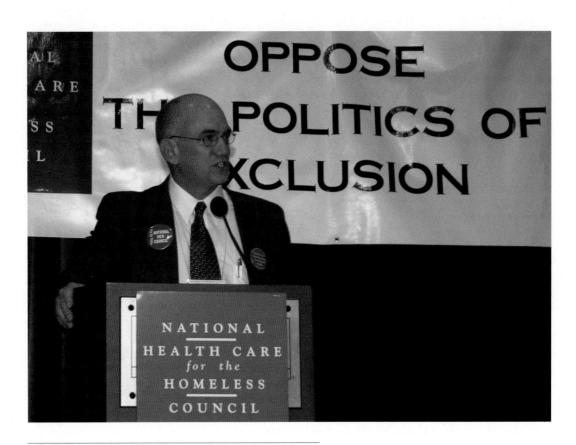

John Lozier, Executive Director of the National Health Care for the Homeless Council, opens the Council's Annual Symposium in Washington, DC, in May 2003.
Photo by James O'Connell MD

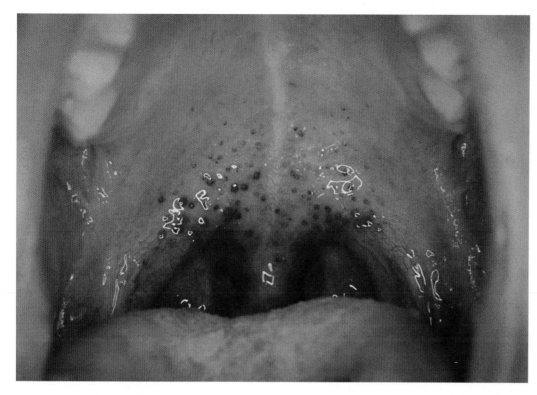

Streptococcal Pharyngitis (Strep Throat)

Maria Pitaro, MD

S ore throat is a very common reason for a visit to a health care provider. While the major treatable pathogen is group A beta hemolytic Streptococcus (GAS), this organism is responsible for only 15-30% of sore throat cases in children and 5-10% of cases in adults. Other pathogens that cause sore throat are viruses (about 50%), other bacteria (including Group C beta hemolytic Streptococci and *Neisseria gonorrhea*), Chlamydia, and Mycoplasma. In this era of increasing microbiologic resistance to antibiotics, the public health goal of all clinicians should be to avoid the inappropriate use of antibiotics and to target treatment to patients most likely to have infection due to GAS.

Clinical Manifestations

Pharyngitis due to GAS varies in severity. The most common presentation is an acute illness with sore throat, fever (often >101°F/38.3°C), tonsillar exudates (pus on the tonsils), and tender cervical adenopathy (swollen glands). Patients may also have headache, malaise, and anorexia. Additional physical examination findings may include petechiae of the soft palate and a red, swollen uvula. Many patients have a milder illness without exudates. Nausea, vomiting, and abdominal pain may be prominent in children. Interestingly, the presence of cough, coryza, runny nose, hoarseness, conjunctivitis, and diarrhea make infection with GAS less likely.

Scarlet fever is caused by certain strains of GAS. These patients have a diffuse, erythematous rash with the texture of sandpaper that blanches when pressed. The rash is most visible on the neck and chest and in the folds of the skin and usually spares the face, palms, and soles. Flushing of the cheeks and pallor around the mouth is common, and the tongue becomes swollen, red, and mottled ("strawberry tongue"). Both skin and tongue may peel during recovery.

Pharyngitis due to GAS is usually a self-limited condition with symptoms resolving in 2-5 days even if untreated. Treatment has been shown to prevent some complications of GAS pharyngitis.

Complications

Two classes of complications exist: suppurative and non-suppurative. Suppurative complications of GAS pharyngitis include the following infections:
- retropharyngeal infections, including cellulitis or abscess;
- otitis media;

Streptococcal Pharyngitis (Strep Throat). Inflammation of the oropharynx with petechiae, or small red spots, on the soft palate. Photo courtesy of the CDC

- sinusitis; and
- rare complications due to bacteremia, such as necrotizing fasciitis, meningitis, or brain abscess.

Some studies have shown that antibiotic therapy of GAS can decrease the incidence of otitis media and sinusitis.

The most common non-suppurative complications are acute rheumatic fever and acute post-streptococcal glomerulonephritis. Acute rheumatic fever (ARF) is an inflammatory disease involving the heart, joints, connective tissue, and nervous system. This usually arises within 2-4 weeks of pharyngitis and can result in progressive rheumatic heart disease. ARF happens in < 3% of untreated cases of GAS during an epidemic and in < 0.5% of sporadic cases. Penicillin therapy for treatment of GAS pharyngitis within 9 days of onset of symptoms has been shown to decrease the incidence of ARF by 75%.

Acute post-streptococcal glomerulonephritis is due to infection with certain strains of GAS that can affect the kidneys and complicates approximately 5% of cases of GAS pharyngitis in children. Most cases occur in children younger than 7 years of age. The glomerulonephritis usually occurs within 10 days following a GAS upper respiratory infection. The clinical presentation is variable, ranging from asymptomatic microscopic hematuria to acute nephrotic syndrome with proteinuria, edema, hypertension, and acute renal failure. Unlike ARF, antimicrobial therapy does not prevent acute post-streptococcal glomerulonephritis. Recurrence is rare, and the disease does not usually lead to residual renal damage. A very rare non-suppurative complication of GAS pharyngitis is streptococcal toxic shock syndrome, a severe systemic illness with shock and organ failure. Recently a new syndrome called PANDAS (Pediatric Autoimmune Neuropsychiatric Disorder Associated with Group A Streptococci) has been described. The syndrome involves obsessive-compulsive disorder or tic disorder with other neurologic abnormalities of abrupt onset in association with GAS infections. A clear-cut relationship of the syndrome with GAS infection has yet to be established.

Prevalence and Distribution

GAS most often affects children and young adults (5-15 years of age). Infection is most common during the winter and early spring. GAS is the cause of approximately 15-30% of acute pharyngitis in children and 5-10% in adults.

Transmission

GAS spreads when a person coughs or sneezes infected droplets into the air that come into contact with another person's mucous membranes. Crowded settings such as schools and shelters heighten the chance of transmission among pupils and guests. On rare occasions outbreaks have been attributed to contaminated food.

The average incubation period is 1-4 days, and the highest risk of transmission occurs during the acute stage. The rate of transmission of GAS in untreated patients is approximately 35% in close contacts, such as family members or schools. After an infected person completes 24 hours of therapy with penicillin, the risk of transmission diminishes significantly.

Sometimes people "carry" the GAS infection, but they are not sick with GAS and pose no risk to spread the disease. Carriers are those in whom GAS has colonized the nose, throat, or skin and who do not have clinical evidence of illness. These persons rarely transmit streptococcal infection and are not at risk for developing rheumatic fever.

Clinical Diagnosis

Since sore throat is such a common problem and distinguishing viral infection from GAS infection can be difficult, several clinical prediction rules have been developed. These rules can help providers predict which patients are likely to have GAS and need treatment, which patients should be tested, and which patients are unlikely to have GAS and in whom antibiotics can be safely withheld. Because of recent overuse of antibiotics and the emergence of antibiotic resistance, some experts recommend that only patients with positive cultures or rapid antigen tests should be treated.

In adults, the Centor criteria are most often used. The 4 criteria are:
- tonsillar exudates;
- tender anterior cervical adenopathy;
- fever by history;
- absence of cough.

Persons with three or four of these criteria may be treated empirically for GAS. Those with zero or one criterion do not need to be tested or treated. If two or three criteria are present, testing should be performed and patients treated only if the test is positive.

The McIsaac modification of the Centor criteria has been studied in children. Points for a patient are added based on the following scoring:

- history of fever or T>101°F (38°C)   +1
- absence of cough   +1
- tender anterior cervical adenopathy   +1
- tonsillar swelling or exudates   +1
- age <15 years   +1
- age > or = 45 years   -1

Children with 0 points are unlikely to have GAS infection and do not need to be tested. Those with 1-3 points should be tested and treatment based on the test result. Those with 4-5 points have a high likelihood of having GAS infection and may be treated empirically or tested and treated if the test is positive.

Laboratory Diagnosis

Throat culture is the gold standard for the definitive diagnosis of GAS pharyngitis. Although it takes 24-48 hours to obtain results from a culture, delaying therapy for this period of time will usually not be harmful to patients. In the shelter settings where follow-up may be difficult, clinicians must make a clinical determination whether to treat empirically or wait for the culture results.

Rapid antigen-detection tests are available in some settings and can provide an immediate diagnosis. If the rapid antigen test is positive, treatment should be initiated. If the rapid antigen test is negative, a throat culture should be obtained. False positive throat cultures and rapid antigen tests may result from a GAS carrier who has pharyngitis due to another organism, such as a virus.

Antibody tests, such as anti-streptolysin O (ASLO), can confirm streptococcal infection in the recent past but do not help with the diagnosis of acute disease.

Treatment

Antibiotic treatment can prevent local complications and limit the spread of disease, an important consideration in the shelter setting. Treatment can reduce the duration and severity of symptoms if begun within 48-72 hours of symptom onset and can also prevent rheumatic fever if begun within 9 days of the onset of illness.

Penicillin is the treatment of choice for those with no history of allergy. Penicillin has a narrow spectrum, low cost, and proven efficacy. An oral regimen of penicillin VK (Pen-Vee K™) 250 mg 2-3 times daily in children and 500 mg 2-3 times daily in adults for 10 days is recommended. Alternatively, intramuscular benzathine penicillin G (Bicillin L-A™), 1,200,000 units for adults and

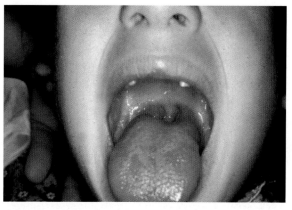

Streptococcal Pharyngitis (Strep Throat). The tonsils are swollen and reddened in this child with a fever, tender anterior cervical lymph nodes, and an absence of cough. Photo courtesy of the CDC

children >60 pounds, and 600,000 units in children < 60 pounds), may be a more practical regimen for those who will have difficulty following the oral regimen. If oral therapy is chosen, completion of the full 10-day course is essential to ensure adequate treatment. Symptoms generally subside before the therapy is complete.

For penicillin-allergic patients, erythromycin (Eryc ™, E-mycin ™) is the recommended therapy. Many broader spectrum antibiotics have been shown to be effective in treating GAS pharyngitis, such as azithromycin (Zithromax™), clarithromycin (Biaxin™), cephalosporins and amoxicillin-clavulanate (Augmentin™). However, the use of these agents is not recommended as they have the potential to increase antibiotic resistance among respiratory pathogens.

Prevention and Control

Prompt diagnosis and treatment of infections can prevent transmission. Caregivers should ensure that patients complete the full course of therapy even when their symptoms have resolved. Patients with a history of rheumatic fever may prevent recurrent bouts by using continuous antibiotic prophylaxis.

Close contacts of an acute case of GAS pharyngitis should have a throat culture if symptoms develop within 2 weeks of exposure to an infectious case. Epidemics of GAS infection must be reported to the local board of health or appropriate health agency.

Summary

Many different organisms cause throat infections. Group A beta-hemolytic streptococci (GAS) account for less than 30% of throat infections, but diagnosis and treatment of GAS pharyngitis is essential to prevent complications.

GAS pharyngitis is most common in children and young adults. GAS spreads when a person coughs or sneezes infected droplets into the air that another person inhales. The symptoms of infection with GAS are sore throat, fever, and neck glands that are swollen and tender. The symptoms usually resolve in several days, even without treatment.

The definitive diagnosis of GAS pharyngitis is by throat culture or rapid antigen testing, although some people should be treated based on clinical signs and symptoms. Infected people receive penicillin or erythromycin treatment for 10 days. Symptoms will disappear before the completion of treatment, but the full 10-day course of therapy is necessary to completely eradicate the infection and to prevent complications.

Infections such as GAS pharyngitis spread easily in shelters. A guest or staff member who has symptoms of strep infection should see a doctor, physician assistant, or a nurse practitioner immediately, since prompt diagnosis and treatment can prevent further infection in this population. ▥

The author would like to acknowledge the critical role of Megan Sandel, MD, in reviewing and editing this chapter.

Streptococcal Pharyngitis Medication List

Generic	Brand Name	Cost
amoxicillin-clavulanate	Augmentin	$$$
azithromycin	Zithromax	$$
benzathine penicillin G	Bicillin	$
clarithromycin	Biaxin	$$$
erythromycin	Eryc, E-Mycin	$
penicillin V	Pen-Vee K	$

References

Bartlett JG. Approach to Acute Pharyngitis in Adults. UpToDate, 2003. http://www.uptodate.com

Bisno AL, Gerber MA, Gwaltney JM, et al. Practice guidelines for the diagnosis and management of group A streptococcal pharyngitis. *Clinical Infectious Diseases* 2002;35(2):113-125.

Boruchoff S, Weinstein MP. Throat Cultures and Other Tests for the Diagnosis of Pharyngitis. UpToDate, 2003. http://www.uptodate.com

Chin J, Ascher MS, eds. *Control of Communicable Diseases Manual.* Washington, DC: American Public Health Association; 2000.

Cooper RJ, Hoffman JR, Bartlett JG, et al. Principles of appropriate antibiotic use for acute pharyngitis in adults: background. *Annals of Internal Medicine* 2001;134(6):509-517.

Ebell MH, Smith MA, Barry HC, et al. Does this patient have strep throat? *Journal of the American Medical Association* 2000;284(22):2912-2918.

Hayes CS, Williamson H. Management of group A beta-hemolytic streptococcal pharyngitis. *American Family Physician* 2001;63(8):1557-1565.

Pichichero ME. Complications of Streptococcal Tonsillopharyngitis. UpToDate, 2003. http://www.uptodate.com

Pichichero ME. Treatment of Streptococcal Tonsillopharyngitis. UpToDate, 2003. http://www.uptodate.com

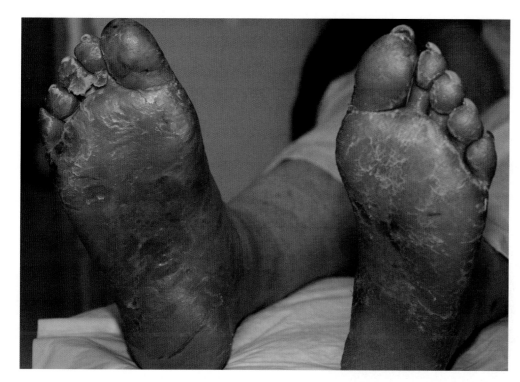

Tinea Pedis (Athlete's Foot)

Claire J. Carlo, MD
Patricia MacWilliams Bowe, RN, MS

Tinea pedis, also called "athlete's foot", is a fungal infection of the foot that is very common among homeless populations. Fungi are plant-like organisms that live as parasites or saprophytes (organisms that rely on dead tissue for their nutrition).

Fungi can exist in two forms:
- yeasts, which are unicellular;
- molds, with branched structures called hyphae.

Fungi that cause superficial infections of the skin and nails are called dermatophytes. These fungi infect the keratin of the top layer of the epidermis as well as the nails and are responsible for tinea pedis.

Dermatophytes grow will in moist, occlusive environments. Conditions such as diabetes and HIV/AIDS interfere with the body's immune function and increase the risk of acquiring dermatophyte infections. These infections are very common among homeless populations, as will be outlined later.

Prevalence and Distribution

Nearly everyone in the population is exposed to the common fungi that cause tinea pedis. Each person's immune system determines whether infection results from such exposure. As adults age, tiny cracks develop in the skin of the feet, increasing the susceptibility to tinea infections. Once acquired, a fungal infection can linger inactively for years and later become active when a person reaches the age of 60-70. More than 70% of the US population will have tinea pedis at some time in their lives. One third of all patients are estimated to have toenail infections as well. Diabetes is a significant risk factor, as diabetics are 50% more likely to have a fungal infection than non-diabetics.

Limited data is available on the prevalence in the homeless population. One study that examined the prevalence of skin disorders among homeless men staying in a 450-bed shelter in Boston in 1992 found 38% of the residents had tinea pedis, and 15.5% had toenail onychomycosis.

Symptoms and Diagnosis

There are three forms of tinea pedis:
- interdigital - macerated, scaly, fissured skin occurs between the toes, especially in the web space between the 4th and 5th toes;
- plantar ("moccasin foot") - fine, powdery scale is present on a reddened background of the sole, heel, and sides of the foot;
- vesicular (bullous) - an acute inflammatory reaction consisting of vesicles and pustules.

Individuals may be asymptomatic or may experience burning, itching, or stinging.

Severe Tinea Pedis. This gentleman lives on Boston's streets and came to McInnis House with this burning and painful rash of both feet. Note the prominent scaling on the reddened soles of his feet.
Photo by James O'Connell MD

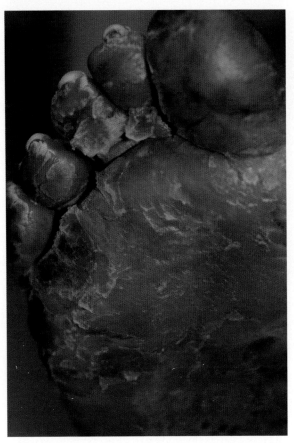

The diagnosis of tinea pedis is usually made clinically and based upon the examination of the affected area. Definitive diagnosis may be made by scraping the skin for a KOH preparation, a skin biopsy, or culture of the affected skin. The KOH preparation is less likely to be positive in severe cases with maceration of the skin. In mild cases the fungus can usually be recovered in a scraping. In severe cases it is recovered less than half the time.

In the evaluation and diagnosis of tinea pedis, clinicians should keep in mind that superinfection with bacteria can occur.

Toenails infected with tinea pedis appear thickened, discolored, and dystrophic.

Treatment and Complications

Treatment modalities come in several forms. Topical agents include creams, powders, and sprays. The creams and sprays are more effective than powders.

Topical agents are generally effective in mild forms of interdigital tinea pedis. Non-prescription, over-the-counter (OTC) topical agents work moderately well. The less expensive OTC creams, such as clotrimazole (Lotrimin™, Mycelex™) and miconazole (Monistat™, Micatin™), work as well as the more expensive OTC cream terbinafine (Lamisil™), but they require 4 weeks of treatment

compared to 1-2 weeks of treatment with terbinafine cream. In our clinical practices, the first choice of treatment is usually an OTC cream. If the tinea pedis is extensive, a prescription topical antifungal would be used. Prescription topical antifungal creams, such as econazole (Spectazole™) and nystatin (Mycostatin™), are fungicidal and achieve a cure in a shorter time. In more extensive tinea pedis or with failure of topical agents, oral medications available by prescription can be used.

The length of treatment with topical agents may be as long as 4 weeks depending on the cream chosen. Duration of therapy with oral agents can be 1-2 weeks depending on the medication used. In cases of tinea pedis with inflammatory signs and symptoms (including erythema, pruritis, and burning), a combination steroid/antifungal cream can be used. The steroid is not necessary when signs of inflammation are lacking.

Onychomycosis requires treatment with oral antifungal medication for an extended period of time.

Modes of Transmission

Warm moist areas are fungi friendly. Optimal environments are dark, damp, and warm. Poor hygiene, closed footwear, minor skin or nail injuries, and prolonged moist skin create ideal environments for transmission.

Tinea pedis is contagious and spread through direct contact with people or objects such as showers, shoes, socks, locker rooms, or pool surfaces. Pets can carry the fungus and may also be a source of transmission.

Prevention

Keeping the feet clean and dry is one of the best methods of prevention. Other methods are well-ventilated shoes that fit properly and are not tight. Alternating shoes daily will allow shoes to dry thoroughly in between wearing. Socks should be dry and changed frequently. Wool socks draw moisture away from feet and are highly recommended. Wearing sandals or flip-flops in public showers or pool areas may also help prevent tinea pedis. The use of foot powders is controversial but may be helpful for persons susceptible to tinea pedis who have frequent exposures to areas where the fungus is suspected.

Special Considerations for Homeless Populations

Regular and thorough skin examinations with emphasis on the feet should be conducted by clinicians caring for homeless persons. Good patient education, with simple instructions as to the importance of good foot hygiene, can help prevent and minimize the progression of tinea pedis. Good education consists of proper hygiene instructions, emphasizing the importance of drying the feet, practicing good nail care, and wearing properly fitting shoes with clean dry socks. Patients should be shown the correct use of any necessary topical or oral treatments.

Clinicians should be vigilant to treat other predisposing factors to tinea pedis that occur in homeless and other populations, including peripheral vascular disease, peripheral neuropathy, alcoholism, and the use of vasoconstrictive drugs such as cocaine.

Summary

Tinea pedis is commonly called "athlete's foot." A fungus that grows predominantly in warm moist environments causes this infection that involves the feet and toes. Shoes, showers, and pool or locker room areas are frequent culprits that foster and spread tinea pedis infections. Nearly everyone is exposed to this fungus, but one's immune system determines whether an individual will develop infection. For example, diabetics are 50% more likely to have tinea pedis.

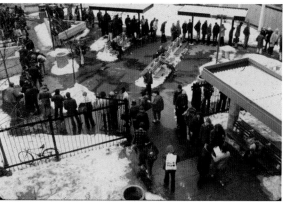

Standing in interminable lines is a daily routine for homeless persons, often exposed to the extremes of temperature and weather. These men are waiting for the doors of a local shelter to open in the late afternoon. Photo by Melissa Shook

Tinea pedis may present between the digits of the toes (interdigital), on the plantar surface (plantar), or as vesicles (vesicular). Patients may be asymptomatic or experience burning, stinging, or itching. Bacterial superinfection, including cellulitis of the lower extremity, is a complication of tinea pedis.

Prevention is the best measure, especially wearing dry shoes and socks, properly fitting shoes, and sandals or flip-flops in the shower areas. Treatment may be a cream, spray, or powder. If the case is extensive or involves the nails (onychomycosis), oral agents may be necessary.

Regular foot exams should be a routine aspect of health care for homeless persons. Clean and dry socks, as well as shoes that are dry and fit properly,

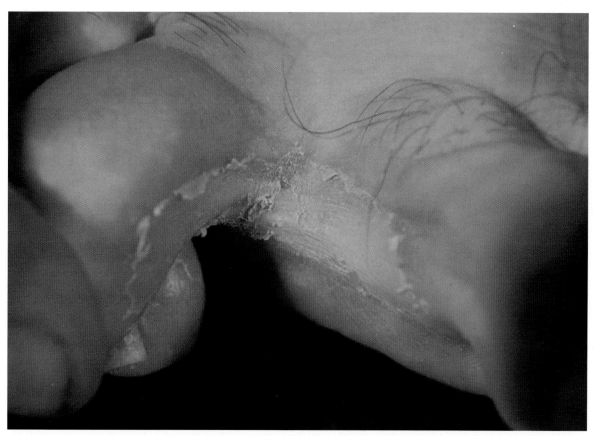

Tinea Pedis of the Toes.
An example of the typical fissured skin and scaling between the toes in tinea pedis.
Photo courtesy of the CDC

are all important for the prevention and treatment of tinea pedis. However, access to socks and shoes is often limited to the majority of homeless persons living in shelters and on the streets. Clinicians should screen carefully for other predisposing factors, such as peripheral vascular disease, peripheral neuropathy, and diabetes. Education about good foot care benefits all involved. ⊞

Tinea Pedis Medication List

Generic	Brand	Cost
Oral agents		
fluconazole	Diflucan	$$$$
griseofulvin	Fulvicin, Grifulvin, Grisactin	$$
itraconazole	Sporanox	$$$$$
ketoconazole	Nizoral	$$$$
nystatin	Mycostatin	$
terbinafine	Lamisil	$$$$$
Topical agents		
clotrimazole	Lotrimin, Mycelex	$
econazole	Spectazole	$$
ketoconazole	Nizoral	$
miconazole	Micatin, Monistat	$
naftifine	Naftin	$$
nystatin	Mycostatin	$
terbinafine	Lamisil	$$$
tolnaftate	Tinactin	$

References

Crawford F, Hart R, Bell-Syer S, Torgerson D, Young P, Russel I. Athlete's foot and fungally infected toenails. *British Medical Journal* 2001;322(7281):288-289.

Markova T. What is the most effective treatment for tinea pedis (athletes's foot)? *Journal of Family Practice* 2002;51(1):21.

Stratigos A, Stern R, Gonzales E, et al. Prevalence of skin disease in a cohort of shelter-based homeless men. *Journal of the American Academy of Dermatology* 1999;41(2 Pt 1):197-202.

Weinstein A, Berman B. Topical treatment of common superficial tinea infections. *American Family Physician* 2002;65(10):2095-2102.

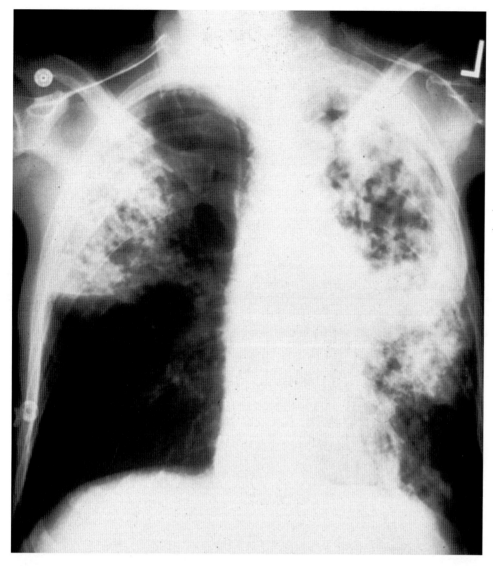

Tuberculosis (TB)

John Bernardo, MD
Jill S. Roncarati, PA-C

Tuberculosis (TB) remains the leading cause of mortality from infectious diseases in humans in the world. In contrast to the world situation, the 14,900 cases of TB reported in the USA in 2003 represent the lowest number of cases ever recorded by public health authorities. However, select populations remain at high-risk for the disease, including people born in countries outside the USA with high prevalence of the disease, persons infected with HIV, and homeless individuals.

Cavitary Tuberculosis. This 50 year old man was brought to the shelter clinic in 1985 with weight loss and a persistent cough. The chest x-ray shows cavitary TB, loss of lung volume, and a right upper lobe pneumothorax. Radiograph courtesy of James O'Connell MD

Following decades of decline, tuberculosis re-emerged in the mid-1980's across the USA as a major public health crisis, including multi-drug resistant disease. This epidemic was due in large part to the disassembly of the categorical public health infrastructure for TB required to maintain control of the disease. Unfortunately, as policy makers and public health authorities attempt to economize budgets, lessons of the past are forgotten. TB program functions are increasingly assigned to generalist public health divisions and to the private sector, where the principles and complexities of TB control are often not well-understood. Recent outbreaks of TB among homeless persons in Seattle, Washington, and Portland, Maine, provide warning signals; public health officials and policy makers must advocate for the maintenance of the principles of TB control to avoid another national epidemic of this disease.

The complexities in the diagnosis and treatment of tuberculosis infection and disease call for close cooperation among public health officials, laboratories, and health care providers, especially those who provide care to people at-risk. New diagnostic and epidemiologic tools, new treatment regimens, and advancements in our understanding of the disease process require all stakeholders in TB control to be continually educated and trained in order to maintain expertise and provide optimal care.

Tuberculosis is preventable and treatable, and most epidemics are avoidable. To prevent TB disease, people infected with TB need to be identified, especially those at increased risk for developing disease, including homeless persons and drug abusers. Early recognition and prompt intervention for TB disease is the key to limiting the spread of TB to others.

Mode of Transmission

Tuberculosis is caused by *Mycobacterium tuberculosis*. These bacteria usually infect people via the respiratory tract. A person with pulmonary TB, the most common form of tuberculosis, can cough the organisms into the air, and others who share the air space may inhale the "droplet nuclei" generated by the cough and become infected. TB can infect other parts of the body after it enters through the lungs, but these infections seldom lead to the transmission of organisms to others.

While the infectiousness of each case varies, TB is not highly infectious in general. People who have had prolonged contact with an infectious person are at highest risk of becoming infected, particularly persons with impaired immune systems, sleeping partners, or those who share close air space for several hours. A person with active pulmonary TB is unlikely to continue transmitting the organism to others once proper therapy has been instituted with clinical and bacteriologic improvement for 14 days.

Tuberculosis Infection

After a susceptible person inhales the organisms responsible for TB infection, the bacteria begin to multiply in the lungs and then spread through the body via the blood and lymph systems. The body's immune system eventually controls the TB organisms in most cases. This immune response, called "sensitization," usually takes from 4-12 weeks. The tuberculin (PPD) skin test and the QuantiFERON (QFT) blood test measure this immune response, or

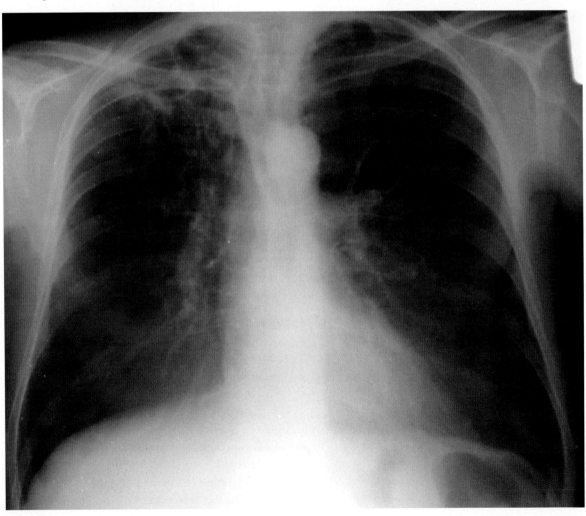

Pulmonary Tuberculosis. 56 year old man was noted to be coughing nightly in the shelter. Note the RUL infiltrate with cavity formation. Sputum was positive for AFB. Culture positive for M. tuberculosis, resistant to INH and SM. Radiograph courtesy of John Bernardo MD

sensitization, to the TB organism.

A positive PPD skin test or QuantiFERON test documents prior infection with *M. tuberculosis.* Most infected persons carry the infection in its "latent," or dormant, form called Latent Tuberculosis Infection (LTBI). This infection may not become active until later in life. Others with a positive PPD or QFT test may have active TB disease. Everyone with a positive test should undergo a proper medical evaluation, including a chest radiograph, to rule out active tuberculosis.

The Centers for Disease Control and Prevention (CDC) and the American Thoracic Society (ATS) recently published revised guidelines for tuberculin skin testing and for use of the QuantiFERON test. The TB skin test is a highly standardized test; it must be placed and read by persons trained in its application and interpretation. QFT is a laboratory test performed on blood drawn from the patient within 12 hours. Criteria for interpretation of the tuberculin skin test are summarized in Table 1.

Persons infected with TB may occasionally not show a positive PPD skin test or QFT test. Provided enough time has passed for "sensitization" to occur following an exposure to an infectious case (i.e. usually 4-12 weeks), certain conditions such as some malignancies, sarcoidosis, infection with HIV, or the use of immunosuppressive medicines (such as prednisone) may suppress the body's response to the test. No methods today enable one to determine TB infection in such circumstances; so-called "anergy" skin test panels have been shown to be unreliable and are not recommended.

Tuberculosis Disease

Tuberculosis disease usually occurs when a latent infection becomes active. Disease may follow the initial infection if the immune response fails to contain the spread of the organisms from the lungs (see above), especially in young children (less than 5 years of age) or persons with compromised immune systems (such as HIV-infected persons). Most TB disease in the USA today represents re-activation of latent TB infection. Symptoms and signs of TB disease often are not specific and may be overlooked easily. Active pulmonary disease may present with a cough productive of sputum, fevers, weight loss, night sweats, and/or general fatigue. Tuberculosis of the lymphatic system may produce swollen lymph nodes; tuberculous meningitis may present as a change in mental status.

Caregivers should suspect active TB in anyone who exhibits these symptoms and has had:

- a recent close exposure to an active case of infectious TB;
- a history of a positive PPD or QFT test;
- an abnormal chest x-ray that suggests the presence of TB.

The presence of any of the following should increase the suspicion of TB:

- people with impaired immune systems, including those at-risk for infection with HIV;
- recent PPD skin test conversion (now "positive," with an increase in size of the reaction of 10 mm or more);
- diabetes mellitus or certain malignancies, such as leukemia or lymphoma;
- prolonged treatment with corticosteroids (more than 15 mg prednisone per day or equivalent, for more than 30 days) or other immunosuppressive drugs;
- malnutrition;
- chronic alcoholism;
- recent immigration from a region of the world where TB is endemic.

Tuberculosis and HIV Infection

People infected with HIV who are at risk for exposure to tuberculosis are at a high risk for TB disease. People with HIV infection and history of prior TB infection are at high risk to reactivate their latent TB infection (estimated at approximately 7-10% per year). Persons with impaired immunity from HIV who are exposed to an infectious case of TB are at great risk of developing active TB, although that risk has not been quantified.

With early diagnosis and appropriate treatment, TB is curable. However, TB can be fatal, especially in people with untreated, or inadequately-managed, advanced disease. Death also may occur in people with poor immunity whose infections can sometimes proceed unchecked and lead to overwhelming tuberculosis.

Diagnosis

The first step in the diagnosis of TB is the suspicion by the provider or the patient for the disease; the disease must be suspected before the appropriate tests are performed to confirm the diagnosis. The clinical picture, including history, signs, symptoms, and chest radiograph, all contribute to establishing a tentative, working diagnosis of TB in the appropriate setting.

The "typical" chest radiograph in pulmonary tuberculosis has infiltrates of the upper lobes (apical

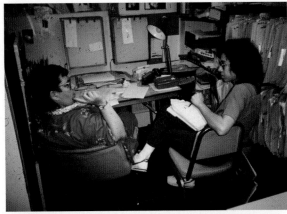

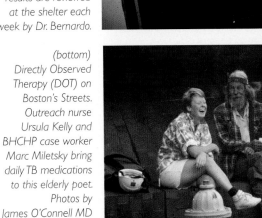

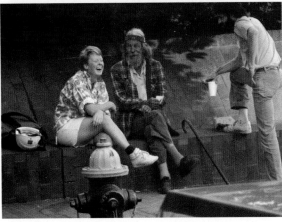

cause of infection in AIDS patients with poor immune systems), identification of the TB organism by culture is necessary to confirm a diagnosis and guide treatment.

The analysis of smears may not lead to a confirmed diagnosis by itself but can help assess the degree of infectiousness. The more organisms seen on a sputum smear, the more infectious the person is likely to be. In general, persons with 3 negative sputum smears for mycobacteria, taken at least 8 hours apart (with at least 1 sputum obtained as a first-morning specimen), are less likely to be very infectious.

While the laboratory culture of *M. tuberculosis* remains the "gold standard" for the diagnosis of tuberculosis disease, conventional culture may take up to 8 weeks before results are obtained. Newer culture methods using liquid media now enable detection of the growth of *M. tuberculosis* in 7–21 days. Molecular tests that detect *M. tuberculosis* DNA or RNA in samples of respiratory secretions (including sputum) enable confirmation of a diagnosis of TB within hours in certain circumstances; however, these tests do not provide drug susceptibility data that are essential to the management of the disease and hence do not replace the culture entirely as a tool.

Since the laboratory may take weeks to confirm a diagnosis of TB, caregivers should consider isolation of the patient and initiation of multiple drug treatment for TB disease without knowing

or posterior segments) or the superior segments of the lower lobes of the lungs with occasional cavity formation. Such a chest x-ray should immediately raise the clinician's suspicion for TB and trigger appropriate actions. However, the radiograph may involve any lobe or segment and may be mistaken for a routine bacterial pneumonia. Many TB cases have been treated inappropriately as community-acquired pneumonia with routine antibiotics for many weeks before TB was suspected and treatment is initiated. The delay in diagnosis created by such errors frequently results in prolonged transmission of TB to others in close environments, such as shelters. Inappropriate treatment of TB with a single antibiotic, such as a fluoroquinolone, which is often used to treat bacterial pneumonias but which also has excellent antituberculosis activity, also may result in drug resistance.

The chest radiograph also may take on other appearances, such as hilar or mediastinal lymphadenopathy or a pleural effusion.

Identification of the TB organism by culture of sputum or tissue biopsies confirms a diagnosis of TB. Because microscopic analysis may confuse other organisms with *M. tuberculosis* on stained sputum smears, fluids, or tissues (such as *Mycobacterium avium* complex, a noninfectious but common

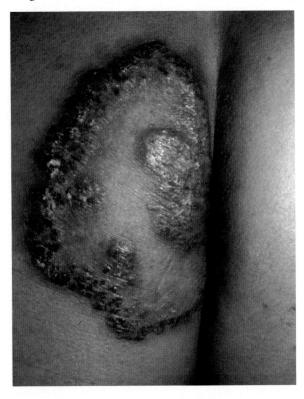

Table 1: Criteria for Tuberculin Skin Test Positivity by Risk Group

TST induration	Risk Group
≥ 5 mm	HIV + Recent close contact of infectious TB case Fibrotic changes on CXR consistent with prior TB Patients with organ transplants or other immuno-suppression (such as >15 mg prednisone/d for >30 days)
≥ 10 mm	Recent immigrants (<5 yr) from high prevalence countries Injection drug users Residents/employees of high-risk congregate settings (e.g. shelters, hospitals, prisons/jails, nursing homes) Mycobacteriology laboratory personnel Persons with high-risk medical conditions (e.g. diabetes mellitus, chronic renal failure, weight loss of ≥10% ideal body weight, certain malignancies, and hematologic disorders Children < 4 yr of age or infants/children/adolescents exposed to adults at high risk
≥ 15 mm	Persons with no risk factors for TB

the culture results whenever the disease is strongly suspected. Sometimes a short course of antituberculosis medications leads to a noticeable improvement in a TB suspect's condition, even when laboratory tests and cultures show no evidence of organisms. This is known as a clinically verified case response.

Treatment

A physician familiar with antituberculosis drugs and their side effects should supervise the treatment of TB infection or TB disease.

Treatment of Latent Tuberculosis Infection (LTBI)

Formerly termed "preventive therapy," treatment of LTBI targets persons with TB infection who are not ill with TB but are at-risk of reactivation of their LTBI to develop active TB disease. These people cannot spread TB to others. Treatment of LTBI destroys the residual organisms of the first infection and prevents reactivation TB disease from occurring. In general, the lifetime risk for reactivation TB disease is approximately 10%; however, this risk is greatest in persons recently infected with the organism (i.e. within the first 2 years of initial infection), in infected close contacts of active cases (with a positive PPD skin test or QFT test), in HIV-infected persons, and in young children.

Recent guidelines for *Targeted Testing and Treatment of Latent Tuberculosis Infection* have

been published, and subsequently revised, by the CDC/ATS. Treatment of LTBI usually consists of a 9-month course of a single medication, isoniazid (INH), administered daily. When taken for the full period, this regimen confers greater than 90% protection against reactivation disease. Where there is a high likelihood of infection with a strain of TB resistant to INH, the prescribing provider may substitute rifampin (Rimactane™, Rifadin™) daily for 4 months or use both INH and rifampin (RIF) for 4 months. A CDC/ATS recommendation for a shorter course of treatment, using 2 months of daily RIF plus pyrazinamide (PZA), another first-line antituberculosis medication, has been withdrawn because of severe hepatic side effects associated with the regimen. *This regimen should not be used to treat LTBI.*

The major side effect of INH and RIF is toxicity to the liver (i.e. drug-induced hepatitis). Clinical liver toxicity from INH is rare, especially in young adults, occurring in less than 1 in 1,000 patients in one study; liver toxicity from RIF is much less common. People older than 35 years, those who abuse alcohol or drugs, and persons with a history of liver disease are at risk for liver toxicity from these medications. People taking either of these medicines should be educated about potential side effects and instructed to stop the medicine and report to their provider immediately should they

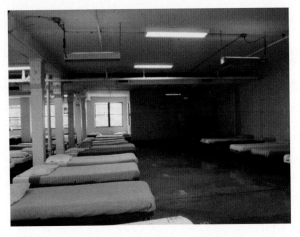

Ultraviolet Lights. Pine Street Inn and other shelters have used UV lights as a means of preventing the spread of TB organisms. Studies are underway to evaluate the clinical usefulness of these lights. Photo by James O'Connell MD

suspect toxicity is occurring.

Caregivers should be alert to symptoms of hepatitis in people taking INH or RIF. These may include nausea, vomiting, fever, jaundice, pain or discomfort in the right upper quadrant of the abdomen, or coffee- or tea-colored urine. Blood tests for liver function (AST/ALT) should be taken at baseline and monitored at least monthly in persons at-risk for liver toxicity from these medications. In most cases, persons with active hepatitis should be referred to an expert for further management before treatment of LTBI is initiated. Persons receiving these medications should be monitored by a health care provider at least monthly for signs and symptoms of toxicity and for adherence. No more than a 1 month supply of medications should be given to the patient at monitoring visits. Approximately 20% of people taking INH will increase their AST up to 5 times the upper limit of normal, with no adverse outcome. If these patients have no symptoms or signs of liver toxicity, the medication may be continued with close monitoring. In persons with signs or symptoms of liver toxicity, the medication should be stopped, and the patient should be evaluated as soon as possible. The CDC/ATS guidelines recommend stopping the medication in persons with signs or symptoms of liver toxicity and whose AST is greater than 3 times normal.

INH interacts with phenytoin (Dilantin™), a common seizure medication, increasing serum levels of both drugs. Patients taking Dilantin™ should have levels monitored during INH treatment.

Rifampin increases the metabolism of a number of drugs, including methadone and warfarin (Coumadin™), an anticoagulant drug. Dosages of these medications may have to be increased during therapy with RIF. Also, RIF may accelerate the clearance of hormones used in oral or implant contraceptives, making them ineffective. Women who use such birth control methods should use an alternative form of birth control to avoid pregnancy while taking RIF. Rifampin also may cause an orange discoloration of urine, sweat, tears, semen, or stool. Permanent discoloration of contact lenses may occur. Rifampin also may result in false-positive urine tests for opiate drugs.

Treatment of Tuberculosis Disease

Guidelines for the *Treatment of Tuberculosis* have been published recently by the CDC/ATS and the Infectious Diseases Society of America (IDSA). Medical treatment of TB disease usually consists of multiple drugs administered daily or intermittently for at least 6 months. The standard recommended treatment regimen includes 4 antituberculosis drugs: INH, RIF, PZA, and either ethambutol (EMB) or streptomycin (SM) given daily for 2 months (60 doses), followed by 4 months of 2 drugs (usually INH + RIF; 120 doses). The length of treatment and the choice of medications depend on drug susceptibility results, the patient's response to treatment, and the presence or absence of cavitation on the initial chest x-ray. Details on individual medications and descriptions of various treatment regimens are provided in the CDC/ATS/IDSA statement.

Isoniazid may cause a condition of the nerves that results in numbness and tingling sensations, especially in people with poor nutrition. This side effect may be avoided by administering pyridoxine (vitamin B6) along with the INH in select patients. Vitamin B6 also should be given to pregnant women who receive INH. Side effects of PZA may include liver toxicity (drug-induced hepatitis), gastrointestinal intolerance, and increased levels of uric acid (which can cause gout). Ethambutol or EMB (Myambutol™) can cause inflammation of the optic nerve, causing decreased visual acuity and impaired red/green color discrimination. Monthly monitoring of patients receiving EMB should include questions about vision and eye tests of acuity and of color vision. Streptomycin is given by injection; major side effects include toxicity to the kidneys and impaired hearing. Pyrazinamide and streptomycin should not be given to pregnant women.

In patients with pulmonary tuberculosis, *sputum cultures should be monitored at least monthly following the start of therapy*. Patients who have a cavity on the initial chest x-ray and fail to convert their sputum culture to negative by the end of 2 months of 4 drug therapy have a high rate of relapse; in these patients, drug susceptibility studies should be monitored and treatment should be extended to 9 months.

Physicians base the combination of drugs and the length of therapy on many factors, and the complexities of case management of patients with active TB should be undertaken with close collaboration among direct care providers, the laboratory, and the local public health authority. In complex cases, such as cases involving young children or patients with HIV infection, care may be best provided with close consultation with a tuberculosis specialist.

Adherence to Therapy

In its recent statement on the *Treatment of Tuberculosis,* the CDC/ATS/IDSA assigned *responsibility for the successful completion of treatment for tuberculosis to the provider and the public health system and not to the patient.* Successful treatment of tuberculosis today requires more than the prescription of medications; the medications must be taken as prescribed, for the appropriate duration, as dictated by each individual case. Treatment for tuberculosis is lengthy, even though symptoms may disappear shortly after therapy is initiated. Patients who feel better are more likely to stop taking their medications, especially when there are other personal priorities. Problems with adherence can lead to treatment failure or relapse, with renewed spread of infection and development of drug resistance. Adherence can be encouraged by a system of patient-centered case management. The responsibility for successful completion of treatment is assigned to a specific provider, usually a nurse or a TB field worker, who is able to tailor the medication regimen as much as possible to the patient's lifestyle. Direct observation of treatment (DOT) by a health care provider is a valuable tool in case management and should be considered the standard-of-care for all newly-diagnosed cases and TB suspects. If all attempts to achieve adherence fail, many jurisdictions provide for involuntary hospitalization under public health law to continue treatment and assure its completion. Fortunately, this measure rarely is required.

When adherence is no longer a concern, clinicians can give a one-month supply of medication at a time. Each person should receive detailed instructions about the symptoms of toxicity, as well as instructions to discontinue therapy and consult with the supervising physician immediately if side effects are suspected. A provider should see the patient at least once a month to assess for adherence, for the response to treatment, and for side

effects. The vicissitudes of survival on the streets can make adherence to a rigid schedule difficult for many homeless persons. No place may be available to safely store the medications. Adherence can be enormously improved by offering DOT intermittently (e.g. 2-3 times per week) at a site frequented by the patient. Incentives or enablers (such as public transportation passes, food coupons, etc.) also may help encourage adherence. Combination medications (e.g. Rifamate™, containing INH + RIF, or Rifater™, containing INH + RIF + PZA) minimize the risk of incorrect dosing of medications. Rifater™ can be used only in daily regimens. Each dose should be documented to reduce possible confusion about adherence over a long course of therapy.

Control of Tuberculosis
General control measures

One of the best measures for controlling the spread of TB (or any infectious disease that is spread by the respiratory route via aerosol) is simple: shelter guests and staff should cover their mouths and noses when they cough or sneeze. Guests can comply with this measure more readily when tissues are easily available.

Another way to reduce the incidence of airborne infections is to provide good ventilation to outside air in all rooms. For smaller shelters this may involve opening windows. Measures such as High Efficiency Particulate Air (HEPA) filters and ultraviolet irradiation of re-circulated and upper room air have been used in an attempt to minimize spread of TB in shelters and in other long-term living spaces. However, the clinical utility of these measures is not yet clear, and we are awaiting the results of studies currently underway.

Some shelters try to assign the same bed to their guests each night. A "bed list" is kept to facilitate contact investigation in the event that an infectious case is found. In addition to promoting a sense of stability, this is excellent public health practice; the fewer persons exposed to an undiagnosed person with active pulmonary tuberculosis, the lower the number of guests at-risk for infection.

Surveillance for tuberculosis can facilitate early case finding. Educating shelter staff and guests about TB and encouraging them to report persons with an unusual or prolonged cough can lead to a diagnosis of TB in an individual with unsuspected TB disease. Criteria for medical evaluation may be based on a "cough log" that records the names of persons who are coughing at night. Shelter staff who have close contact with guests should be tested for TB infection (PPD or QFT) regularly, at least every 6 months in facilities where TB is a problem. Ideally, guests in such a facility should undergo testing for LTBI at least every 6 months. Limited numbers of qualified staff and large numbers of guests may make this latter goal a difficult one to achieve.

Contact Investigation

When a guest in a shelter has been diagnosed with active tuberculosis, the local health department usually carries out an investigation to identify and test contacts to the case. Infected contacts to an active case are among the highest risk groups for development of active disease (see above). The "contact investigation" usually is based on PPD skin testing and chest radiography of high-risk close contacts. A PPD is placed immediately, and if negative, the PPD is repeated again 8-12 weeks following the last exposure to the person with TB. QuantiFERON has not been studied adequately yet in contacts, although a positive QFT test has the same significance as a positive (5mm) PPD skin test in this setting. Infected contacts should receive treatment with INH or RIF to prevent disease.

Close contacts may include:
- friends;
- family members or co-workers who have spent hours sharing airspace with the TB patient;
- people who have slept next to the patient during the infectious period.

Shelter bed lists may help identify those sleeping next to the TB patient. If investigators find that many close contacts are infected, the circle may have to be widened, and persons less closely associated with the patient also may need an evaluation.

Molecular epidemiologic tools, such as RFLP (called "DNA fingerprinting"), can identify individual strains of TB organisms in a given case. Linked with conventional epidemiological investigations, these methods are being used by public health authorities to track transmission of tuberculosis in communities and are able to distinguish the transmission of a single strain from reactivation disease.

Summary

Tuberculosis (TB) is a disease caused by bacteria. The TB organism infects people through the lungs. A person ill with TB can infect others by coughing or sneezing droplets containing live TB germs into the air. However, in most circumstances TB is not highly infectious.

Once the droplets are breathed into the lungs, the TB bacteria multiply slowly. After a few weeks, the TB organisms spread through the body, and the immune system gradually develops a response to stop the spread over the ensuing 4-12 weeks. During this time, the person may or may not feel sick but cannot spread TB to anyone else. TB organisms that remain viable are contained in a "latent", or dormant, state by the now-sensitized immune system.

The infection may become active in later life and lead to tuberculosis disease. The PPD skin test or the QuantiFERON (QFT) test helps identify people who have latent TB infection (LTBI), allowing caregivers to treat them with medicine to kill the bacteria before their infection becomes active. Because TB usually spreads to others when the infection becomes active, early identification and treatment of LTBI prevents the spread of TB in the community.

A person who tests PPD or QFT positive should undergo a medical evaluation, including a history, a physical examination, and a chest radiograph. If the evaluation reveals no signs of illness, medication can prevent the development of disease. Daily doses of a single anti-TB drug are used to treat LTBI: isoniazid (INH) for 9 months or rifampin (RIF) for four months, with monitoring at least monthly.

People with active TB disease usually have varied signs and symptoms of illness, although rarely some persons can be without symptoms. Cough with or without sputum, fevers, weight loss, sweats at night, swollen lymph glands, and general tiredness can be symptoms of TB. These are non-specific, and many other systemic illnesses may show these same signs or symptoms. If TB is suspected in a shelter staff person or guest, prompt evaluation by a clinician, including a chest x-ray, should be performed. Treatment of active TB requires multiple drug therapy (usually 2 to 4 medications) taken for 6 to 12 or more months.

Anti-TB drugs work well to cure TB when taken according to directions. Patient centered case management, using direct observation (and recording) of treatment doses by a health care worker (called DOT) is the standard of care. Therapy can be tailored to the patient's lifestyle and priorities in order to maximize adherence and assure successful completion of therapy. When all attempts to achieve adherence fail, many jurisdictions impose legal measures to hospitalize the patient involuntarily to continue treatment.

All anti-TB drugs can have side effects, such as

nausea, vomiting, fevers, or skin rashes. The most serious side effects of some of the medicines (e.g. INH, RIF, PZA) involve the liver. Signs of jaundice (yellow eyes or skin, tea-colored urine) or discomfort over the liver (right upper quadrant of the abdomen) are reasons to stop the drugs immediately and refer the patient to a TB specialist.

Diagnosis of a case of active and potentially infectious TB should lead to a contact investigation to identify and treat infected close contacts of the TB patient. The local board of health usually conducts or provides assistance with these activities. ■■

Tuberculosis Medication List

Generic	Abbreviation	Brand Name	Cost
isoniazid	INH	INH	$
rifampin	RIF	Rimactane, Rifadin	$$$
ethambutol	EMB	Myambutol	$$$$$
pyrazinamide	PZA	PZA	$$$
pyridoxine	B6	Vitamin B6	$
streptomycin	SM		$$$$$
Combination Pills			
INH + RIF		Rifamate	$$$$
INH + RIF + PZA		Rifater	$$$$$

References

Centers for Disease Control. Tuberculosis outbreak in a homeless population - Portland, Maine, 2002-2003. *MMWR* 2003;52:1184-1185. www.cdc.gov/mmwr/preview/mmwrhtml/mm5248a5.htm

Centers for Disease Control. Tuberculosis outbreak among homeless persons - King County, Washington, 2002-2003. *MMWR* 2003;52:1209-1210. www.cdc.gov/mmwr/preview/mmwrhtml/mm5249a4.htm

American Thoracic Society/Centers for Disease Control. Targeted tuberculin testing and treatment of latent tuberculosis infection. *American Journal of Respiratory and Critical Care Medicine* 2000;161:S221-247. www.cdc.gov.nchstp.tb/

Centers for Disease Control. Guidelines for using the QuantiFERON®-TB test for diagnosing latent *Mycobacterium tuberculosis infection. MMWR* 2003;52:15-18. www.cdc.gov/mmwr/preview/mmwrhtml/rr5202a2.htm

Update: adverse event data and revised American Thoracic Society/Centers for Disease Control recommendations against the use of rifampin and pyrazinamide for treatment of latent tuberculosis infection. *MMWR* 2003;52:735-739. www.cdc.gov/mmwr/preview/mmwrhtml/mm5231a4.htm

Nolan CM, Goldberg SV, Buskin SE. Hepatotoxicity associated with isoniazid preventive therapy: a 7 year survey from a public health tuberculosis clinic. *Journal of the American Medical Association* 1999;281:1014-1018.

ATS/CDC/IDSA: Treatment of tuberculosis. *American Journal of Respiratory and Critical Care Medicine* 2003;167:603-662. www.cdc.gov/mmwr/preview/mmwrhtml/rr5211a1.htm

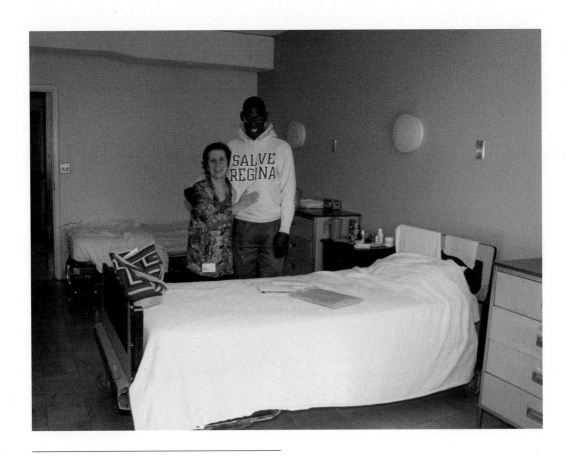

Street Team nurse Sharon Morrison with a grateful and beaming patient in his room at Barbara McInnis House.
Photo by James O'Connell MD

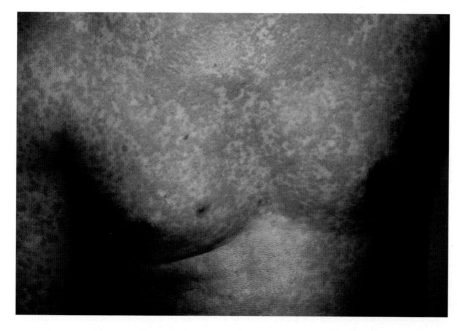

Upper Respiratory Infection (URI/Common Cold)

Kathly M. Jean-Gilles,
MSN, RN, RRT-NPS, FNP
Gregory A. Wagoner, MD, MBA

An upper respiratory infection (URI) generally refers to the common cold. Infection may involve any of the airways and air passages above the lungs, including the bronchi, trachea, throat, nose, and sinuses. Other ailments included in this category are acute bronchitis, chronic bronchitis, pharyngitis, and acute sinusitis.

The common cold, the most frequently acquired illness in the USA, is caused by more than 200 known viruses. Rhinovirus causes the largest number of viral URI's, but other etiologies include:

- parinfluenza virus;
- adenovirus;
- coronavirus;
- coxsackievirus;
- echovirus; and
- respiratory syncytial virus (RSV).

URI is a self-limited illness, generally resolving on its own without major complications or specific treatment. A thorough review of the published information indicates that antibiotics are rarely beneficial.

Symptoms

Typical symptoms of an upper respiratory infection include nasal discharge and congestion, coughing, sneezing, headache, sore or scratchy throat, chills, and general malaise. Some people experience burning eyes and pressure in the ears and sinuses. Adults rarely have fever with URIs, and when present the fever is often less than 101°F (38.3°C). Children can experience fevers as high as 102°F (38.9°C).

URIs generally last about one week. One in four people will have symptoms for 2 weeks or longer. When these signs and symptoms are focal, particularly severe, or persist for longer than two weeks, clinicians must evaluate for more serious conditions such as tonsillitis, otitis media, sinusitis, pharyngitis, or pneumonia.

The common cold must be differentiated from streptococcal pharyngitis, or strep throat, which requires early antibiotic treatment. As noted in the chapter on streptoccal pharyngitis, early treatment of strep throat can prevent rheumatic fever but not the glomerulonephritis caused by immune complex deposition. People with streptococcal infection may show a higher fever (to 104°F/40°C), and the physical examination may show tender anterior cervical lymph nodes and large inflamed tonsils with gray-white exudate. Cough is often absent in strep throat but almost always present in URI.

Complications

The common cold rarely leads to secondary bacterial infections that require antibiotic treatment. Persistent signs and symptoms, including progressive dyspnea (shortness of breath) and the production of purulent sputum, may indicate a specific bacterial infection (tonsillitis, otitis media,

Viral Exanthem. This fine reddish macular rash is diffuse and typical of many viral illnesses. This man developed a URI several days later, which resolved within one week. Photo by Howard Koh MD

sinusitis, pharyngitis) that requires treatment with antibiotics.

Prevalence and Distribution

Upper respiratory infection is the most common and the most expensive illness in the USA, representing 9% of the practice of the average family physician or pediatrician. Each year, adults get an average of 2-4 colds, while children get an average of 6-8 colds. Although most cases are mild and usually last about a week, colds are the leading cause of lost days at work and at school.

URIs are very common because large numbers of viruses are able to cause these signs and symptoms. Because the human body does not develop effective immunity, these organisms cause reinfection of humans. Adults with children in the home have more colds than those without children, presumably due to the children's exposure to a wide variety of organisms at school. Cigarette smokers have the same incidence of colds as nonsmokers, but the illness is usually more severe in smokers. Children of smokers have a higher incidence of URIs than children of non-smokers.

Transmission

Upper respiratory infections can be transmitted by direct contact, infection from surface particles, or inhaling infectious viral particles. Young children may serve as the reservoir of these infections, passing infection to one another at school and into homes. URIs are thought to spread when infected people cough, sneeze, or rub secretions onto their hands. They then pass the disease to others who infect themselves when they rub their eyes or touch their noses or mouths.

Infected people may also sneeze or cough infected droplets into the air. The droplets can then land directly on other people's mucous membranes or on surfaces (such as toys) mouthed by others. Secretions generally lose their infectivity if allowed to dry, but they can stay infectious for hours or even days on skin, nylon, and surfaces such as stainless steel and Formica™.

Diagnosis

Patients usually recognize the typical symptoms of the common cold and diagnose themselves. Clinical examination does not help to identify the specific virus. It is important to rule out streptococcal infection by throat culture if this diagnosis is considered in the differential. Either throat cultures or one of the "rapid-strep" tests can be used to confirm Streptococcus presence.

Direct complications of the URI, such as bacterial bronchitis, sinusitis, and otitis media, need to be identified and treated with the proper antibiotic. Clues to the occurrence of secondary bacterial infection include:

- fevers over 101°F (38.3° C) in adults and 102°F (38.9°C) in children;
- green or yellow purulent drainage from the nose accompanied by headache or facial pain;
- cough that produces green or yellow sputum;
- pain in one or both ears (more than a sensation of pressure).

These symptoms often show the need for laboratory tests to confirm the diagnosis. Useful tests include a throat or sputum culture, a sinus or chest x-ray, and a complete blood count (CBC). An elevated white blood count almost always points to something other than the common cold.

Treatment

The common cold is caused by viruses and should never be treated with antibiotics. Taking antibiotics unnecessarily can lead to antibiotic resistance, a potentially dangerous situation in which infection-causing bacteria become immune to the effects of certain antibiotics. Unnecessary antibiotic use also increases the potential for adverse drug reactions. Symptomatic therapy remains the mainstay of common cold treatment.

Drinking plenty of fluids will help prevent dehydration from coughing and low-grade fevers. Bedrest, if the shelter setting permits, can help with the general fatigue that accompanies a cold, hasten recovery, and minimize transmission of the virus. Saline gargles can reduce the pain of a sore throat. Decongestants such as pseudoephredrine (Sudafed™) are designed to decrease nasal secretions and decrease the swelling of sinus passages. Patients should not take decongestants for more than 3 to 4 days to avoid a rebound of symptoms. Cough preparations containing suppressants such as dextromethorphan, codeine, or terpin hydrate can help reduce a cough. Aspirin, acetaminophen (Tylenol™), or an anti-inflammatory agent such as ibuprofen can help with general achiness. Aspirin should not be used in children under 18 years because of the risk of Reye syndrome.

Inhalants, such as cromolyn sodium or the intranasal use of ipratropium, may improve cold symptoms also. Both therapies are generally well-tolerated and shown to reduce the severity of symptoms and/or reduce the duration of illness.

Other treatments, such as vitamin C, echinacea, or zinc, have not been consistently shown to be beneficial to cold sufferers.

Prevention and Control

The common cold evades prevention, cure, and treatment. Researchers have tried many methods, such as vaccines, nasal interferon, ultraviolet light, and high dose vitamin supplements. None of these studies has yet proven conclusive for the general population.

The best way to prevent a cold is to avoid contact with the virus. In a shelter, viruses can spread easily within a large group of people. To curtail transmission, shelters should be well ventilated, and guests and staff should have the basic tools of hygiene readily available. For the common cold, this means an adequate supply of tissues and receptacles for their disposal. Both guests and staff should be aware of how the use of tissues can limit the spread of viruses. Hand washing is an additional preventative step. Use of a disinfectant such as phenol (as contained in Lysol™) may decrease transmission of virus left on hard surfaces.

Parents and caregivers should discourage children (and other adults) from touching their eyes and noses. Careful handwashing with warm water and soap is also especially important before preparing, serving, or eating food.

Complications

Occasionally, upper respiratory infections are associated with subsequent complications, especially in immunocompromised patients. Sinusitis caused by either bacteria or virus can occur in association with a URI. The vast majority of these infections are viral in nature. Lower respiratory tract infections are uncommon sequelae, including pneumonia caused by respiratory syncytial virus and other types of pneumonia.

Other complications include asthmatic exacerbations, aggravation of congestive heart failure, and otitis media.

Summary

An upper respiratory infection (URI), or the common cold, can come from many different viruses. Colds are most likely spread by coughing and sneezing infected droplets into the air. Others can then inhale these droplets. Transmission also

occurs when infected people touch secretions from their noses or throats and then touch other people's hands, other objects, or surfaces. Crowded shelters can promote the spread of many infections, especially when children are present.

No specific treatment exists for the common cold. Certain measures can relieve the symptoms, such as:

- bedrest for fatigue;
- fluids for dehydration;
- saltwater gargling for sore throats;
- medications including Tylenol for aching or Sudafed™ for nasal congestion.

People who have fevers over 101°F (38.3°C), coughs that produce sputum, or green or yellow discharge from the nose or throat should see a health care provider. These might be signs of a more severe illness.

Good hygiene can help prevent the spread of cold viruses. Shelters should be well ventilated and have an adequate supply of tissues, soap, and paper towels for guests and staff. ■

The authors of this chapter gratefully acknowledge the invaluable contribution of Joan Lebow, MD, who authored this chapter in the original Manual.

References

Bauman KA. The family physician's reasonable approach to upper respiratory tract infection care for this century. *Archives of Family Medicine* 2000;9(7):596-597.

Hirschmann JV. Antibiotics for common respiratory tract infections in adults. *Archives of Internal Medicine* 2002;162(3):256-264.

Hwang MY. JAMA patient page: the common cold. *Journal of the American Medical Association* 1998;279(24):2066.

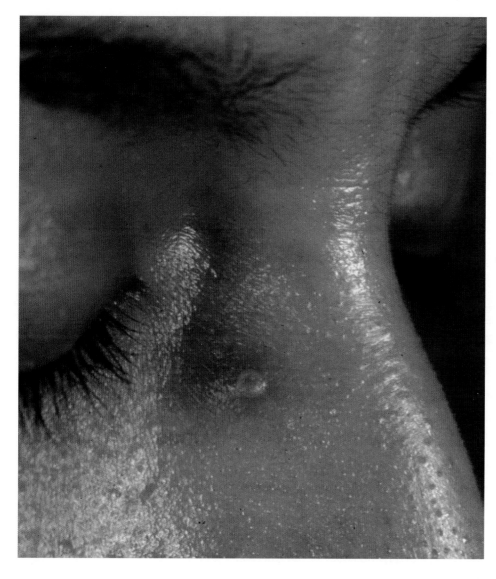

Varicella (Chickenpox)

Sarah McSweeney-Ryan, MD
Megan Sandel, MD

V aricella, or chickenpox, is caused by the varicella-zoster virus (VZV). This same virus is also responsible for herpes zoster, or shingles. Most people in the past were infected with this virus in childhood and developed chickenpox. In 1995, the varicella vaccine became licensed in the USA and is now recommended for children at one year of age, as well as for other healthy people who have not yet been infected with chickenpox.

Chickenpox. A typical vesicle (blister) on a red areola. History and physical examination can usually distinguish this rash from that of other herpes viruses, including zoster or simplex. Photo by Irwin Freedberg MD

Chickenpox typically appears as a generalized rash with itchy, blister-like lesions. Symptoms also include fever as high as 102°F (38.9°C), tiredness, and slight body discomfort. The symptoms usually resolve over 4 to 6 days. Once the rash crusts over, a person is no longer infectious.

After infection with chickenpox, the virus lies dormant in nerve cells and can reactivate years later as herpes zoster. Shingles, the common name for herpes zoster, typically appears in one limited area of one side of the body, such as along the thoracic spine or the ophthalmic division of the trigeminal nerve. This rash is blister-like and itchy and can be very painful as well.

VZV is highly contagious, and nearly every non-immunized person who is exposed to this virus develops chickenpox. Children usually have a mild illness, although serious complications can occur. Chickenpox is more severe in adults, who may experience fatigue, muscle aches, joint pain, and headache. Adults also have a higher risk of complications from chickenpox, primarily viral

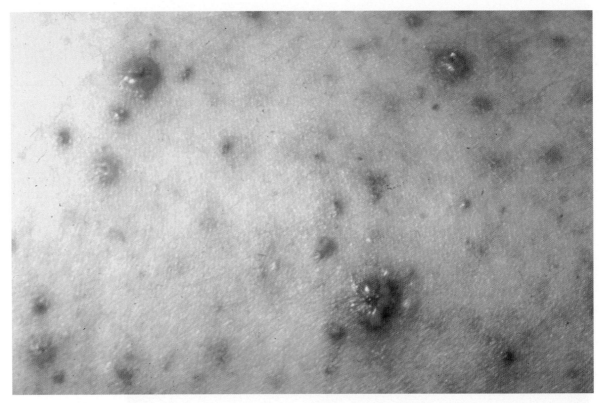

pneumonia. Both adults and children commonly develop bacterial superinfections of the viral skin lesions.

In the late 1990's approximately 12,000 people were hospitalized for chickenpox each year in the USA, and approximately 100 people died of complications from chickenpox infection annually.

Varicella infection early in pregnancy, particularly during the first and early second trimester, can in rare cases lead to severe congenital manifestations in the child, involving the central nervous system, skin, extremities, and eyes. Children exposed to varicella in utero can develop herpes zoster at a young age without having previous chickenpox. If a mother is ill with varicella during the period from 5 days before delivery until 2 days afterwards, the newborn risks developing severe generalized chickenpox, with a mortality rate as high as 30 percent. Death is most often due to pneumonia.

Varicella infection in an adult or child with a poor immune system also can be a very serious event. The lesions can be extensive and patients may have continuous eruption of the lesions with persistently high fevers into the second week of illness. The infection may progress and involve the liver, lungs, brain and meninges.

Prevalence and Distribution

Almost all adults in the USA have a history of chickenpox infection. Chickenpox occurs most commonly in the late winter and early spring months. Most cases of chickenpox in the USA occur in children less than 10 years old. Since the introduction of the varicella vaccine in 1995, significant decreases in the incidence of chickenpox have been demonstrated in some areas of the USA. Over time it is anticipated that the prevalence of chickenpox will decrease as a result of universal vaccination.

Transmission

Humans are the only source of infection with the varicella virus. The virus is transmitted from person to person through the air and through direct contact with the drainage of a rash. When an infected person coughs or sneezes, secretions from the nose and throat become airborne and may infect persons who have not previously been infected or who have not been vaccinated. Infection can also occur from contact with contaminated items, such as towels, sheets, and clothing. Additionally, contact with the drainage from zoster lesions can cause chickenpox in persons with no history of chickenpox and who have not been vaccinated. Such contact does not cause zoster or shingles, although any person who has had chickenpox can later develop herpes zoster.

People infected with chickenpox are contagious for as many as 5 days before the chickenpox rash appears, and for up to 6 days afterwards. Lesions are thought to be infectious until they crust over.

Generally, people with no prior history of exposure or immunization will show symptoms anytime from 10 days after the first day of presumed exposure until 21 days after the last day of possible exposure, or one incubation period. This latter period of 21 days can stretch to 28 days if the person has received varicella zoster immune globulin (see below). Patients with poor immune systems and generalized varicella are able to spread the virus for as long as new lesions are forming.

Persons who have been infected with chickenpox typically have lifelong immunity to the virus.

When people who have received the varicella vaccine are exposed to chickenpox, approximately 85% of them do not acquire chickenpox. Of vaccinated individuals who do develop chickenpox, the illness typically has a mild course.

Less than 8% of people develop a mild rash after vaccination with varicella. These chickenpox-like lesions do contain varicella virus, but transmission of the virus from such lesions is rare and typically leads to a mild course of chickenpox. In a shelter setting where healthy children who receive the vaccine may be in contact with people who have weak immune systems, no precautions need to be taken unless the child or recently immunized person develops a rash. Vaccinated persons who develop a rash should avoid contact with immunocompromised individuals for the duration of the rash.

Diagnosis

The itchy, blister-like rash characteristic of chickenpox is the easiest way to identify the disease. The vesicle is usually surrounded by a red circle or areola. Lesions often start on the scalp or trunk and may spread to the face and proximal limbs. Lesions can appear in the mucous membranes of the conjunctiva or oropharynx, particularly in adults. A typical infection in a child results in 100 to 300 lesions.

The lesions may continue to form over a period of 3 to 5 days; they will not all appear at the same stage of development. This is an important consideration when trying to distinguish chickenpox from impetigo, in which the lesions are uniform in appearance.

Chickenpox can also be confused with other forms of disseminated herpes viruses, including zoster and simplex.

During the first 3 to 4 days of the rash, microscopic examination of scrapings from the lesions can demonstrate the presence of multinucleated giant cells, a finding typical for any of the herpes virus family.

Treatment

The treatable symptoms of uncomplicated chickenpox include fever and itching. Acetaminophen (Tylenol™) should be used for fever. Aspirin and salicylate-containing products should be avoided, because aspirin (salicylate) use during varicella illness increases the risk of developing Reye syndrome, which is a progressive swelling of the brain along with liver complications.

Studies also suggest that the use of some non-steroidal anti-inflammatory agents, such as ibuprofen (Advil™), may increase the risk for a more severe course of chickenpox in healthy children.

Calamine lotion may be used to provide relief from itching. Daily cleansing of the lesions with soap and water is recommended to prevent infection of the lesions. Clipping of the nails should be encouraged to minimize damage to the skin from scratching.

Chickenpox can be treated with acyclovir (Zovirax™), an antiviral drug. However, there is a very limited time period during which acyclovir can affect the outcome of the infection. When acyclovir is started within 24 hours of onset of the chickenpox rash, a modest decrease in symptoms can be seen. Acyclovir is not recommended for routine use in children who are otherwise healthy.

Individuals with weak immune systems will need treatment with intravenous antiviral medications. Physicians may consider using oral acyclovir for otherwise healthy people who may be at risk for moderate to severe varicella: children older than 12 years of age; people with chronic skin or lung disorders; people receiving treatment with steroids; or people receiving long-term treatment with aspirin or salicylates. Pregnant women infected with chickenpox should speak with a physician immediately to see if acyclovir is indicated.

Prevention and Control

The varicella vaccine was licensed by the US Food and Drug Administration in March of 1995 and is recommended for all healthy persons over one year of age who have no history of chickenpox infection. The decision to administer the varicella vaccine universally in the USA was based upon the effectiveness and safety of the vaccine, the financial burden incurred by chickenpox infection on society, and the risk of complications and death after chickenpox infection.

The vaccine has been shown to be approximately 85% effective for preventing infection with chickenpox. When vaccinated people do get chickenpox, it is usually very mild with fewer lesions, lower fevers, and a shorter course of illness.

Current immunization guidelines:

- all healthy toddlers should be given one dose of the vaccine between 12 and 18 months of age;
- all healthy children less than 13 years of age with no history of chickenpox infection should receive one dose of the vaccine;
- healthy children over 13 years of age and healthy adults with no history of chickenpox infection should receive two doses of the vaccine four to eight weeks apart;
- the vaccine should NOT be given to people with weak immune systems, people receiving steroid treatments, or pregnant women;
- there are no current recommendations for booster immunizations, though this will be reassessed in the future.

For individuals who may be unsure of prior infection with chickenpox, a blood test to check antibody titers may be performed to assess immunity. Vaccinating someone who is immune to chickenpox, however, is not harmful.

In Massachusetts, as in most states, cases of varicella must be reported to the local health department. Local health departments are a source of information and support concerning prevention and control measures.

When a case of chickenpox occurs in a shelter, all persons should be evaluated for their risk of infection. Close contacts are considered to be those who have lived in the same house or shelter as the person with chickenpox and those who have been indoors with the infected person for more than an hour. All close contacts should be interviewed concerning their chickenpox history, vaccination history, and other factors that would make them candidates for treatment with either the varicella vaccine or varicella-zoster immune globulin (VZIG).

Post-Exposure Immunization

People who have not had a chickenpox infection or have not received the vaccine are considered susceptible to infection. Susceptible children and adults who are otherwise healthy should receive the varicella vaccine within 3 days (and up to 5 days) of exposure to prevent or significantly decrease the severity of chickenpox. Vaccination after exposure may not prevent infection, particularly if the exposure has occurred earlier than realized.

Post-Exposure Treatment with VZIG

VZIG (varicella zoster immune globulin) is a preparation containing high levels of antibodies to the chickenpox virus. Prepared from the plasma of normal blood donors, VZIG may not prevent disease, but it can lessen the severity of illness. VZIG must be given within 96 hours of exposure to be effective. VZIG should be given to susceptible people at a high risk for complications. VZIG can often be obtained from local chapters of the American Red Cross, as well as local and state health departments.

In the setting of chickenpox exposure, candidates for VZIG include:

- children or adults with immune system problems;
- pregnant women with no history of chickenpox infection or vaccination;
- infants born to mothers infected from 5 days before delivery until 2 days afterwards;
- hospitalized premature infants (28 weeks gestation or more) whose mothers lack a prior history of chickenpox infection or vaccination; and
- hospitalized premature infants (less than 28 weeks gestation or 1000 grams) regardless of the mother's history.

If a pregnant woman with an unclear chickenpox history becomes exposed close to term, obtaining varicella titers before administering VZIG is recommended. Titers can clarify whether the newborn will be at risk if born during the mother's incubation period.

The exact duration that VZIG recipients are protected against chickenpox is unknown. Another dose is indicated if a second exposure occurs to a susceptible person more than 3 weeks after receiving VZIG and the person has not yet shown symptoms.

Staff members and shelter guests with a prior history of chickenpox infection do not risk re-infection. Those staff members and guests who have received the chickenpox vaccination have a less than 15% risk of mild chickenpox infection. To reduce anxiety and confusion whenever there is a chickenpox outbreak in a shelter, we recommend that each staff or volunteer routinely document his or her chickenpox history in the health section of the personnel file.

Special Considerations for Family Shelters

When a case of chickenpox occurs in a family shelter, all new guests should be questioned about a history of chickenpox or vaccination before admission to the shelter. From the first day the rash appears on the initial case until 21 days after the last possible exposure, only individuals with a history of chickenpox infection or vaccination should be admitted to the shelter. This will protect unexposed individuals and hopefully will contain the outbreak to within one incubation period.

In some situations, admissions should be screened for 2 incubation periods, such as when the staff cannot be sure that all susceptible guests and staff have been exposed from the initial case. Screening people with unknown histories by one of the blood tests for immunity is an option if time permits. If an exposed guest has received VZIG, the incubation period should be extended to 28 days after the last possible exposure to the first case.

The incubation period also serves as a reminder not to discharge a guest who has no history of chickenpox infection or vaccination to other group settings until the time has elapsed. If a susceptible person is exposed to an active case, he or she may spread the virus to another setting during the incubation period.

Staff and guests should always wear gloves when handling linen and clothing of guests who have draining lesions of chickenpox or zoster. Everyone should be encouraged to wash his or her hands thoroughly following any contact with soiled items or draining lesions.

Special Considerations for Adult Shelters

If an infected person cannot be isolated from other guests, separate accommodations should be sought. Isolation is important until the lesions crust over and form scabs. If housing with an immune relative or friend is not available, an acute care facility may be another choice. We strongly recommend that any guest sent to alternative housing be closely followed for signs of complications of chickenpox.

Close contacts may be identified through bed lists and by interviews with the infected person. Vaccination or VZIG is recommended for all close contacts without a history of chickenpox. Such a thorough investigation may be difficult or impossible in the larger adult shelters. Those at particularly high risk should be the priority in those situations, such as people known to have HIV infection or other immune system problems.

Infected children or adults may have exposed others outside the shelter in day care, school, or work. Shelter staff and health care providers should work closely with the local board of health to help identify all other persons at risk.

Summary

Chickenpox, or varicella, is caused by the varicella-zoster virus, a virus that also causes shingles (herpes zoster). Chickenpox most commonly occurs in young children. Infection with the virus results in an itchy, blister-like rash that spreads over the entire body. A fever of up to 102°F (38.9°C) is also common. Both fever and rash usually disappear over 4 to 6 days. The virus then "goes to sleep" on nerve endings. Years later, the virus may reappear as zoster or shingles.

A safe and effective vaccine is available to prevent chickenpox, which all healthy non-immune persons and toddlers over one year of age should receive. Chickenpox can spread when an infected person breathes germs into the air or an uninfected person comes into contact with the fluid from open blisters of the rash.

In most cases, the symptoms of chickenpox are easy to treat. Itching can be relieved with calamine lotion and cool baths. Fever can be controlled with acetaminophen (Tylenol™). Aspirin and aspirin containing products should be avoided because they can have dangerous side effects when used for chickenpox symptoms. Always consult a doctor or nurse for proper diagnosis and treatment.

The illness is usually mild in young children who have no other health problems. However, adults and people with other medical problems can have very serious complications from the disease, such as infections of the lung or brain. Pregnant women and their babies are at particular risk.

Shelters and other places where many people live closely together may promote the spread of chickenpox. Shelter staff should discuss the potential dangers of exposure with a health provider familiar with the shelter. The local board of health should be contacted and will help to assess the risk to guests and staff in addition to instituting control measures to prevent further spread within the shelter. ■

*The authors of this chapter gratefully acknowledge
the invaluable contribution of Janet Groth, RN, MS,
who authored this chapter in the original Manual.*

Varicella Medication List

Generic	Brand Name	Cost
acyclovir	Zovirax	$
ibuprofen	Advil, Motrin	$

References

Pickering LK, Peter G, Baker CJ, et al., eds. *The 2000 Red Book: Report of the Committee on Infectious Diseases.* Elk Grove Village, Illinois: American Academy of Pediatrics; 2000:624-638.

American Academy of Pediatrics. Committee on Infectious Diseases. Recommendations for use of live attenuated varicella vaccine (RE9524). *Pediatrics* 1995;95(5):791-796.

American Academy of Pediatrics. Committee on Infectious Diseases. Varicella vaccine update (RE9941). *Pediatrics* 2000;105(1):136-141.

Chartrand SA. Childhood immunizations 2000; varicella vaccine. *Pediatric Clinics of North America* 2000;47(2): 373-394.

Chen TM, George A, Woodruff CA, et al. Clinical manifestations of varicella-zoster virus infection. *Dermatologic Clinics* 2002;20(2):267-282.

Seward JF, Watson BM, Peterson CL, et al. Varicella disease after introduction of varicella vaccine in the United States, 1995-2000. *Journal of the American Medical Association* 2002;287(5):606-611.

Watson B, Seward JF, Yang A, et al. Postexposure effectiveness of varicella vaccine. *Pediatrics* 2000;105(1):84-88.

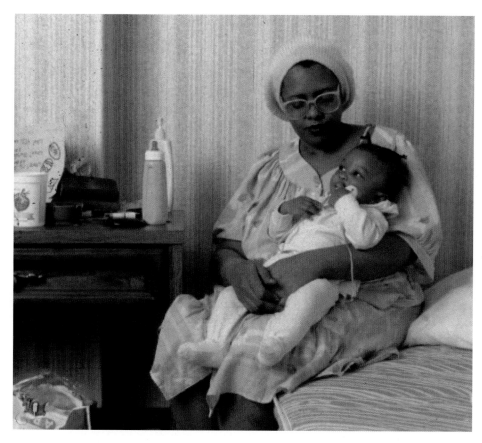

Viral Meningitis

Virginia A. Triant, MD, MPH

Viral meningitis is a central nervous system (CNS) infection characterized by signs and symptoms of meningeal inflammation in the absence of positive bacterial cultures. The incidence varies with season, and the clinical presentation often includes fever, headache, and nuchal rigidity (stiffness of the neck) accompanied by symptoms typical of the specific causal virus. Viral meningitis is usually self-limited and resolves without treatment, although case reports suggest that treatment is indicated and beneficial in certain clinical scenarios.

Viral meningitis should be differentiated from the broader category of aseptic meningitis. Although patients with aseptic meningitis by definition have negative bacterial cultures, the clinical picture of meningitis is not always caused by a virus and is not always infectious.

Diagnosing viral meningitis is complex for two reasons. First, a multitude of viruses can cause meningitis, each with its own characteristic mode of transmission, presentation, and work-up. Second, and more importantly, the presentation of viral meningitis may only differ slightly from that of bacterial meningitis, a life-threatening and highly contagious disorder that requires immediate recognition and treatment.

Prevalence and Distribution

Viral meningitis occurs with a peak monthly incidence of 1 per 100,000 persons in temperate climates. Reported cases are highest during the summer and early fall. The exact incidence is difficult to determine since many cases of viral meningitis are not reported to public health authorities. Many cases are probably undiagnosed because this self-limited disorder often resolves without progression of symptoms.

Enteroviruses are the most common cause of viral meningitis, accounting for 75-90% of cases. The enterovirus genus includes coxsackievirus, echovirus, poliovirus, and human enteroviruses 68 to 71. Other common causes of viral meningitis include herpes simplex virus-2 (HSV-2), human

Mother comforts her child despite the hardships of living in a sparse motel room. Photo by David Comb

Table 1: Causes of Viral Meningitis

Common	Less common	Rare
Enteroviruses	HSV-1	Influenza
HSV-2	CMV	Parainfluenza
HIV	EBV	Rotavirus
LCMV	VZV	Vaccinia
Arbovirus	Adenovirus	Encephalomyocarditis
Mumps	Measles	virus
	Rubella	

Note: HSV=herpes simplex virus;
HIV=human immunodeficiency virus;
LCMV= lymphocytic choriomeningitis virus;
CMV=cytomegalovirus; EBV=Epstein Barr virus;
VZV=varicella zoster virus

immunodeficiency virus (HIV), lymphocytic choriomeningitis virus (LCMV), arbovirus, and mumps virus. Less commonly, HSV-1, cytomegalovirus (CMV), Epstein Barr virus (EBV), varicella zoster virus (VZV), adenovirus, measles, and rubella cause viral meningitis. Rare causes of viral meningitis include influenza, parainfluenza, rotavirus, vaccinia, and encephalomyocarditis virus. Most cases of recurrent viral meningitis are caused by HSV-2. HSV-1 typically causes encephalitis rather than meningitis. Table 1 lists the causes of viral meningitis by frequency.

Enteroviruses are estimated to cause approximately 75,000 cases of viral meningitis in the USA annually. The rising prevalence of HSV-2 in the USA has led to recognition of this virus as a common cause of meningitis, with some estimates ranking it the second leading cause. LCMV is thought to account for 10-15% of cases of viral meningitis. The incidence of mumps meningitis has fallen by more than 95% since initiation of widespread vaccination measures. In the past, as many as half of the cases of aseptic meningitis were of unknown etiology, but better laboratory techniques have resulted in improved identification of a causal agent.

Some forms of viral meningitis occur with seasonal variation. Cases in the summer or early fall are most likely to be caused by enteroviruses or arboviruses. LCMV or mumps are the most probable causes during the winter months. Cases of HIV- and HSV-associated meningitis are not seasonal.

Depending on risk factors, certain groups are more likely to develop a particular form of meningitis or experience a more severe illness. For example, sexually active populations are more likely to develop HSV-2 or HIV meningitis. Unvaccinated individuals are at risk for meningitis caused by mumps, measles, or rubella. Finally, neonates (especially those less than 2 weeks of age) and adults with agammaglobulinemia who contract enteroviral meningitis tend to develop more severe cases.

Mode of Transmission

The mechanism of transmission of viral meningitis depends upon the specific viral etiology. Ninety percent of cases in which a specific virus is identified are caused by enteroviruses, which are transmitted via the fecal-oral route or through infected respiratory secretions.

HSV-2 is transmitted through contact with an active ulcerative lesion or contact with an infected host shedding HSV from a mucosal surface. HIV is transmitted via sexual contact or contact with infected blood. LCMV is contracted through contact with infected rodents or through contaminated environmental surfaces. Arboviruses are transmitted in the setting of tick bites, and mumps virus is spread via respiratory droplets.

Symptoms and Diagnosis

Classic symptoms of meningitis include fever, headache, and nuchal rigidity. Viral meningitis can present more sub-acutely than bacterial, with malaise, lethargy, myalgias, anorexia, nausea, vomiting, abdominal pain, or diarrhea. The headache in viral meningitis is often frontal or retro-orbital and can be associated with photophobia or

Figure 1:

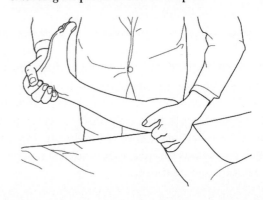

KERNIG'S SIGN

Elicitation: Flexing the patient's hip 90 degrees then extending the patient's knee causes pain.

pain on eye movement. While nuchal rigidity is usually present, it is frequently mild, occurring only near the limit of neck anteflexion (bending the neck forward so that the chin touches the upper chest).

Diagnosis can be confirmed by lumbar puncture and analysis of cerebrospinal fluid (CSF). CSF findings in viral and bacterial meningitis both reflect the presence of meningeal irritation but are otherwise quite distinct. Viral meningitis is characterized by an increased WBC count with a lymphocyte predominance, slightly elevated protein, and normal glucose. Early viral meningitis can show a neutrophil predominance, but the differential shifts towards lymphocytes within eight to 24 hours. Glucose is usually normal (greater than 50 percent of serum value) but can be moderately decreased in some cases of enterovirus, mumps, HSV, and LCMV. Assuming a non-traumatic tap, red blood cells are typically absent; however, they can be present in HSV-1 meningitis. In contrast, CSF findings in bacterial meningitis typically include a very high WBC count with neutrophil predominance, higher protein, and low glucose.

Polymerase chain reaction (PCR) is increasingly used to diagnose viral meningitis when routine viral cultures are negative. On average, CSF cultures are positive in only half of aseptic meningitis cases. In two-thirds of culture-negative cases, the specific viral etiology can be identified by PCR. With the present technology, PCR is routinely used to diagnose enterovirus, HSV, CMV, EBV, and VZV meningitis.

A brief discussion of the clinical presentations of some of the common viral causes of meningitis is merited, as identification of a specific viral etiology can direct treatment.

Enterovirus

In addition to an abrupt onset of headache, fever, nausea, vomiting, malaise, photophobia, and nuchal rigidity, enteroviral meningitis may present with herpangina, pleuritic chest pain, conjunctivitis, or abdominal pain. Enterovirus CSF cultures are positive in 40-80% of patients who undergo lumbar puncture, but incubation time ranges from 4-12 days. Enteroviruses can also be isolated from throat or stool specimens but can yield false positive results. CSF PCR for enterovirus, with a sensitivity of over 97% and a specificity of close to 100%, is the diagnostic test of choice.

HSV-2

Primary HSV-2 infection results in meningeal

Figure 2:

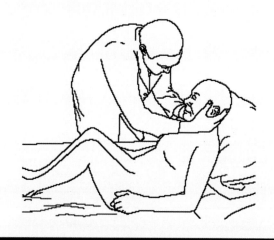

BRUDZINSKI'S NECK SIGN

Elicitation: Flexing the patient's neck causes flexion of the patient's hips and knees.

involvement in 13-36% of patients. Some studies have indicated that 25% of women and 11% of men with initial HSV-2 infection develop meningitis. On rare occasions, HSV-2 meningitis can present with severe but atypical symptoms of meningitis, such as urinary retention, paresthesias, focal weakness, or signs of ascending myelitis. The majority (85%) of patients with HSV-2 meningitis also have genital lesions that typically precede CNS symptoms by 7 days. While viral cultures are positive in 80% of cases of HSV-2 meningitis, HSV PCR is the diagnostic test of choice.

HIV

In 5-10% of new HIV diagnoses, meningitis is a component of the initial viral illness. This mononucleosis-like syndrome is characterized by fever, malaise, lymphadenopathy, rash, and pharyngitis. In contrast to other types of viral meningitis, HIV meningitis can present with seizures or cranial nerve palsies. Cranial nerves V, VII, and VIII are most commonly affected. While CSF cultures for HIV are often positive, diagnosis is more typically made by standard HIV testing. HIV meningitis tends to be self-limited.

LCMV

In LCMV meningitis, flu-like symptoms can accompany headache and meningeal signs. Rarely, patients can present with a rash, pulmonary infiltrates, alopecia, orchitis, parotitis, myopericarditis, or arthritis. CSF findings are typical of viral

Table 2: Differential Diagnosis of Viral Meningitis

Broad Category	Example
Bacterial meningitis	Leptospira sp. Borrelia burgdorferi Treponema pallidum Mycoplasma pneumoniae Rickettsia sp. Ehrlichia sp. Brucella sp. Chlamydia sp.
Fungal meningitis	Cryptococcus neoformans Coccidiodes immitus Histoplasma capsulatum
Parasitic meningitis	Toxoplasma gondii Angiostrongylus
Mycobacterial meningitis	
Bacterial endocarditis	
Parameningeal infections	Epidural or subdural abscess
Neoplastic	Carcinomatous meningitis Leukemias Lymphomas
Autoimmune	Sarcoid Behcet's disease SLE
Drug-induced	Nonsteroidal anti-inflammatory drugs (ibuprofen most common) Sulfa drugs Phenazopyridine Azathioprine Anti-CD3 monoclonal antibody Intravenous immune globulin

meningitis, with the exception of occasionally lower glucose and higher cell counts.

Mumps

Common features of mumps infection include orchitis, parotitis, and laboratory evidence of pancreatitis. However, the characteristic parotitis is present in only half of patients with mumps meningitis. Infection is more common in males, and documented prior infection excludes the possibility of current infection. In contrast to other viral meningitides, the CSF can show a neutrophilic pleocytosis and a decreased glucose.

Arbovirus

Arbovirus infections typically occur in clusters in a localized geographic region during the summer or fall. In addition to typical symptoms of viral meningitis, a history of tick exposure is often present.

The differential diagnosis of viral meningitis is critical because the signs and symptoms can be very similar to other forms of meningitis that are life-threatening if not treated promptly. It is critical for the clinician to distinguish bacterial and non-bacterial causes of meningitis. The severity of the clinical presentation and the analysis of the CSF findings are helpful in making this distinction. The presence of either or both of two classical signs, called the Kernig and Brudzinski signs, suggests a non-viral etiology of the meningitis. When a patient is supine or seated, a positive Kernig sign is the inability or reluctance to fully extend the knee when the hip is flexed 90 degrees as illustrated in Figure 1. Patients who spontaneously flex the hip during passive flexion of the neck have a positive Brudzinski sign as illustrated in Figure 2. Both tests were initially developed as diagnostic tools in chronic (e.g. tuberculous) meningitis but are now used to demonstrate the nuchal rigidity that is characteristic of acute bacterial meningitis. Profound alterations in consciousness, seizures, or focal neurological deficits are suggestive of a parenchymal rather than meningeal process.

Viral meningitis should also be differentiated from West Nile meningoencephalitis. From an epidemiological perspective, the risk of contracting West Nile virus increases more than twenty-fold in those over 50 years of age. In contrast, viral meningitis is common in the young as well as the elderly. While West Nile virus in its mild form can present with symptoms that resemble viral meningitis – malaise, headache, and gastrointestinal symptoms – it has several distinct clinical features. Unlike viral meningitis, meningoencephalitis caused by West Nile virus is characterized by severe muscle weakness, a diffuse flaccid paralysis, and diminished reflexes. In some cases it can resemble Guillain-Barre syndrome. In addition, nearly 20% of patients with West Nile virus have an erythematous rash. The differential diagnosis of viral meningitis is outlined in Table 2.

Treatment and Complications

Most cases of viral meningitis are self-limited and require only symptomatic treatment. Hospitalization is not usually necessary. Treatment with intravenous immunoglobulin is indicated in persons with humoral immunity deficiency and neonates with severe infection. Patients whose CSF or other clinical findings are ambiguous or suggest the possibility of non-viral meningitis should be treated promptly with antibiotics.

Anecdotal evidence supports the use of acyclovir (Zovirax™) to treat HSV meningitis and severe EBV or VZV meningeal infection. Controlled trial data are unavailable, and whether treatment decreases the severity or duration of symptoms or reduces complications remains unknown. Antiviral therapy is considered to be appropriate in the setting of primary HSV meningitis (versus recurrent) or for patients with severe neurological symptoms and signs. Therapy consists of IV acyclovir or oral acyclovir (Zovirax™), famciclovir (Famvir™), or valacyclovir (Valtrex™). Prophylaxis with acyclovir is indicated in patients who have frequent recurrences of HSV meningitis.

A new antiviral agent, pleconaril, is currently being investigated for the treatment of enteroviral meningitis. Previous trials have suggested that pleconaril shortens the duration of symptoms. Although a randomized placebo-controlled trial has shown the agent to be effective and safe for enteroviral meningitis, indications for its use are still being defined.

Prevention and Control

Prevention of viral meningitis can be achieved by reduction of risk factors and by vaccination strategies. The spread of HSV-2 and HIV can be reduced through education on how the viruses are transmitted and the promotion of strategies for preventing transmission, such as barrier protection during sexual contact and needle exchange programs. Meningitis from mumps, measles, and rubella, as well as VZV, can be prevented by vaccination.

Control of the spread of viral meningitis depends on the specific viral agent. Transmission of enterovirus meningitis, for example, can be decreased through basic hygiene techniques such as hand washing.

Special Consideration for Homeless Populations

Homeless populations living in shelters are at an increased risk of developing communicable diseases because of the large number of individuals with diverse exposures living in close quarters. Given the easy transmissibility of infectious diseases in shelter settings, it is imperative to identify serious and treatable infections early to prevent spread to co-habitants. Any individual with symptoms of meningitis should be emergently directed to medical attention so that bacterial meningitis can be ruled out by lumbar puncture. Despite signs of systemic viral infection, symptoms of meningitis should not be automatically ascribed to a viral etiology, as a concurrent bacterial infection may still be present.

Shelters are unique settings that can facilitate the screening of risk factors for preventable infections. Upon intake to a shelter, guests can be screened for a vaccination history and current medical conditions. Depending on the risk factor or medical history, guests can be offered education, counseling, or access to vaccinations.

Summary

- The differential diagnosis of viral meningitis is broad: always rule out non-viral causes first, as the untreated mortality rate of bacterial meningitis is very high.
- If there is any question about the etiology of meningitis, start antibiotics.
- Viral meningitis is usually self-limited.
- Cases vary seasonally, with enterovirus being the most common cause.
- A detailed history and physical exam help to hone the diagnosis.
- Hallmark symptoms include fever, headache, and stiff neck.
- Diagnosis is by lumbar puncture and CSF analysis.
- Viral PCR studies of the CSF are more sensitive and specific than routine cultures.
- Treatment is usually not indicated.
- Acyclovir (Zovirax™) is used for treatment and prophylaxis of HSV meningitis.
- New antiviral therapies are under investigation.
- Shelter settings can increase transmission of meningitis but facilitate risk factor assessment and prevention strategies. ■

The author of this chapter gratefully acknowledges the invaluable contribution of Jean Molloy, RN,C, MS, who authored this chapter in the original Manual.

Viral Meningitis Medication List		
Generic	**Brand Name**	**Cost**
acyclovir	Zovirax	$
famciclovir	Famvir	$$$
valacyclovir	Valtrex	$$$$

References

Johnson RP. Aseptic meningitis. UpToDate, 2003.

Johnson RP, Gluckman SJ. Overview of viral infections of the central nervous system. UpToDate, 2003.

Petersen LR, Roehrig JT, Hughes JM. West Nile virus encephalitis. *New England Journal of Medicine* 2002;347(16): 1225-1226.

Redington JJ, Tyler KL. Viral infections of the nervous system 2002: update on diagnosis and treatment. *Archives of Neurology* 2002;59(5):712-718.

Rotbart HA, Webster AD, Pleconaril Treatment Registry Group. Treatment of potentially life threatening enterovirus infections with pleconaril. *Clinical Infectious Diseases* 2001;34:72-77.

Tyler KL. West Nile virus encephalitis in America. *New England Journal of Medicine* 2001;344(24):1858-1859.

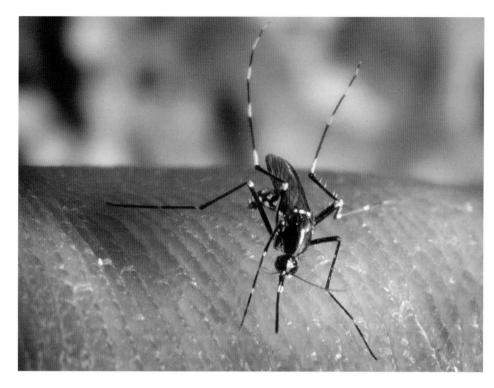

West Nile Virus & Other Mosquito-borne Infections

Emily Zielinski-Gutiérrez, DrPH

West Nile virus (WNV) can cause serious and sometimes fatal illness. This virus has been documented in the USA since 1999 and is most often spread through the bite of an infected mosquito. In 2002, WNV caused the largest epidemic of a mosquito-borne viral meningoencephalitis (severe neurological disease) ever recognized in the Western Hemisphere. In the USA, more than 4100 human WNV disease cases were reported from 740 counties in 39 states and the District of Columbia. The epidemic was focused in the central USA, from the Great Lakes to the Gulf Coast. Approximately 3000 individuals were hospitalized with central nervous system infection, with 284 fatalities. Intensive West Nile virus activity continued in 2003, with most cases reported in the Great Plains and immediately west of the Rocky Mountains. Updates on WNV activity can be found at: http://www.cdc.gov/westnile.

Other mosquito-borne viral infections in the USA include: St. Louis encephalitis (SLE); Eastern and Western equine encephalitis (EEE and WEE); and LaCrosse (LAC) encephalitis. Human illness due to these other viruses is less common than WNV, though occasional large outbreaks can occur. Dengue fever is a mosquito-borne virus that is an important health concern in Latin America and Asia. This disease has been seen on rare occasions in Hawaii as well as in Texas, usually along the border with Mexico.

Prevalence and Distribution

First seen in the greater New York City area in 1999, WNV has now become established throughout much of the USA and North America. By 2002, only 6 states (including Alaska and Hawaii) had not reported any WNV activity. It is likely that all lower 48 states will eventually report WNV activity. High levels of WNV activity with shifting geographic focal points are expected in the future. WNV transmission has also been reported in parts of Canada, Mexico, and the Caribbean. Less than 1% of all people exposed to a WNV-infected mosquito develop severe disease; the remainder show no or only mild symptoms. Based on surveys in which blood samples were taken in areas of virus activity, it is estimated that 60-2000 human WNV infections occurred for each reported hospitalized case. This suggests a total of 180,000 to 600,000

A female Aedes albopictus mosquito, also known as the Asian Tiger Mosquito, feeding on a human host. Photo courtesy of the CDC

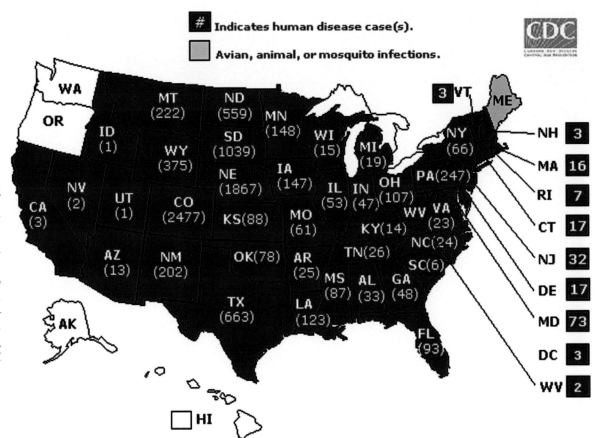

# Indicates human disease case(s).

Avian, animal, or mosquito infections.

CDC

WA

OR

MT (222)

ND (559)

MN (148)

ID (1)

SD (1039)

WI (15)

MI (19)

3 VT

ME

WY (375)

NE (1867)

IA (147)

NY (66)

NH 3

NV (2)

UT (1)

CO (2477)

KS(88)

IL (53)

IN (47)

OH (107)

PA(247)

MA 16

CA (3)

MO (61)

KY(14)

WV VA (23)

RI 7

CT 17

AZ (13)

NM (202)

OK(78)

AR (25)

TN(26)

NC(24)

SC(6)

NJ 32

DE 17

MS (87)

AL (33)

GA (48)

MD 73

TX (663)

LA (123)

DC 3

AK

FL (93)

WV 2

HI

WNV Map. Distribution of WNV infection during 2003. If WNV infection in any area of a state is reported to CDC Arbonet, that entire state is shaded accordingly, with the total number of human cases in parentheses. Courtesy of the CDC

human WNV infections in the USA during 2002 alone. Once infected with WNV, individuals probably develop long-lasting, if not lifelong, immunity to the virus.

Other mosquito-borne viral diseases in the USA have tended to be more regional. Between 1964 and 2000, there were 2776 cases of California serogroup virus infections (mainly LAC encephalitis) reported in 27 states, all in the eastern half of the USA. LAC encephalitis is traditionally active in the upper Midwest and Great Lakes states, with an increasing number of cases in Mid-Atlantic states. Only 182 human cases of Eastern equine encephalitis (EEE) were reported from 1964 to 2000, with an average of 5 cases each year, mostly occurring in the eastern half of the country. During that same period, 640 cases of Western equine encephalitis (WEE) have been reported; however, in the past 10 years less than 1 case per year has been reported. Like WNV, St. Louis encephalitis (SLE) is an "epidemic" arbovirus that has been responsible for more disease than the other domestic arboviral diseases: 4482 cases were reported from 1964 to 2000, with almost 2000 of those reported in 1975 alone. Cases have been reported in most states, with concentrations in the Midwest, Texas, and California. A significant outbreak of SLE occurred in northeastern Louisiana

in 2001. Maps, charts, and other information detailing the arboviral encephalitides can be found at: http://www.cdc.gov/ncidod/dvbid/arbor/arbocase.htm

Mode of Transmission

The most important route of WNV transmission, as well as other mosquito-borne viral diseases discussed here, is through the bite of an infected mosquito. The main cycle of WNV is between mosquitoes and birds. Mosquitoes become infected with the virus when they feed on a bird infected with WNV. Approximately 10 to 14 days after the mosquito bites the infected bird, the mosquito can transmit the virus to another bird or mammals, including humans. The mosquito injects the virus into the bird, animal, or person while taking a blood meal. As of 2002, WNV had been found to infect 36 species of mosquitoes and more than 160 species of birds. Many of these mosquito species are most likely to bite between dusk and dawn.

Other modes of WNV transmission are also possible but represent a very small percentage of cases. While the bite of an infected mosquito remains the most important means of transmission, investigations have confirmed that WNV can be spread through blood transfusion and transplanted

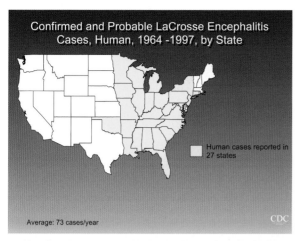

Confirmed and Probable LaCrosse Encephalitis Cases, Human, 1964 -1997, by State

Human cases reported in 27 states

Average: 73 cases/year

CDC

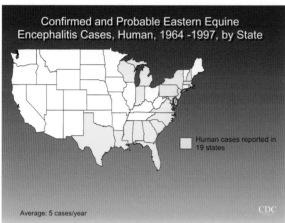

Confirmed and Probable Eastern Equine Encephalitis Cases, Human, 1964 -1997, by State

Human cases reported in 19 states

Average: 5 cases/year

CDC

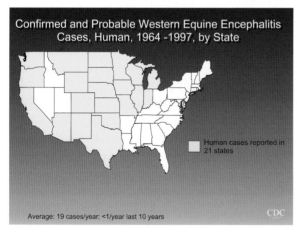

Confirmed and Probable Western Equine Encephalitis Cases, Human, 1964 -1997, by State

Human cases reported in 21 states

Average: 19 cases/year; <1/year last 10 years

CDC

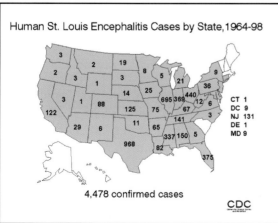

Human St. Louis Encephalitis Cases by State, 1964-98

CT 1
DC 9
NJ 131
DE 1
MD 9

4,478 confirmed cases

CDC

organs. Beginning in July 2003, all donated blood is screened for the presence of WNV. Transplacental (mother-to-child) WNV transmission has been reported, and possible transmission through breastfeeding (mother-to-child) has also been reported. Transmission of WNV and similar viruses to laboratory workers has also occurred on very rare occasions.

While no person-to-person transmission of WNV has been documented, transmission through shared, contaminated needles is a possibility. Touching or sharing utensils with a person infected with WNV does not pose a risk of infection. Evidence also suggests that mosquitoes are unlikely to become infected with WNV by biting a person infected with the virus, most likely because humans do not develop sufficient viremia (circulating virus in the bloodstream) to continue the transmission cycle.

Symptoms and Diagnosis

The incubation period for WNV, the time between infection from a mosquito bite until symptoms appear in humans, appears to range from 3 days to 2 weeks. About 80% of human WNV infections do not result in any symptoms or illness. 20% of infected individuals develop West Nile fever (WNF), but only 1 in 150 infected persons develops severe disease such as encephalitis or meningitis.

WNF can be difficult to distinguish from other viral infections. Symptoms of mild WNV disease include fever, headache, body aches, occasionally a skin rash on the trunk of the body, and swollen lymph glands. Symptoms of mild disease will generally last a few days and then resolve without treatment.

Severe disease associated with WNV outbreaks includes meningitis (inflammation of the membranes surrounding the brain), encephalitis (inflammation of the brain), or meningoencephalitis (inflammation of the brain and the surrounding membranes). More recent investigations have also described a polio-like syndrome associated with WNV, involving cases of acute flaccid paralysis. The symptoms of severe WNV disease include headache, high fever, neck stiffness, stupor, disorientation, coma, tremors, convulsions, muscle weakness, and paralysis.

Advanced age is by far the most significant risk factor for developing severe disease after infection. The risk of severe disease is greatest among people age 50 years and older.

CDC Arbonet Maps. These maps show the distribution of infection of LAC, EEE, WEE, and SLE during 2003. Updated maps are available from the CDC at http://www.cdc.gov/ ncidod/dvbid/arbor/ arbocase.htm.

Treatment and Complications

No specific treatment is yet available for WNV infection. Patients with severe disease often require hospitalization, which may involve intensive care and even mechanical ventilation. Although several potential treatments have been suggested for WNV encephalitis, no evidence is available yet to document the efficacy of these treatments.

Fatality rates among persons with severe WNV disease in the USA have remained constant at approximately 10% in 2000, 2001, and 2002. Advanced age is the most important risk factor for death, with patients older than 70 years of age at highest risk. In New York, persons 75 years and older were nearly nine times more likely to have a fatal outcome than younger persons. Encephalitis with severe muscle weakness and a change in the level of consciousness were also prominent clinical risk factors predicting fatal outcome. Some limited data suggest that certain pre-existing conditions, such as diabetes mellitus or immunosuppression, may be independent risk factors for death.

Many individuals hospitalized for severe WNV disease have substantial long-term complications. Among patients hospitalized in New York and New Jersey in 2000, more than half did not return to their previous level of function by the time of release from the hospital and only one-third were fully ambulatory. The New York City Department of Health performed a one-year follow-up of persons hospitalized with WNV disease in 1999 and found frequent and persistent symptoms, such as fatigue, memory loss, difficulty walking, muscle weakness, and depression.

Prevention and Control

Prevention and control of WNV and other arboviral diseases requires the education and use of protective measures by individuals, the control of breeding sites on the household or facility level, and the implementation of an Integrated Mosquito Management (IMM) Program on a community-wide level. IMM involves the monitoring of WNV activity in birds, animals, mosquitoes, and humans, and the use of mosquito control measures when appropriate.

The most effective way for individuals to avoid infection is to prevent mosquito bites. This can be accomplished in several ways:

- regular use of insect repellent on exposed skin and clothing when outdoors. Repellents containing DEET (N,N-diethyl-m-toluamide) are the most effective for use on exposed skin. Repellents containing permethrin or DEET can be used on clothing, as mosquitoes may bite through thin clothing;
- repellents containing DEET are very safe when used according to product instructions. Do not spray repellent with DEET under clothing;
- do not use permethrin directly on skin;
- products with a higher percentage of DEET (up to 50%) give longer protection. Products with more than 50% DEET do not offer additional protection;
- wearing protective clothing - long sleeves, long pants, and socks (especially when sprayed with repellent) - can further limit mosquito bites;
- avoiding exposure to mosquitoes during prime biting hours is another prevention step. Many species of mosquitoes actively bite between dusk and dawn. People should use precautions (repellent, protective clothing) especially during these hours or avoid the outdoors if possible.

Additional steps can be taken to limit mosquito populations by eliminating or controlling mosquito-breeding sites, such as containers with standing water. In specific areas where homeless persons spend significant periods of time, campaigns can be conducted to reduce disposable containers that breed mosquitoes. In addition, local mosquito control authorities can conduct larviciding or adulticiding (control of immature or mature mosquitoes) in those areas. Possible breeding sites located near shelters should be controlled. Even a small amount of standing water can be sufficient to allow mosquitoes to breed.

Keeping mosquitoes from indoor areas is another step in prevention. The installation or repair of window and door screens in shelters and soup kitchens, as well as other places frequented by homeless persons, can help limit the risk of mosquito-borne disease.

Special Considerations for Homeless Populations

Homeless populations may be at higher risk for WNV and other mosquito-borne diseases due to their increased exposure to the outdoors and their limited access to preventive measures. Health care providers should vigorously promote the use of insect repellents, especially for homeless persons over the age of 50. Repellent use for homeless

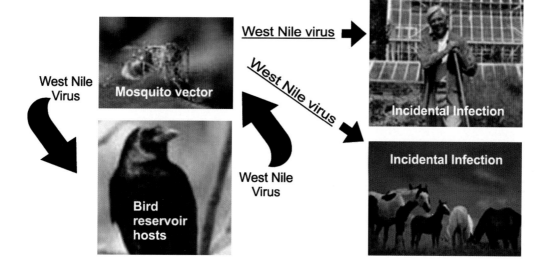

West Nile Virus Transmission Cycle

West Nile Virus

West Nile virus

West Nile virus

West Nile Virus

Mosquito vector

Bird reservoir hosts

Incidental Infection

Incidental Infection

WNV Cycle. Mosquitoes are the vector for WNV and birds are the usual reservoir. People, horses, and most other mammals are infected incidentally and are not reservoirs. Courtesy of the CDC

populations requires several special considerations:

- cost: access to insect repellents among persons with limited financial resources may be problematic. Some local or state health departments or mosquito control programs may be able to assist with repellent supplies or may have recommendations for lower cost products. Businesses that sell repellents may also be able assist shelters in obtaining repellents;
- personal hygiene: an additional concern for homeless populations may be limited opportunities to bathe between repellent applications. DEET is a very safe product when used as directed. While DEET can be reapplied when a person is still outdoors, most products recommend bathing when returning indoors. The availability of showering facilities is often limited for homeless persons, and this should be taken into consideration. The ability to follow directions and use the product safely is also a concern, if the product is made available for personal use;
- use of repellent on clothing: repellents with DEET or permethrin can be used on the clothing, which may be particularly useful for homeless populations. Protec-

tion from one permethrin application can last as long as 6 weeks, even through several launderings. As noted previously, permethrin should not be used directly on skin;

- For more information on safe use of repellents please consult:
  - Centers for Disease Control and Prevention: http://www.cdc.gov/ncidod/dvbid/westnile/qa/insect_repellent.htm
  - National Pesticide Information Center: http://npic.orst.edu/

Summary

West Nile virus and other mosquito-borne viral diseases, while relatively low in incidence, pose a significant risk to homeless populations due to their potential for mosquito bites and extensive exposure to the outdoors. Increased mosquito control and frequent application of repellent are considered critical for all vulnerable populations. All persons over the age of 50 are at higher risk for severe disease, which typically results in hospitalization. ■

The author would like to acknowledge the critical role of Ilanit Kateb, CDC, in reviewing and editing this chapter.

References

Campbell GL, Marfin AA, Lanciotti RS, et al. West Nile virus. *Lancet Infectious Diseases* 2002;2(9):519-529.

Centers for Disease Control and Prevention. Acute flaccid paralysis syndrome associated with West Nile virus infection -- Mississippi and Louisiana, July -- August 2002. *MMWR* 2002;51(37):833-836.

Fradin MS, Day JF. Comparative efficacy of insect repellents against mosquito bites. *New England Journal of Medicine* 2002;347(1):13-18.

Mostashari F, Bunning ML, Kitsutani PT, et al. Epidemic West Nile encephalitis, New York, 1999: results of a household-based seroepidemiological survey. *Lancet* 2001;358(9278):261-264.

New York Department of Health. West Nile virus surveillance and control: an update for healthcare providers in New York City. *City Health Information* 2001;20(2).

Petersen LR, Marfin AA. West Nile Virus: a primer for the clinician [review]. *Annals of Internal Medicine* 2002;137(3): 173-179.

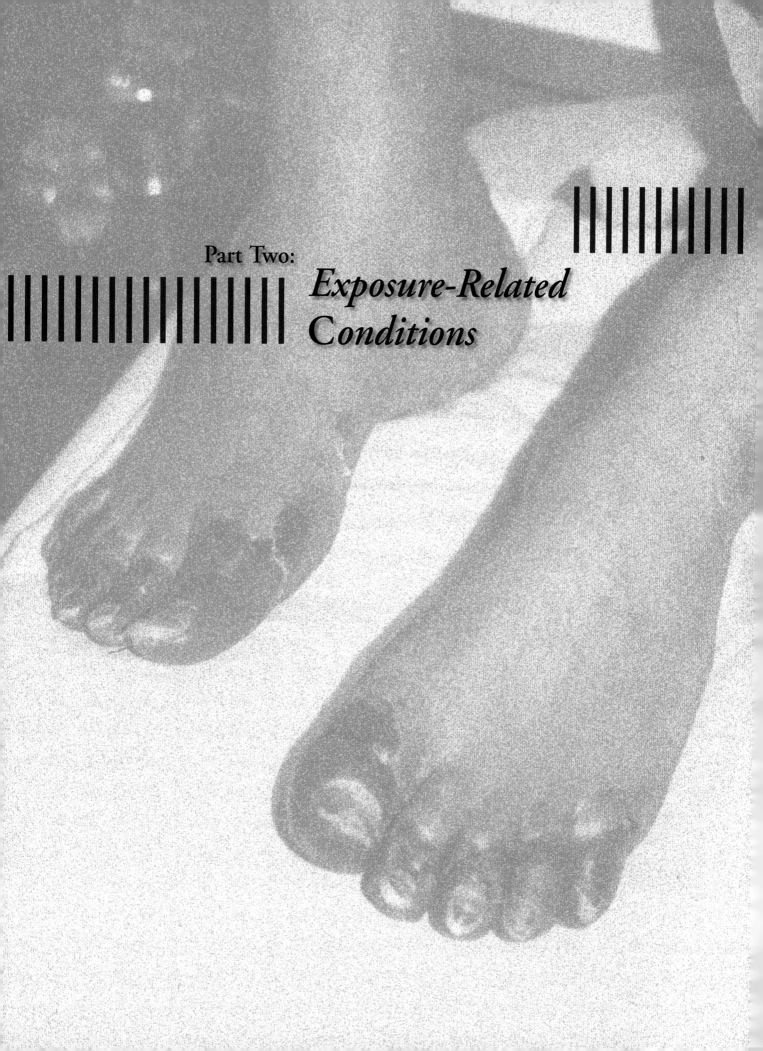

Part Two:
Exposure-Related Conditions

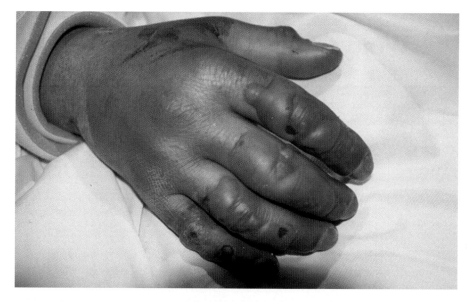

Accidental Hypothermia & Frostbite: Cold-Related Conditions

James J. O'Connell, MD
Denise A. Petrella, RN, CS, ANP
Richard F. Regan, PA-C

Mankind has struggled with injuries from the extremes of weather throughout history. While ancient physicians such as Hippocrates and Galen wrote extensively about hypothermia, most reports of cold injuries in the literature come from military history. Hannibal lost half of his army crossing the Alps in 218 B.C. During Napoleon's retreat from Moscow in the fall and winter of 1812, as many as 50,000 soldiers died of hypothermia. During the Great World Wars of the first half of the 20th century, ground troops on the march and in the trenches of Europe succumbed to the severe effects of the cold. High altitude frostbite was described in 1943, accounting for more injuries to heavy bomber crews in World War II than all other causes combined. And during the Korean War, 10% of the total US casualties were due to the cold.

Homeless persons who wander our urban cities and rural areas are vulnerable to the extremes of weather and exposure. Our goal in this chapter is to review how best to recognize, evaluate, and treat the common but preventable cold-related injuries of hypothermia and frostbite.

Hypothermia

During the twenty-year period from 1979-1998, hypothermia was the cause of death for approximately 700 persons annually in the USA, with half of these deaths attributed to extremely cold weather. Mortality rates in accidental hypothermia have ranged from 30-80%.

Hypothermia occurs not only during the bitter cold. Other important contributing factors include wind speed, moisture, alcohol, drugs, and the duration of exposure to the cold. Our worst case of hypothermia among Boston's homeless population occurred in early October several years ago, when a sunny day of 55°F (13°C) was followed by rain and a fall in temperature to 34°F (1.1°C) in the evening. Our patient's body temperature was 59°F (15°C), and he survived after undergoing cardio-pulmonary bypass therapy at Massachusetts General Hospital.

Definition and Pathogenesis

Hypothermia is defined as a core body temperature below 95°F (35°C), and can be helpfully categorized as follows:

- mild hypothermia: 90°-95°F (32°-35°C)
- moderate hypothermia: 82°-90°F (28°-32°C)
- severe hypothermia: below 82°F (28°C)

The body generates heat through the metabolism of food and water, the work of the muscles, and certain chemical reactions. The body's heat is lost primarily through the skin and lungs in four important ways:

- *radiation* accounts for 65% of heat loss.

Early Frostbite of the Hand. This man left the Accident Floor at Boston Medical Center on a clear January morning with a temperature of 18°F and no wind. We found him one hour later with frostbite of his fingers. This picture was taken several days later. The blisters are bloody, and he eventually lost two fingers. Photo by James O'Connell MD

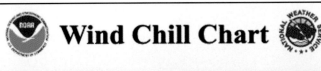

Wind Chill Chart

Wind (mph) \ Temperature (°F)	40	35	30	25	20	15	10	5	0	-5	-10	-15	-20	-25	-30	-35	-40	-45
5	36	31	25	19	13	7	1	-5	-11	-16	-22	-28	-34	-40	-46	-52	-57	-63
10	34	27	21	15	9	3	-4	-10	-16	-22	-28	-35	-41	-47	-53	-59	-66	-72
15	32	25	19	13	6	0	-7	-13	-19	-26	-32	-39	-45	-51	-58	-64	-71	-77
20	30	24	17	11	4	-2	-9	-15	-22	-29	-35	-42	-48	-55	-61	-68	-74	-81
25	29	23	16	9	3	-4	-11	-17	-24	-31	-37	-44	-51	-58	-64	-71	-78	-84
30	28	22	15	8	1	-5	-12	-19	-26	-33	-39	-46	-53	-60	-67	-73	-80	-87
35	28	21	14	7	0	-7	-14	-21	-27	-34	-41	-48	-55	-62	-69	-76	-82	-89
40	27	20	13	6	-1	-8	-15	-22	-29	-36	-43	-50	-57	-64	-71	-78	-84	-91
45	26	19	12	5	-2	-9	-16	-23	-30	-37	-44	-51	-58	-65	-72	-79	-86	-93
50	26	19	12	4	-3	-10	-17	-24	-31	-38	-45	-52	-60	-67	-74	-81	-88	-95
55	25	18	11	4	-3	-11	-18	-25	-32	-39	-46	-54	-61	-68	-75	-82	-89	-97
60	25	17	10	3	-4	-11	-19	-26	-33	-40	-48	-55	-62	-69	-76	-84	-91	-98

Frostbite Times: ▢ 30 minutes ▢ 10 minutes ▢ 5 minutes

$$\text{Wind Chill (°F)} = 35.74 + 0.6215T - 35.75(V^{0.16}) + 0.4275T(V^{0.16})$$

Where, T = Air Temperature (°F) V = Wind Speed (mph)

Effective 11/01/01

The most glaring example is the uncovered head, which can dissipate up to 50% of the body's heat;

- *conduction* is the direct transfer of heat to a nearby object that is cooler than the body. This is usually only a small fraction of the heat lost by the body, but wet clothing causes a 20-fold increase in heat loss from the body, and submersion in cold water increases the heat loss by 32 times;

- *convection* occurs when the warm layer of heat near the body is lost by the movement of air, and the degree of heat loss is dependent on the speed of the wind. For example, a wind of 12 mph increases heat loss by 5 times;

- *evaporation* is the heat lost when liquids are converted to gas. The evaporation of water cools the body at the rate of 0.6 kcal per gram. This occurs through sweating and respiration, which together account for about 20% of the body's heat loss.

When hypothermia occurs, cell membranes allow intracellular fluid to leak out, and enzymes begin to malfunction. Electrolyte imbalance occurs, especially hyperkalemia (increased potassium in the bloodstream). Water inside and outside the cells begins to crystallize, and cell death results. The hypothalamus attempts to stimulate heat production through shivering and by increasing catecholamine and adrenal activity. To minimize heat loss, blood flow to the peripheral tissues is reduced by vasoconstriction.

Causes of Hypothermia

In a study of 85 consecutive patients with hypothermia at San Francisco General Hospital, underlying infection or sepsis was the primary cause in 33 (39%) and alcohol ingestion in 27 (32%). Exposure accounted for only 9 cases. Almost half (49%) of these cases of hypothermia resulted in death.

Thus the differential diagnosis of hypothermia is important to keep in mind. In addition to environmental exposure, several medical conditions can either cause or increase the risk of hypothermia, including: sepsis, hypoglycemia, neuromuscular disease, malnutrition, hypothyroidism, and adrenal insufficiency. Some medications can hinder the body's response to the cold and increase the risk of hypothermia, such as beta-blockers (e.g. propranolol or Inderal™), clonidine (Catapres™), meperidine (Demerol™), and neuroleptics (e.g. haloperidol or Haldol™). Alcohol is particularly dangerous because it not only alters the ability to feel the cold

Table 1: Factors that predispose to hypothermia		
Environment		
	Time of year	
	Ambient temperature	
	Wind chill	
	Water chill	
Behavior		
	Inadequate or wet clothing	
	Immersion	
	Prolonged exposure	
	Lack of fitness	
	Fatigue	
	Inadequate shelter and heat	
Drugs		
	Alcohol	
	Nicotine	
	Opiates	
	Barbiturates	
	Benzodiazepines	
	Tricyclic antidepressants	
	Phenothiazines	
Decreased thermoregulation		
	Age extremes	
	Central nervous system trauma	
	Stroke	
	Wernicke's encephalopathy	
	Burns	
	Sepsis	
	Acute myocardial infarction	
	Chronic renal failure	
	Pancreatitis	
	Neoplasms	
Decrease heat production		
	Hypothyroidism	
	Hypoglycemia	
	Hypoadrenal states	
	Anorexia	

occur. Cardiac arrhythmias are common;

- *severe hypothermia*, below 82°F (28°C): hypotension, slow pulse, pulmonary edema, coma, ventricular arrhythmias (including ventricular fibrillation). The heart can stop beating completely (asystole or "flat line" on the EKG).

Diagnostic Evaluation

Early recognition is critical. Clinicians caring for homeless persons should maintain a high degree of suspicion for hypothermia whenever the weather turns cold. The astute clinician needs to be alert to any of the signs and symptoms described above. Most standard thermometers are not accurate below 93°F (34°C) and are not suitable for measuring the degree of hypothermia. The tympanic thermometers that are commonly used are unproven to date for assessing hypothermia.

The physical examination can be perplexing, especially in moderate and severe hypothermia. Patients can appear dead: comatose, the blood pressure difficult to hear, respirations shallow to absent, the pulse not palpable, the pupils dilated, deep tendon reflexes absent, and when shivering stops (usually around 85°-89°F or 30°-32°C) the muscle tone increases and can appear similar to rigor mortis. Helpful findings are signs of frostbite, sites

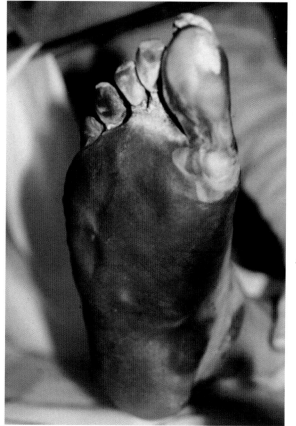

Plantar Frostbite. This elderly man slept for several cold nights in an abandoned car in South Boston. He has severe frostbite involving the toes and soles of his feet. Photo by James O'Connell MD

and impairs judgment, but also causes peripheral vasodilation that further enhances the loss of heat.

Symptoms and Clinical Presentation

Everyone caring for homeless persons in shelters and on the streets should become familiar with the signs and symptoms of hypothermia:

- *mild hypothermia*, 90°-95°F (32°-35°C): increased heart rate and respiratory rate, hyperventilation, difficulty walking, slurred speech, impaired judgment, pronounced shivering, and frequent urination due to the "cold diuresis";
- *moderate hypothermia*, 82°-90°F (28°-32°C): the pulse drops, breathing becomes shallow with a slowed respiratory rate, shivering stops, the reflexes are slowed, and the person can become very confused and disoriented. Paradoxical undressing may

Table 2: Interesting Hypothermia Facts
The half life of morphine is 1.5 hours at 98.6°F (37°C), but 36 hours at 77°F (25°C).
Pancreatitis is seen in about 50% of patients after they are warmed.
At core temp of 86°F (30°C), urine flow is three times normal.
With every 1°C drop in core body temperature: • blood flow in the brain decreases 7% • viscosity of blood increases 5% • hematocrit increases 2%
Advance life support protocols, especially defibrillation, may be ineffective when the core temperature is less than 86°F (30°C).

of insulin or drug injection, and evidence of head trauma. The rule is to assume that no one is dead "until warm and dead"; thus resuscitation efforts should continue until the body temperature reaches 90°-95°F (32°-35°C).

The medical complications of hypothermia are legion, and space limits our discussion. Laboratory studies should look for evidence of lactic acidosis, rhabdomyolysis, and bleeding disorders. Conduction is very slow through the cold myocardium, and the EKG can show prolongation of all intervals and a variety of arrhythmias, from atrial fibrillation to ventricular fibrillation. The characteristic elevation of the J point, called the Osborn wave, is a classic sign of hypothermia. Seen best in leads V2-V5, the height of the Osborn wave roughly corresponds to the degree of hypothermia.

Management

The management of hypothermia begins with an initial evaluation and, if indicated, CPR should be initiated. 911 should be called immediately. The prevention of further heat loss is paramount, such as removing wet clothing and covering the head with a hat.

Rewarming the person is the next step. However, the appropriate techniques are somewhat controversial and a subject of much debate. The three basic techniques are as follows:

- *Passive external rewarming.* This is the treatment of choice for mild hypothermia. After wet clothing is removed, the person should be covered with blankets or other insulation. This will limit further heat loss and allow the patient's body to generate heat and increase the core body temperature. Persons with mild hypothermia

should be able to generate heat through shivering.

- *Active external rewarming.* This means the utilization of warm blankets, warm baths, or heating pads to warm the patient. This is generally sufficient in moderate hypothermia, as well as for anyone who has failed to respond to passive external rewarming. There is a risk with this process which is called "afterdrop". When both the extremities and the trunk are warmed together, the cold blood which has been pooled in the extremities returns to the central circulation and can cause a drop in the core temperature. At the same time, peripheral vasodilation begins as the extremities are warmed, and this flow of blood away from the core can cause a sudden drop in blood pressure and result in dangerous arrhythmias. For these reasons, rewarming of the trunk should routinely be undertaken before the extremities.

- *Active internal rewarming.* Several treatment modalities are available for rewarming persons with severe hypothermia, and the most common include irrigation of the pleural and peritoneal spaces with warm fluids, hemodialysis, and cardiopulmonary bypass. These techniques can be augmented by the use of warm humidified oxygen, warm intravenous fluids, and bladder irrigation with warm saline.

CPR should be started on site and continued during transportation for anyone found with severe hypothermia and cardiac arrest. Since the cold has a protective effect on the brain during anoxia, attempts at rewarming should wait until after arrival at the hospital. Remember that persons with core temperatures as low as 57°F (14°C) have survived.

Hypothermia may be an insidious cause of death among homeless persons that is often overlooked. Mild hypothermia causes poor coordination and clumsiness, stiff joints and muscles, and confusion; this can lead to stumbling and falling as well as poor judgment that may cause accidents, drownings, and falls that result in death. The sequence of events leading to death can often be complex, and hypothermia should always be considered when the weather is cold.

Frostbite

Frostbite refers to local tissue freezing and injury that can occur with any degree of hypo-

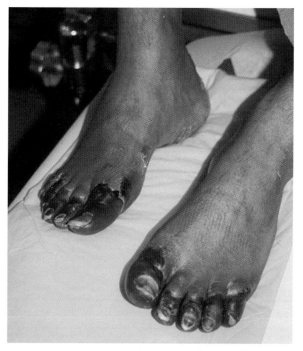
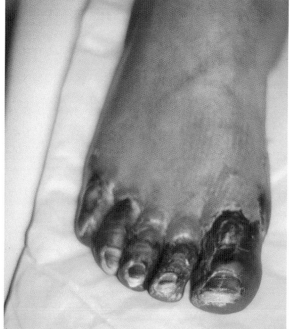
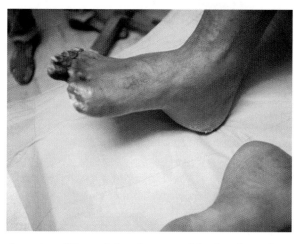
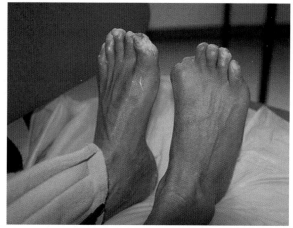

The Devastation of Frostbite.
This young man slept in the snow and sustained frostbite of all toes. These pictures show the course of his ordeal over a very painful 18 months at McInnis House.
Photos by James O'Connell MD

(clockwise)
1. Two Weeks. The toes are blackened and necrotic with marked eschar. Viable tissue is likely beneath this eschar, but the line of demarcation between dead and living tissue is not known at this time. The current standard of care is to wait for auto-amputation in order to preserve as much of the toes as possible.
2. One Month. The wound is clean and dry without evidence of infection. The eschar is beginning to separate from the viable tissue beneath.
3. Three Months. The eschar and necrotic tissue of the great toe are now separating in the process of auto-amputation. The metatarsal head is visible, and surgery was necessary to cover the exposed bone.
4. Eighteen Months. Resolution of the frostbite and the remaining viable toes.

thermia. "Frostnip" refers to cold-related tingling and numbness that is not associated with any tissue damage. The hands and feet are the most common sites (almost 90% of the time), followed by the ears, nose, cheeks, and penis. While most texts note that the very young and the elderly are at highest risk, frostbite is most common in adults from 30-50 years old. In extensive studies from the Scandinavian countries, frostbite has been associated with wet and improper clothing, a history of previous hypothermia or frostbite, wound infection, diabetes, and smoking. All of these factors are commonplace among persons struggling with homelessness, and clinicians need to be vigilant for frostbite during the cold weather.

Mechanisms of Tissue Injury

We now have a better understanding of the pathways that cause injury in frostbite. Three processes - *tissue freezing, hypoxia, and the release of inflammatory mediators* - occur at essentially the same time.

- The freezing of the tissue is accompanied by the formation of ice crystals that damage the cell membranes. Water then leaks out of the cells, leading to cellular dehydration and death.
- Peripheral blood vessels constrict in response to the cold, depriving the tissue of oxygen. The flow of blood in the capillaries ceases, leading to clotting or thrombosis within small arterioles and venules. This further exacerbates the hypoxia in the tissue.
- Inflammatory mediators are released in response to all of these insults: local tissue damage, hypoxia, and thrombosis. The most potent are the prostaglandins PGF2

Adapted from
Heggers JP,
McCauley RL, Phillips LG.
Cold-induced injury:
frostbite.
In: Herndon DN, ed.
Total Burn Care.
Philadelphia:
WB Saunders; 1996:
408.

Table 3.	Treatment of Frostbite
Patients with frostbite injuries are admitted to the hospital	
On admission, the affected area(s) will be rapidly rewarmed in circulating warm water, 104-108°F (40-42°C) for 15-30 minutes. Patients presenting 24 hours after injury will not be rewarmed.	
On completion of rewarming, the affected parts will be treated as follows:	

a. debride white blisters and apply topical aloe vera (e.g. Dermaide Aloe Cream™) every 6 hours to prevent further synthesis of thromboxane;

b. bloody or hemorrhagic blisters should be left intact and aloe vera (e.g. Dermaide Aloe Cream™) applied every 6 hours;

c. splint and elevate the injured area;

d. tetanus prophylaxis;

e. IV narcotics as needed;

f. ibuprofen 400 mg every 12 hours orally;

g. IV penicillin G 500,000 units every 6 hours for 48-72 hours to decrease potential streptococcal infection during the edema phase;

h. daily hydrotherapy for 30-45 minutes at 104°-108°F (40°-42°C);

i. avoid smoking, which causes vasoconstriction and can further aggravate the cold injury.

and thromboxane A2. These cause further vasoconstriction, depriving the tissue of yet more oxygen, and also cause platelet aggregation, exacerbating the thrombosis. The peak time for the release of these mediators is during the rewarming process.

The goal of treatment is to reverse or limit each of these processes. Rewarming can stop the tissue from freezing and reverse the vasoconstriction, while medications can block the release of the inflammatory mediators.

Diagnosis and Clinical Manifestations

The American College of Surgeons categorizes frostbite by the degree of tissue injury. This determination cannot be made until after rewarming, and sometimes it may take up to two weeks before the extent of damage is known.

- *First degree frostbite* is superficial and characterized by numbness, swelling, and a central white area surrounded by redness.
- *Second degree frostbite* is also superficial and accompanied by clear or cloudy blisters that develop over the first 24 hours after the injury. These blisters are usually surrounded by redness and swelling.
- *Third degree frostbite* involves bloody or hemorrhagic blisters that are a sign of deeper tissue injury. These blisters blacken and slough off about two weeks after the injury.
- *Fourth degree frostbite* affects muscle and bone and causes necrosis, gangrene, and

eventual loss of tissue. The long term sequellae are devastating, including amputation, chronic pain, and osteoarthritis.

Many clinicians prefer only two classes of frostbite: superficial (first and second degree) and deep (third and fourth degree). This practical approach acknowledges that the treatment of frostbite is the same for all degrees until the demarcation between the viable and non-viable tissue occurs 3-6 weeks later.

Regardless of the degree of injury, most persons with frostbite experience similar initial symptoms. The involved area feels cold and numb and can become clumsy. With rewarming, the numbness gives way to a severe throbbing pain that can last for many weeks. Some patients also describe a sensation of an "electric shock" running through the affected area. The frostbitten area often develops sensory loss and an increased cold sensitivity which can last for years. Arthritis and chronic neuropathic pain can occur after deep frostbite in an area.

Treatment

The goal of treatment is to salvage tissue by reversing the effects of tissue freezing, hypoxia, and the release of inflammatory mediators. The three phases of treatment for frostbite are described in this section.

Pre-Thaw Phase

The aim of this initial phase is to avoid thawing and re-freezing, which magnifies tissue damage. Wet clothing should be removed from the affected area. In urban areas with hospital availability, do not try to thaw in the field. The affected area should be wrapped in lose clothing and splinted to avoid trauma. Try to minimize movement of the area. Never rub or massage the area. Do not use heating pads or heat lamps because the frostbitten area is without sensation, and serious burns can easily occur.

Hospital Care Phase

Rapid rewarming is the cornerstone of treatment in this phase. The affected area should be warmed in water at 104°-108°F (40°-42°C). Mild antibacterials such as hexachlorophene or providine-iodine may be added. The rewarming process can be very painful, especially if this is done too quickly. Narcotics should be used for pain control as needed. Rewarming is complete when the skin becomes pliable and has a reddish-purple color.

Once rewarming is completed, continued immediate treatment is crucial to minimize tissue damage. Unfortunately, many homeless persons present for care of frostbite long after the initial damage and after the affected area has been warmed. No treatment protocol has been uniformly endorsed for the immediate treatment of frostbite after rapid rewarming. Many clinicians have adapted aspects of McCauley's protocol:

- debride white blisters, and apply topical aloe vera (e.g. Dermaide Aloe Cream™) every 6 hours to prevent further synthesis of thromboxane;
- bloody or hemorrhagic blisters should be left intact and aloe vera (e.g. Dermaide Aloe Cream™) applied every 6 hours;
- splint and elevate the injured area;
- tetanus prophylaxis;
- IV narcotics as needed;
- ibuprofen 400 mg every 12 hours orally;
- IV penicillin G 500,000 units every 6 hours for 48-72 hours to decrease potential streptococcal infection during the edema phase;
- daily hydrotherapy for 30-45 minutes at 104°-108°F (40°-42°C);
- avoid smoking, which causes vasoconstriction and can further aggravate the cold injury.

Early surgery is not indicated for the treatment of frostbite unless a fasciotomy is required to treat a compartment syndrome.

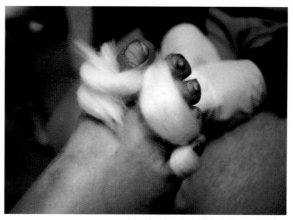

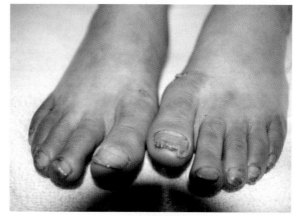

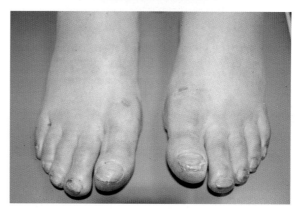

Early Frostbite. (top) BHCHP nurse practitioner Denise Petrella noted early frostbite on the toes of a man who came to the shelter clinic with a cold. He was admitted to McInnis House for care. (middle) Improvement at one week. (bottom) Resolution at two weeks. Photos by James O'Connell MD

Post-Thaw Care Phase

The goal of this phase is two-fold: 1) to prevent secondary infection and 2) to support the homeless patient through a painful period of difficult medical decisions and great psychological stress, especially for those with severe frostbite who await the possible auto-amputation of digits or fingers.

In severe frostbite, an eschar forms in 9-15 days that is hard, black, and leathery. Over time (usually 22-45 days) the underlying tissue demarcates, and the viable tissue begins to separate from the non-viable eschar.

Patients should be monitored carefully for purulent drainage, which can be a sign of cellulitis or a deeper infection of the bone called osteomyelitis. Wound care is needed for the shallow ulcers caused by blister formation. At our Barbara McInnis House in Boston, we have found that a thin coat of silver sulfadiazine cream (Silvadene Cream™) with a clean dressing twice each day protects and quickly dries the wound.

Severe frostbite can cause a very painful peripheral neuropathy. Narcotics are usually required for pain control, but with time these can be tapered if other neuropathic pain medications such as gabapentin (Neurontin™) are effective.

Amputation is often the most vexing problem, primarily because of the difficulty in predicting the severity of underlying injury. There is much wisdom to the adage: "freeze in January, amputate in July." In our experience at McInnis House, most fingers and toes that have suffered severe frostbite will mummify and autoamputate in 3-6 weeks, but some have taken far longer. To avoid this prolonged and stressful period of watching and waiting, there is considerable hope that certain imaging techniques will be able to accurately measure the extent of damage within the first week or two of injury. The use of technetium scintigraphy and MRI are among the possible future approaches, and the goal remains to maximize stump length while guiding early surgical intervention.

The complications of frostbite include residual pain, cold and heat intolerance, hyperhydrosis (increased sweating in the area), atrophy of the skin, and pigment changes.

We have seen a broad range of these complications at McInnis House, where we have admitted over 100 persons with frostbite over the past decade. One patient complained bitterly of severe "phantom pain" in the left foot for several months after losing three toes to frostbite. We initially suspected drug-seeking, but he underwent surgical sympathectomy in which several sympathetic nerves were severed. He almost immediately stopped asking for further pain medication. Several years later he returned to McInnis House with another episode of frostbite and lost several more toes during a six-month admission. He again suffered intense pain, which resolved when he underwent a new procedure called spinal cord stimulation. In this operation, an electrode is placed directly in the spine and a wire tunneled under the skin to a transducer. This gentleman is now able to directly stimulate the spine whenever the pain occurs, and this has replaced all of his previous pain medication.

Summary

Accidental hypothermia can be a life-threatening condition that affects virtually every organ system in the body. Hypothermia is defined as a body temperature below 95°F (35°C).

Hypothermia does not occur only during the bitter cold. Other important contributing factors include the wind speed, moisture, alcohol and other drugs, and the duration of exposure to the cold.

Several risk factors can cause homeless and other people to be more susceptible to hypothermia, including malnutrition, underlying infection, low blood sugar, neuromuscular disease, and certain medications.

Early recognition of hypothermia is very critical, and the treatment includes resuscitation and rewarming. Anyone with hypothermia should be brought to the hospital as soon as possible.

Frostbite is cold-induced tissue injury that usually affects the hands and feet, but can also involve the ears, cheeks, nose, and penis.

Frostbite can be superficial or deep. Deep frostbite can result in the amputation of fingers or toes or other affected areas.

The best treatment of both frostbite and hypothermia is prevention. Wear a hat and gloves in the cold, as well as layered clothing. Remember that frostbite occurs much more rapidly on windy and wet days. ∎

Frostbite Medication List

Generic	Brand Name	Cost
sulfadiazine cream	Silvadene	$
aloe vera	Dermaide Aloe Cream	$
gabapentin	Neurontin	$$$$

References

American College of Surgeons, Committee on Trauma. *Advanced Trauma Life Support.* Chicago, IL: American College of Surgeons; 1997.

Centers for Disease Control and Prevention. Hypothermia-related deaths - Philadelphia, 2001, and United States, 1999. *MMWR* 2003;52(5):86.

Heggers JP, McCauley RL, Phillips LG. Cold-induced injury: frostbite. In: Herndon DN, ed. *Total Burn Care.* Philadelphia: WB Saunders; 1996:408.

Mechem CC. Accidental hypothermia. UpToDate, 2004. http://www.uptodate.com

Morris DL, Chambers HF, Morris MG, Sande MA. Hemodynamic characteristics of patients with hypothermia due to occult infection and other causes. *Annals of Internal Medicine* 1985;102:153-157.

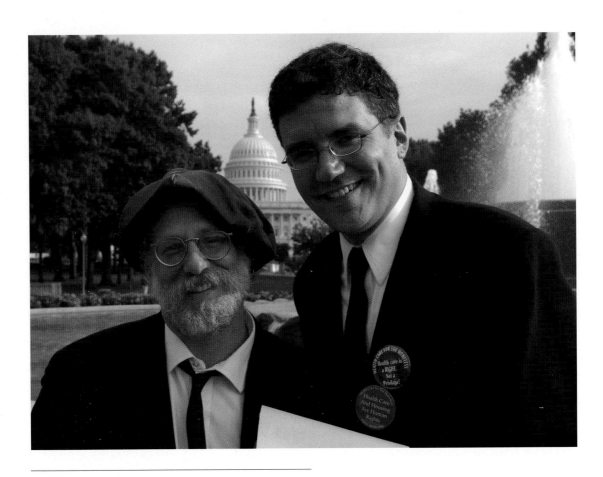

Jeff Singer, President and CEO of Maryland's Health Care for the
Homeless, Inc., with Kevin Lindamood, Director of Community
Relations, at the 2003 National Health Care for the Homeless
Council Rally in Washington, DC.
Photo by James O'Connell MD

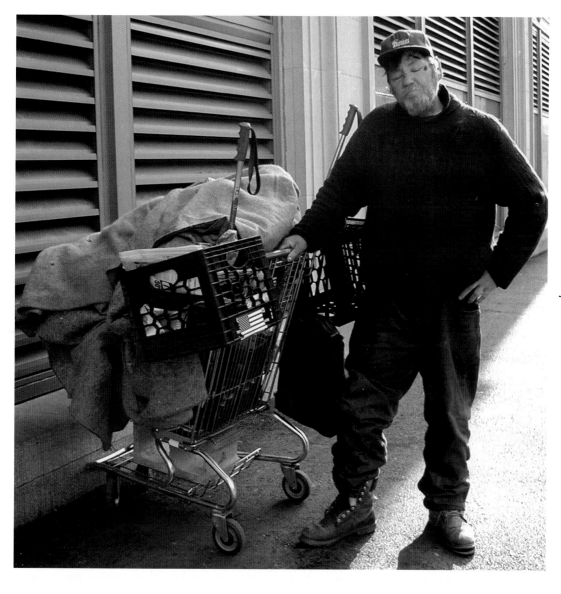

Hyperthermia & Heat Stroke: Heat-Related Conditions

Joseph Rampulla, MS, APRN,BC

H eat-related conditions occur when excess heat taxes or overwhelms the body's thermoregulatory mechanisms. Heat illness is preventable and occurs more commonly than most clinicians realize. Heat illness most seriously affects the poor, urban-dwellers, young children, those with chronic physical and mental illnesses, substance abusers, the elderly, and people who engage in excessive physical activity under harsh conditions. While considerable overlap occurs, the important syndromes are: heat stroke, heat exhaustion, and heat cramps. Heat stroke is a life-threatening emergency and occurs when the loss of thermoregulatory control results in hyperpyrexia (very high fever) and severe damage to many internal organs.

The exposure to the heat and the concrete during the hot summer months places many rough sleepers at great risk for heat stroke and hyperthermia. Photo by Sharon Morrison RN

Epidemiology

Heat illness is generally underreported, and the true incidence is unknown. Death rates from other causes (e.g. cardiovascular, respiratory) increase during heat waves but are generally not reflected in the morbidity and mortality statistics related to heat illness. Nonetheless, heat waves account for more deaths than all other natural disasters combined in the USA. The elderly, the very poor, and socially isolated individuals are disproportionately affected by heat waves. For example, death records during heat waves invariably include many elders who died alone in hot apartments. Age 65 years, chronic illness, and residence in a poor neighborhood are all associated with higher risk of death during heat waves.

From 1979 through 1999, 8015 deaths in the USA were directly attributed to excessive environmental heat exposure. During the 7-day Chicago heat wave of 1995, the death rate increased by 85%, with the majority of deaths among the poor and socially isolated. Interestingly, northern cities have greater increases in death rates during hot weather than southern cities. Northern cities have wider swings in temperature, fewer air conditioners, and the citizens are not as well acclimated to the heat.

Thermoregulation

Metabolism, muscle activity, and the environmental temperature all contribute to the generation and maintenance of body heat. When the body temperature rises, peripheral vessels dilate and cardiac output increases, shunting blood flow closer to the surface of the skin where it can be cooled. Sweating provides water on the skin's surface, which then evaporates and further cools the body. This cooling process by evaporation depends on the gradient between the body temperature and the atmospheric temperature. Humidity and high environmental temperatures hinder heat dissipation. Behavioral factors play an important role in cooling, including seeking a cooler environment or shade from the sun, reducing physical activity, and replacing the water and salt lost through sweating. People with impaired mobility or impaired judgment may not be able to engage in these behaviors, and are at risk for heat illness.

After 7-14 days of persistent heat exposure, the body becomes acclimated and adjusts to the heat through increased sweating, avid retention of salt by the kidneys, and an increase in cardiac stroke volume. Even with adequate water and salt intake, homeostatic mechanisms may break down and cause severe hyponatremia and cerebral edema.

Heat Disorders

When the body's ability to dissipate heat is overwhelmed and/or too much water and salt are lost, the core body temperature rises and several distinct heat syndromes may develop (see Table 1). Many risk factors can increase a person's susceptibility for developing a heat syndrome, including: generalized skin conditions (e.g. sunburn, psoriasis) that interfere with sweating; dehydration; alcoholism; mental illness; cardiopulmonary disease; and age

greater than 65. In addition, children absorb more heat relative to their body mass and do not sweat as much as adults, thereby rendering them particularly vulnerable to heat disorders. Asphalt and concrete in cities absorb and retain heat, creating the "urban heat phenomenon" which also interferes with nighttime cooling in cities. Numerous drugs affect heat dissipation and heat production, most notably anticholinergics, beta-blockers, antipsychotics, tricyclic antidepressants, lithium, ethanol, and diuretics. Stimulants also generate excess heat: cocaine, amphetamines, MDMA (Ecstasy), and supra-therapeutic doses of thyroxine (see Table 2).

Heat Stroke

Heat stroke is a life-threatening febrile illness due to the breakdown of the body's heat control systems and the subsequent acute immunologic and metabolic reactions to elevated body temperatures. When simple exposure to high environmental temperature overwhelms thermoregulatory mechanisms, the condition is called "classic" or non-exertional heat stroke. When the body temperature rises in a healthy person who exercises strenuously in a hot environment, this is referred to as "exertional heat stroke."

Risk factors may be present but are not requisite. The onset of heat stroke is rapid, and patients may have a prodrome of weakness, headache, chills, ataxia, and nausea. Chest pain may be present, as well as shortness of breath and abdominal pain. Thirst is not a reliable indicator of impending heat stroke. The body temperature rises rapidly, sweating ceases, and multiple system failure ensues (usually heralded by neurological problems). An acute phase inflammatory reaction appears to be involved in the progression from heat exhaustion to heat stroke.

During heat stroke fever is 104°F (40°C) or greater. Sweating usually ceases and the skin becomes hot and dry. Confusion, delirium, and ataxia are followed by loss of consciousness. Some patients will have seizures that usually occur during cooling. Tachycardia and hyperventilation are common vital sign changes. Laboratory examination reveals an elevated hematocrit (secondary to hemoconcentration), electrolyte and acid-base disturbances (typically hyponatremia, metabolic acidosis, and hypokalemia), and evidence of muscle, renal, and hepatic damage. The electrocardiogram and cardiac enzymes may indicate myocardial injury. Thrombocytopenia can be profound if disseminated intravascular coagulation has occurred.

Table 1: Major Heat Syndromes

Disorder	Mechanism	Clinical	Treatment	Comments
Heat Stroke				
Classic: Inability to compensate for hot environment. Occurs in patients with impaired homeostatic mechanisms Exertional: Failure to dissipate the heat generated by strenuous exercise. Occurs in otherwise healthy persons who overexert under heat stress conditions	Failure of thermoregulatory systems resulting in severe hyperthermia and multi-system damage Usually accompanied by electrolyte imbalance and cardiac arrythmias. Often seizures, neurological damage, DIC, rhabdomyolysis, renal and hepatic failure	Often rapid onset May be preceded by headache, nausea, weakness, and myalgias High fever 105°-107°F (40.6°C - 46.7°C) Dilated pupils Hot dry skin Lack of sweating (classic) Confusion, ataxia and/or loss consciousness Fast thready pulse Hypotension Heart failure	Support airway, breathing, & circulation Patient must immediately be moved to a cooler environment and transported to the hospital Hospital treatment consists of aggressive cooling, fluid and electrolyte replacement, and support of vital functions	Highly lethal 20% or more have residual neurological damage Patients with exertional heatstroke may continue to sweat
Heat Exhaustion				
Fluid and electrolyte imbalance due to sweating resulting in hypovolemia	Water and/or salt depletion from excessive sweating that is inadequately replaced Hypovolemia causes weakness and collapse	Insidious or sudden onset Weakness, lightheadedness, syncope, sweating, nausea Low-grade fever Pale, cool, clammy skin Sweating Thready pulse Low BP May be ataxic and confused	Patient should lie down in a cool area Fluid and salt should be replenished. Slightly salty or sports drinks can be given in sips over 2-4 hours. IV's needed if very ill or unable to take oral fluids	May be similar in presentation to insulin shock, alcohol/drug abuse/withdrawal, or hypovolemia from occult blood loss Usually benign, but may progress to heat stroke

Therapy includes immediate cooling, support of failing organ systems, and repletion of fluids with correction of electrolyte abnormalities. Time is critical, and patients should be immediately transported to a hospital. If possible, remove the patient from the hot environment while awaiting the ambulance. Once airway, breathing, and circulation are secure, cooling should begin as soon as possible. This includes removal of clothing, applying water and ice to the skin, and fanning. The initial target temperature is 102°F (38.9°C).

Any individual with a history of heat stroke is at increased risk for future episodes.

Heat Exhaustion

Heat exhaustion is profound weakness caused by the loss of water and salt due to sweating during heat exposure. The manifestations of heat exhaustion can be similar to several other conditions, including insulin shock, hyperthyroidism, toxic ingestions, alcohol withdrawal, arrhythmias, and hypovolemia from bleeding or diarrhea. The major signs and symptoms of heat exhaustion are thirst, malaise, headaches, myalgias, shortness of breath, and nausea. Most patients with heat exhaustion are alert, although anxiety is common and some people become slightly confused. The vital signs may show

Table 2: Medications Affecting Heat Regulation

Drug	Mechanism	Comments
Anticholinergics benztropine (Cogentin™) atropine	Decreases cholinergic mediated sweating Increases heart rate	Often given to counteract the side-effects of antipsychotics
Antihistamines diphenhydramine (Benadryl™)	Anticholinergic Antihistamine	Newer antihistamines less of a problem
Tricyclic Antidepressants amitryptiline (Elavil™) imipramine (Tofranil™)	Anticholinergic	
Antipsychotics **Phenothiazines** chlorpromazine (Thorazine™) fluphenazine (Prolixin™) **Butyrophenones** haloperidol (Haldol™) **Atypical Antipsychotics** clozapine (Clozaril™) risperidone (Risperdal™) olanzapine (Zyprexa™)	Anticholinergic Antihistamine Dopamine blocking	Specific antipsychotics vary in anticholinergic properties Often taken together with other anticholinergics with an additive effect Increased involuntary muscle activity can increase body temperature Increased thirst can lead to water intoxication Neuromuscular Malignant Syndrome is a febrile idiosyncratic reaction to antipsychotics that is similar to heat stroke
Beta-blockers	Reduced cutaneous blood flow	
Diuretics hydrochlorthiazide (HCTZ™) furosemide (Lasix™)	Increased excretion of salt and water	Patients with underlying cardiovascular disease at higher risk from heat stress
Ethanol	Dehydration from diuresis Impaired judgement and awareness	Adrenergic and muscle hyperactivity occur during alcohol withdrawal increasing heat production
Lithium	Increased excretion of salt and water	Patients on lithium should increase both salt and fluid intake during hot weather
Stimulants cocaine amphetamine	Increases adrenergic and muscle activity with increased heat production	Deaths from cocaine overdose increase during heat waves

a normal or slightly elevated temperature with a thready pulse and orthostatic hypotension. The exam generally reveals cool and moist skin, and the legs may be swollen if prolonged standing preceded the episode.

The patient should lie down in a cool area. Fluid and electrolytes can usually be replaced with small frequent sips of slightly salty fluid over several hours. Salt, juice, and water can be added to ginger ale to give it a salty taste. Premixed sports drinks such as Gatorade™ are adequate. Intravenous saline is needed for acutely ill patients and those unable to take oral fluids. Untreated heat exhaustion can progress to heat stoke if sweating stops. Patients should be advised to avoid heat and exertion for at least 24 hours after an episode of heat exhaustion. Eating salted foods and drinking enough fluid can prevent heat exhaustion.

Heat Cramps

Heat cramps are deep and painful spasms in the most actively used muscles and are a direct result of salt depletion. The affected muscles harden and become tender. Spasms of the upper or lower extremities can be debilitating, and abdominal muscle spasms may mimic an acute abdomen. Patients should move to a cool area and replenish salt and fluid. Eating salted foods and drinking enough fluid in the heat can usually prevent heat cramps.

Sunburn

Sunburn is not considered a heat disorder but occurs with overexposure to ultraviolet (UV) sunrays. The skin becomes tender and reddened several hours after exposure and may blister and later peel. Limiting skin exposure to direct sunlight, especially at midday, and the application of a sunscreen are the best ways to prevent sunburn. Para-aminobenzoic acid (PABA) and/or benzophenone-containing sunscreens, with a sun protection factor (SPF) rating of 15, should be applied 30-45 minutes prior to exposure to the sun. Opaque zinc oxide and titanium oxide creams can be used to completely block sunrays in highly exposed areas like the bridge of the nose. Cool moist compresses are soothing, and aspirin or non-steroidal anti-inflammatories help relieve mild to moderate discomfort. Corticosteroids may be needed for more severe sunburns.

Special Considerations for Homeless Populations

Simple community and individual measures, based on the awareness of keeping cool and drinking plenty of fluids during hot weather, can effectively prevent heat disorders. Shelter and street outreach nurses should be trained to detect the early signs of heat illness and intervene promptly. Educational materials for staff and shelter guests can be very effective. All clinicians should ask their patients how they cope with the heat and discuss with them how to seek cool places and drink fluids during hot days. Ideally, vulnerable homeless persons should go to shelters with air-conditioning when the weather is hot. Formerly homeless individuals who live alone in hot rooms are more vulnerable to heat illness than persons living outdoors or in shelters. These vulnerable individuals include those living in group homes for the mentally ill or congregate living programs, as well as families with young children housed in motels. Whenever possible, we recommend that clinicians schedule at least one office visit and possibly a home assessment in the spring or early summer for all newly-housed patients. Plans to deal with the heat can be reviewed at that time. The vulnerability for heat-related illness should be an essential part of the risk assessment performed by clinicians who visit families housed in hotels. Cool baths or showers can help dissipate heat for those living in rooms without air-conditioning. Individuals suffering from paranoia or impaired temperature perception frequently wear heavy winter clothes on hot days and are extremely susceptible to heat-related illness. Many of these individuals are amenable to a creative discussion about dressing more lightly. Remind patients taking psychotropic medications to avoid excess heat. Advise parents not to leave children alone in hot rooms or vehicles. Counsel patients to avoid swimming when intoxicated.

Local regions vary in the specific criteria for instituting public health warnings and activating response systems. In Boston, community cooling centers are opened whenever the temperatures are expected to reach 90°F (32.2°C) or more for 3 consecutive days.

Hydration is clearly critical during hot weather. Individuals with poorly controlled diabetes and alcoholism are often chronically dehydrated. Remind patients to drink water, sodas, or sports drinks throughout the day. Many patients restrict their fluid intake because of a lack of bathroom facilities in the city, and a discussion about safe and available places to urinate is helpful.

Excess sun exposure and heavy physical exertion should always be avoided in the hot weather and especially during the hours before and after noon. Sun-blocking creams should be readily available in clinics as well as in the shelters.

Many homeless people obtain daily work through labor pools and often this requires strenuous work for many hours. These individuals should be counseled about ways to keep hydrated while avoiding overheating at their job sites. ▓

Heat-Related Syndromes Medication List

Generic	Brand Name	Cost
amitryptyline	Elavil	$
benztropine	Cogentin	$
chlorpromazine	Thorazine	$
clozapine	Clozaril	$$$$$
diphenhydramine	Benadryl	$
fluphenazine	Prolixin	$$
furosemide	Lasix	$
haloperidol	Haldol	$
hydrochlorothiazide	HCTZ	$
imipramine	Tofranil	$
olanzapine	Zyprexa	$$$$$
risperidone	Risperdal	$$$$$

References

Bouchama A, Knochel JP. Heat stroke. *The New England Journal of Medicine* 2002;346(25):1978-1988.

Centers for Disease Control and Prevention. Heat-related deaths - four states, July-August 2001, United States, 1979-1999. *MMWR* 2002;51(26):567-570.

Centers for Disease Control and Prevention. Heat-related mortality - Chicago, July 1995. *MMWR* 1995;44(31): 577-579.

Curriero FC, Heiner KS, Samet JM, et al. Temperature and mortality in 11 cities of the eastern United States. *American Journal of Epidemiology* 2002;155(1):80-87.

Weisskopf MG, Anderson HA, Foldy S, et al. Heat wave morbidity and mortality, Milwaukee, Wis, 1999 vs. 1995: an improved response? *American Journal of Public Health* 2002;92(5):830-833.

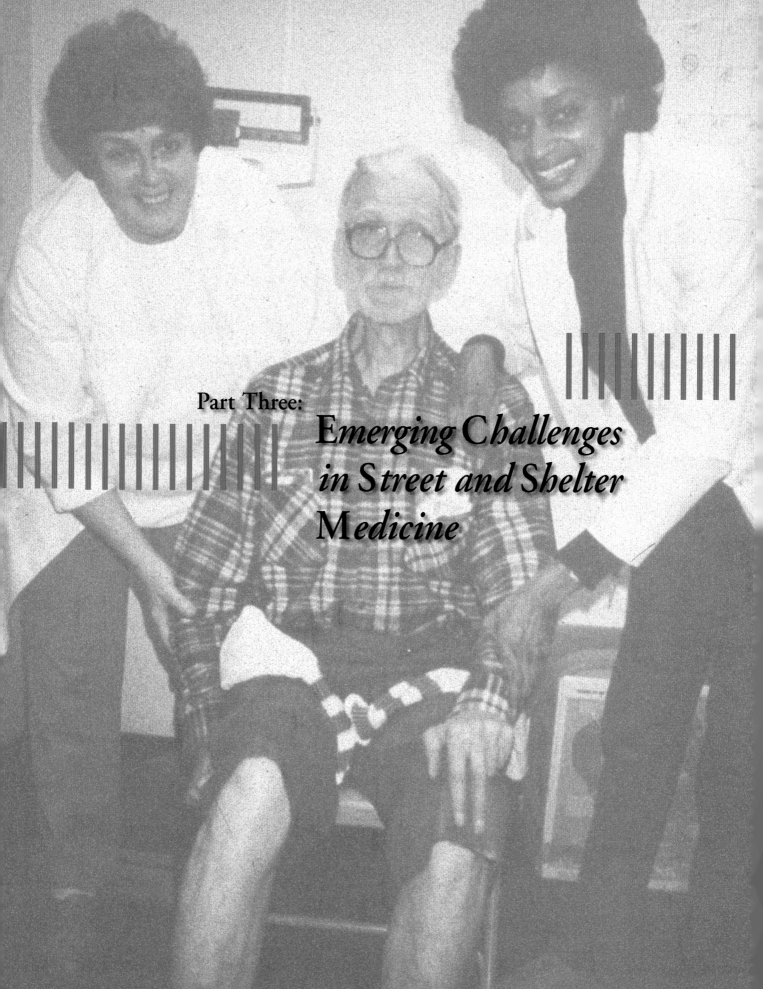

Part Three:

Emerging Challenges in Street and Shelter Medicine

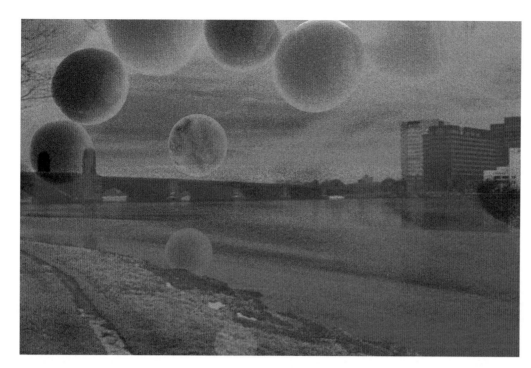

Bioterrorism

M. Anita Barry, MD, MPH
Suzanne Strickland, MPH

The anthrax attacks in 2001 left many providers concerned about the impact of future attacks on their clients and their facilities. What was once a remote possibility became a stark reality for many in the United States. Even though relatively few people were directly affected by the anthrax incidents, concern about safety was widespread.

Since the anthrax attacks, much has been reported about other possible threats involving nuclear, biological, and chemical agents. This chapter is an overview of the major infectious agents most likely to be utilized for bioterrorism. Some common organisms such as Salmonella have not been included, although this bacteria has been used in terrorist events in the USA. Providers of services for homeless persons should be on the alert for any unusual clusters of illness and consult with medical and/or public health providers if they suspect a patient has been infected with any of the organisms or agents discussed in this chapter.

While the exact nature and time of any future terrorist attempts cannot be predicted, several steps can be taken to identify and respond to any unexpected emergency, whether man made or a natural disaster.

Prevention and Control: Emergency Preparedness

Education

All clinical staff should be educated about the biologic agents of concern as described in Table 1. Likewise, staff members should be familiar with the infectious diseases that are reportable to local or state health departments. For any suspected case that is reportable, contact the appropriate public health authorities immediately, even though the likelihood of diseases such as smallpox, plague, or botulism occurring is low. Public health authorities will conduct an epidemiological investigation to determine the causative agent and to identify anyone who may have been exposed to the patient during the infectious period. Obtaining a list of places the patient has stayed will assist greatly in determining possible exposures.

The Emergency Operations Plan (EOP)

- *Create an emergency operations plan (EOP)*
  An EOP spells out actions to be taken when any given situation exceeds the program's capability or routine response, clarifies lines of authority, outlines how all actions will be coordinated, and provides guidelines about internal and external communications. The EOP identifies people, resources, and mutual aid agree-

Illustration by Pat Mullaly

Table 1: Biologic Agents of Concern

Agent	Incubation	Symptoms	Transmission	Precautions	Treatment*
Anthrax *Bacillus anthracis*	Usually<7 days but can occur up to 60 days post-exposure	Cutaneous: raised itchy bump initially; progresses to ulcerated blister with necrotic center Inhalation: initially, nonspecific flu like illness, characterized by fever, myalgia, headache, nonproductive cough, and mild chest discomfort; followed by marked high fever, dyspnea, stridor, cyanosis, and shock	Person-to-person spread extremely unlikely Person-to-person	Standard precautions	Multiple antibiotics including doxycycline, fluroquinolones and others effective for both types
Botulism *Clostridium botulinum*	Usually 12-36 hours (range of 6 hours-2 weeks)	Double vision, blurred vision, drooping eyelids, slurred speech, and difficulty swallowing and dry mouth	Not spread person-to-person	Standard precautions	Antitoxin effective if diagnosed early; supportive care
Plague *Yersinia pestis*	2-4 days	Fever, chills, headache, severe debilitation, rapidly developing shortness of breath, and chest pain	Person-to-person	Airborne, droplet, and contact precautions recommended	Early treatment crucial. Streptomycin, gentamicin when streptomycin not available. Other antibiotics also effective.
Smallpox *Variola major*	7-17 days	Initially, high fever, fatigue, headache and backaches; rash usually develops 2 to 3 days after onset of symptoms. Rash appears first on the mouth, face, and forearms, then spreads inward to trunk of the body	Person-to-person	Airborne and droplet precautions recommended	Supportive therapy; antibiotics to treat secondary infections
Tularemia *Francisella tularensis*	Usually 3-5 days (range of 1-14 days)	Insect bite, slow-healing sore and swollen lymph nodes Inhalation: high fever, chills, headache, fatigue, cough and chest pain Ingestion: sore throat, abdominal pain, diarrhea, and vomiting	Not spread person-to-person		Streptomycin; gentamicin also effective.
Viral Hemorrhagic Fevers	Usually <2 weeks (range of 4-21 days)	Fever, fatigue, dizziness, muscle aches, loss of strength, and exhaustion. Severe cases often show signs of bleeding under the skin, in internal organs, or from body orifices. Severely ill patients may also experience shock, nervous system malfunction, coma, delirium, and seizures. Some types of VHF are associated with renal (kidney) failure	Person-to-person	Airborne and droplet precautions recommended	Supportive care; some types responsive to antiviral medication

*Consult local or state health department for most up to date guidelines.

ments for responding to an emergency before it happens.

- *Find out what's already in place in your organization*
The first step in creating an EOP is to do research. Find out if your organization already has a plan, what the plan says, and if it needs to be updated. Look into what others have done in facilities that are similar to yours. Find out about assistance available through a partner hospital (if you have one), affiliated health care providers, your local or state health department, and from your local, state, or federal emergency management agency.

- *Build a planning team*
The team should consist of a broad spectrum of people from your organization who will bring different perspectives and provide expertise in various areas. The team can consist of medical and mental health clinicians, case managers, outreach workers, and others. The team should also include administrators, as well as human resources and fiscal representatives who have knowledge of contractual and compensation issues so that costs associated with an emergency can be tracked. Facilities and operations staff have knowledge of the layout of the building, have access to all areas of the building, and can help manage flow of people. Once the team is formed, identify a group leader who is responsible for managing the project.

- *Format the plan*
Although causes of emergencies differ, many consequences are the same, so an "all-hazards" format is suggested. This format provides a basic framework to respond to various emergencies and a foundation from which to build hazard specific plans. It consists of the following sections: purpose; roles and responsibilities of an emergency response team; conditions under which the plan will be activated; and phases. Phases of the plan are as follows.
  - identification of the emergency: how will the emergency be identified?
  - assessment of situation: how will the urgency of the situation, the proxim-

ity of the event to your facility, and the seriousness of the potential impact be determined?
  - notification of team members: how will you get in touch with those charged with responding to an emergency?
  - meeting of team and planning of response: where will your team meet to plan its response in a crisis? Planning should take into account issues such as staff skills, building capacity, possible need for isolation and/or quarantine, patient flow/crowd control, security, supply source and availability, and communications to staff, to clients, and to other agencies included in your plan. Isolation and quarantine may pose a significant challenge for those with chemical dependence, post traumatic stress disorder, or other psychiatric conditions, so special consideration of security/crowd control, detoxification, and mental health counseling may be needed. Scenarios should include either the need to shelter in place or to evacuate your building;
  - communication and execution of response plan: are those people identified to report in an emergency aware of the roles they are expected to play? Do they have a plan in place for their own families that will allow them to respond to an emergency?
  - monitoring and adjustment of plan during an event: how will changes in the situation and effectiveness of the

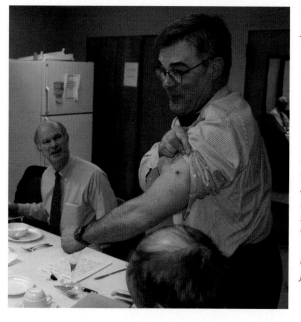

John Noble MD, Director of the Center for Primary Care at Boston University School of Medicine and longtime advocate of the HCH Program, demonstrates his recent small pox vaccination at McInnis House. Dr. Noble worked on small pox eradication with the CDC in the 1960s.
Photo by James O'Connell MD

response be assessed in order to determine if adjustments need to be made?

- post-emergency review: discuss elements of the response that worked well, those that needed improvement, how you can take what was learned from a particular situation, and how to improve your plan.

- *Exercise the plan*
  Once you have developed a plan, make sure that all staff members are familiar with it. It is important to exercise your plan to identify areas for improvement and to integrate it into your agency's culture so that the plan can be successfully executed when needed.

Summary

Disasters can affect all segments of a community, including homeless individuals and families living in shelters or on the streets. Unfortunately, bioterrorism is a threat that must now be faced. Planning for a bioterrorism threat will enable those who work with homeless populations to respond more effectively to a range of emergencies, whether manmade or natural.

Providing health care to homeless persons during a crisis requires responding to many of the same issues providers deal with each day, some of which may be magnified by the crisis. When formulating a plan for your agency, utilize your expertise with this population by considering issues that are specific to working with transient populations, persons with substance abuse issues, those dealing with post-traumatic stress disorder, and those with other mental health issues. ▦

References

Chin J, ed. *Control of Infectious Diseases Manual.* 17th ed. Washington, DC: American Public Health Association; 2000:520-535.

Pickering LK, Peter G, Baker CJ, et al., eds. *The 2003 Redbook: Report on the Committee on Infectious Diseases.* Elkgrove Village, Illinois: American Academy of Pediatrics; 2003:677.

State and Local Guide (SLG) 101. *Guide for All-Hazard Emergency Operations Planning.* Federal Emergency Management Agency; 1996. http://www.fema.gov/rr/gaheop

Viral Hemorrhagic Fevers. Special Pathogens Branch, Centers for Disease Control and Prevention. http://www.cdc.gov/ncidod/dvrd/spb/mnpages/dispages/vhf.htm

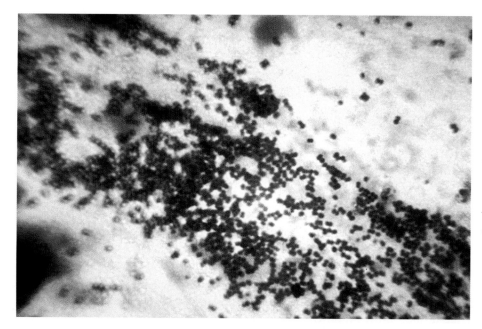

Nosocomial Infections

Adi Gundlapalli, MD, PhD
Louise J. Eutropius, RN, BSN, CIC

"We are discharging Mr. SR to your facility for recuperation and transition after his third admission to our hospital. He was in our hospital for 8 days with a leg wound that is now stable but is still draining a little and will require daily dressing changes. The infection is under control, and he will require a full course of antibiotics. Oh, by the way, he has 'MRSA' in the wound!"

The Latin word "nosocomium" means "hospital." Nosocomial infections are acquired by patients during an admission to a hospital or other health care facility. These microorganisms are usually resistant to several commonly used antibiotics. These organisms were once limited to large hospitals but have now become ubiquitous in health care facilities throughout the USA. To make matters much worse, some of these organisms are now seen in the general community with alarming frequency.

Methicillin Resistant Staphylococcus Aureus. This sputum smear shows Gram positive organisms in clusters, and the culture and sensitivity later showed Staphylococcus aureus resistant to methicillin. Photo courtesy of the CDC

Nosocomial Infections and Homeless Persons

The rising number of homeless and marginally housed individuals in our urban and rural communities has been mirrored by increasing numbers of homeless individuals admitted to hospitals. These individuals are often discharged to skilled nursing care facilities, group homes, homeless shelters, and the streets. It is very likely that your facility has an individual recently discharged from a hospital or other health care setting, often with continuing and complicated health care needs.

In most homeless service facilities, individuals have contact with others, often in crowded living conditions. Such overcrowding, combined with less than optimal hygiene practices, fosters the spread of resistant nosocomial organisms to other individuals.

In these situations, clinicians should be familiar with the possible organisms the patients may have acquired while in the hospital or other health care settings (e.g. a nursing home) and how they can affect you, your staff, and other residents of your facility.

Mode of Transmission

A review of the concept of the "Chain of Infection" helps to explain how patients acquire nosocomial organisms.

A causative or infectious agent is a "bug" that causes disease. This can be a bacteria, virus, parasite, or fungus. The agent usually requires a reservoir in which it survives and multiplies. For most nosocomial infections, the reservoirs for infectious agents are other patients in the hospital or nursing

Figure 1:

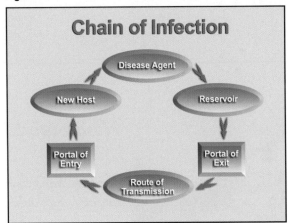

home. The "reservoir" patients may have signs and symptoms of the infection or may be silently colonized with the organism and exhibit no symptoms. Infectious agents can survive for long periods of time in certain environmental reservoirs (e.g. water supply, hands, surfaces of objects).

The infectious agent can be found in body secretions such as wound drainage, in excretions such as stool or urine, or in other body fluids such as blood. The agent escapes the reservoir through a portal of exit. Such portals can be any of the openings of the human body, especially the nose, mouth, and rectum. After exiting the reservoir, the organism must find another person or host in which to live. This passage is called the mode of transmission. For most nosocomial infections discussed in this chapter, the common mode of transmission is direct spread from person to person by infectious agents carried on the hands. Some organisms may be indirectly spread through contact with contaminated objects, such as medical equipment or personal care items. These organisms enter the new host via a portal similar to the portal of exit (e.g. mouth, nose).

The fate of the infectious agent is determined by the competency of the host's immune system. The nosocomial organism infects the new host and either causes disease or results in colonization. Signs and symptoms accompany disease, while colonization does not make people feel ill. In either case, the newly infected or colonized host harbors the agent and serves as a reservoir. The chain of infection can thus continue.

The chain of infection can easily propagate in shelters and respite care programs. Guests, residents, visitors, and staff members can unknowingly harbor nosocomial organisms. Close direct contact and exposure to body fluids or contaminated equipment can result in the transfer of the organism from one person to another if proper infection control precautions are not followed.

Diagnosis

Patients with symptomatic infections are diagnosed in the usual manner, with cultures and specific tests to isolate and identify the causative agents. In contrast, colonization with nosocomial organisms is detected by performing surveillance cultures, since these individuals are unaware that they have been infected. Specific microbiological tests are able to detect the presence of these organisms in body fluids and excretions. Most hospitals now perform routine surveillance testing of asymptomatic inpatients to specifically look for these organisms. Infected patients are identified and appropriate infection control measures instituted.

We recommend that clinicians seek specific information about possible nosocomial organisms whenever someone is discharged to a respite care program or shelter setting after a long and complicated hospitalization. These individuals have a very high likelihood of acquiring nosocomial infections.

Common Nosocomial Organisms

Methicillin Resistant Staphylococcus Aureus (MRSA)

MRSA is a cousin of the regular "staph" that causes many skin and soft tissue infections. This organism has acquired resistance to commonly used antibiotics such as dicloxacillin (Dynapen™) and cephalexin (Keflex™). In many parts of the country, the number of patients in the hospital either colonized or infected with MRSA has grown dramatically in the last two decades.

MRSA is commonly found on the skin, in wounds, and in the nose. The organism is spread by direct contact with body secretions and is rarely transmitted via contaminated surfaces. MRSA is most frequently carried from one patient to the next on the unwashed hands of health care workers.

Infection with MRSA is commonly treated with intravenous antibiotics such as vancomycin (Vancocin™). Newer (and very expensive) antibiotics, such as linezolid (Zyvox™), can be used to treat this organism when vancomycin fails. Active infection is usually treated initially with intravenous antibiotics, followed by a course of oral antibiotics. These oral antibiotics include minocycline (Minocin™), trimethoprim-sulfamethoxazole (Bactrim™, Septra™), clindamycin (Cleocin™), and rifampin (Rifadin™, Rimactane™).

Several outbreaks of MRSA skin and soft tissue infections have occurred among people who have neither been hospitalized nor had any formal contact with any health care facilities. This "community-associated MRSA" is on the rise in several places around the country and represents a shift in how we approach this organism. It is important to keep this in mind when dealing with infections that are not healing or worsening while the patient is being treated with commonly used antibiotics.

Vancomycin Resistant Enterococcus (VRE)

VRE is a Gram positive bacterium that can cause serious infections in hospitalized patients. In the past, virtually all Enterococcus organisms were sensitive to vancomycin. However, resistance to this antibiotic has been increasing, and VRE has become a major nosocomial organism.

VRE is less common than MRSA and usually colonizes the intestines (gut) without causing any disease. Commonly found in stool, VRE is spread in a similar way to MRSA through direct contact via the unwashed hands of health care workers. VRE can also be spread by contact with contaminated surfaces or medical equipment. Rarely, VRE can be found in other bodily fluids such as urine and wounds.

VRE can cause life-threatening infections in patients who are already ill from other diseases. These infections are notoriously difficult to treat. Certain new and very expensive antibiotics, such as quinupristin/dalfopristin (Synercid™) and linezolid (Zyvox™) have been used with some success.

Clostridium Difficile (C. diff)

- *Clostridium difficile (C. diff)* is a bacterium that causes diarrhea. These bacteria are most commonly associated with diarrhea that occurs during or after the use of anti-biotics.
- In many instances, the gut is colonized with *C. diff* and causes no symptoms. The presence of the bacteria is found only when the stool is specifically cultured for it. In some instances, the bacteria secrete a toxin that causes severe diarrhea.
- *C. diff* is also spread by direct contact via the hands of health care workers that have been in contact with contaminated feces or surfaces.
- Diarrhea from *C. diff* can be treated with a commonly used antibiotic, metronidazole (Flagyl™). Occasionally, this treatment

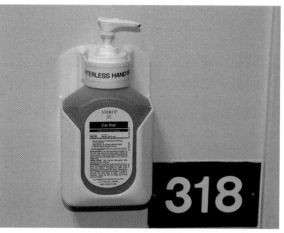

Handwashing as Prevention. Alcohol-based gel solutions are more effective and easier-to-use than soap and water. Staff members at McInnis House use Calstat™ upon entering and leaving each patient room.
Photo by James O'Connell MD

fails, and the oral preparation of vanco-mycin (Vancocin™) may have to be used. The treatment of *C. diff* diarrhea is the only current indication for the use of oral vancomycin.

Prevention and Control

National guidelines have been issued by the Centers for Disease Control and Prevention (CDC) and other agencies concerning the control of infections caused by these nosocomial organisms.

The most effective preventive technique is the practice of excellent hand hygiene. This refers to the age-old method of washing hands with soap and water and the newer method of disinfecting the hands with an alcohol-based gel solution, such as Calstat™, GelSan™, and Purell™. The gel solutions have become very popular in hospitals and nursing homes, as recent studies have demonstrated their effectiveness in the prevention of transmission of organisms. The hands can be cleansed and air-dried in a very short period of time. The gel solutions appear to be more effective than washing hands with soap and water, and we are more likely to use the gel rather than the traditional soap and water. At Massachusetts General Hospital and at the Barbara McInnis House in Boston, dispensers of Calstat™ are placed at the entry to each patient care room, and clinicians are expected to perform hand hygiene when entering and leaving each room.

"Contact Precautions" are the most common practice utilized for the control of nosocomial organisms in hospitals and other health care facilities. Patients are usually placed in a private room with a "Contact Precautions" sign on the door. All visitors and health care workers entering the room are required to wear gowns and gloves while interacting with each patient and the immediate environment. Hand hygiene is performed after removing gowns and gloves and upon leaving the room. Wounds are kept covered, and exposure to body fluids is minimized. Daily cleaning of each room helps to minimize contamination. Certain items, such as rectal thermometers, blood pressure cuffs, and stethoscopes are used exclusively for one patient and are kept in the room.

Considerable controversy surrounds the effectiveness of current prevention and control methods used in hospitals and health care facilities. First, surveillance cultures on all (or a random selection) of inpatients is recommended by some authorities to screen for the presence of nosocomial organisms. This is very expensive and time-consuming, and not all hospitals have the capacity and resources to follow this recommendation. Second, contact precautions have been met with some mixed reactions. While many experts embrace contact precautions as the most appropriate way to control these resistant organisms, others have remained skeptical and have been less stringent in following all the recommendations. It is appropriate to check with your hospital and local health care providers regarding the precautions and protocols utilized for the prevention and control of nosocomial organisms.

Special Considerations for Homeless Populations

Many different facilities care for homeless individuals and families, including shelters, transitional programs, and respite care programs, as well as hospitals and nursing homes. Only basic infection prevention and control activities can be performed in the large adult shelters that are common in many urban cities. Following a discharge from an acute care hospital, respite care programs and nursing homes may frequently care for homeless persons recovering from acute medical and surgical problems. Thus the incidence of nosocomial infections is undoubtedly higher in these facilities than in homeless shelters, and the need for infection control interventions is critically important.

The first principle of infection control is to practice good techniques for ALL patients, regardless of background, risk behaviors, or diagnosis. Surveillance cultures look specifically for nosocomial organisms such as MRSA or VRE and are very helpful in identifying specific patients who are colonized. Clinicians must nevertheless assume that all patients in any health care facility are potential carriers of these resistant organisms.

The level and intensity of infection control depends upon the staffing and resources available at each facility. If available, a private room is ideal for any patient with MRSA, VRE or *Clostridium difficile,* especially when the care of the patient will involve exposure to bodily fluids. However, private rooms are often not available and impractical, and these patients may still be managed in multi-bed rooms as long as careful precautions are in place.

Only rudimentary or basic infection control techniques are possible in most shelter and other homeless settings. All staff members should be educated in the proper techniques for hand hygiene as well as the handling of bodily fluids.

The first and foremost step is to educate guests, residents, staff members, and visitors regarding infectious agents and cleanliness techniques. Everyone should become familiar with the "chain of infection" and the vocabulary surrounding nosocomial organisms. Open wounds should always be kept covered, and appropriate measures should be taken to dispose of soiled dressings. Patients with incontinence of stool and urine must be carefully managed, including the use of diapers whenever possible as well as not sharing personal care items. Housekeeping staff should use standard cleaning agents (with bleach) and should also have access to hospital-grade disinfectants. Soiled laundry should also be carefully handled (preferably with gloves) and can effectively be cleaned with standard laundry protocols. If procedures are performed in your facility, take appropriate precautions in anticipation of possible exposure to blood and other bodily fluids.

Last, and perhaps most importantly, hand hygiene remains the most important intervention and the cornerstone of infection control.

Remember…it's in your hands!!

We would like to thank our colleagues at Wasatch Homeless Health Care, Inc. and University of Utah Hospitals and Clinics who reviewed the chapter and made helpful suggestions. ▓

Nosocomial Infections Medication List

Generic	Brand	Cost
dicloxacillin	Dynapen	$
cephalexin	Keflex	$
linezolid	Zyvox	$$$$$
minocycline	Minocin	$
trimethoprim-sulfamethoxazole	Bactrim, Septra	$
clindamycin	Cleocin	$$
rifampin	Rifadin, Rimactane	$$$
vancomycin	Vancocin	$$$$
quinupristin + dalfopristin	Synercid	$$$$$
metronidazole	Flagyl	$

References

Infection Control and Body Substance Precautions Manual. University of Utah Hospitals & Clinics:
http://uuhsc.utah.edu/hospepi/icmanual.cfm

Guidelines and Recommendations. Centers for Disease Control and Prevention.
http://www.cdc.gov/ncidod/hip/Guide/guide.htm

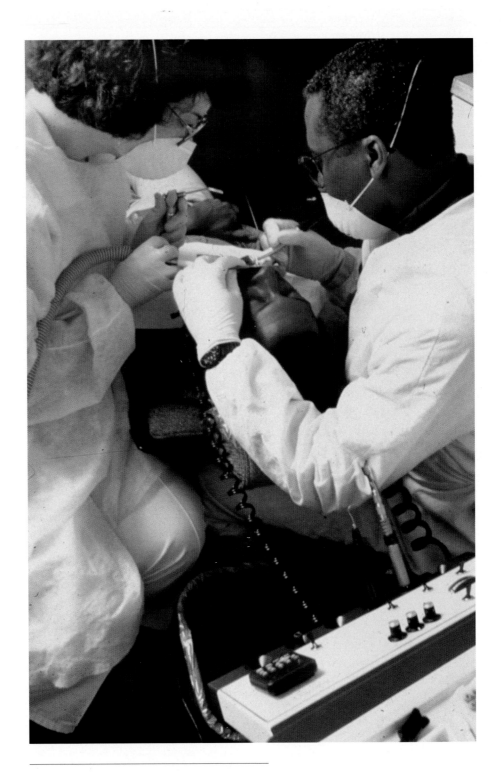

Comprehensive oral health care is provided by BHCHP's
Dental Team at several locations in Boston, including
a new 5-chair clinic that is shared with the South End
Health Center. Here Al Bolden DMD works with dental
assistant Sylvia Roman at St. Francis House.
Photo by David Comb

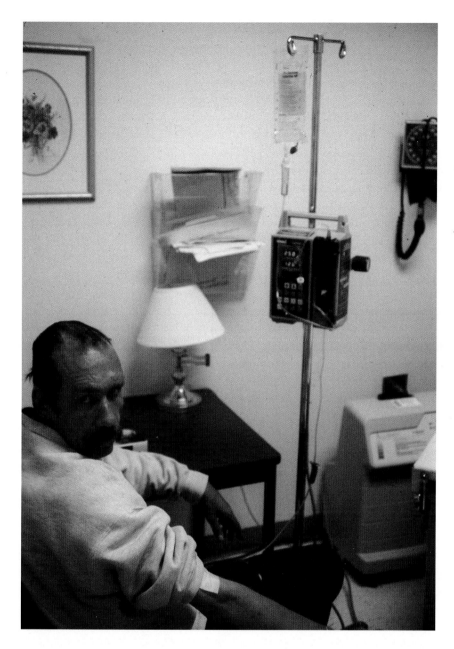

Proper Use of Antibiotics

Monica Bharel, MD

R esistance to antibiotics continues to rise. Over the past decade antibiotic resistance has emerged for common pathogens like *Streptococcus pneumoniae* and *Campylobacter jejuni*. Several factors contribute to antibiotic resistance, including antibiotic overuse and inappropriate use of broad-spectrum antibiotics.

Restricting the use of antibiotics has been shown to decrease the incidence and the spread of antibiotic resistance. By using available evidence to determine etiologies of symptoms and choosing antibiotics based on the most likely pathogens involved, we may be able to narrow our inappropriate antibiotic use.

Based on our population needs and practice setting, we are often faced with treating patients empirically. Although this practice increases the tendency to use broader spectrum antibiotics, we can still do our part to restrict unnecessary antibiotic use. The following common diseases are reviewed to illustrate methods for antibiotic choice.

Upper Respiratory Tract Infections (URI)

The common cold is one of the leading reasons patients seek medical attention. An average adult has 2-3 colds a year, and the average child has 6-10 colds a year. The typical symptoms of a common cold

This man had methicillin-resistant Staphylococcus aureus bacteremia from a scalp laceration. He required several weeks of IV antibiotics at McInnis House after discharge from the hospital. Photo by James O'Connell MD

include nasal obstruction, rhinorrhea (runny nose), and sneezing. Most colds are caused by viruses and require no antibiotic therapy. Some common viral pathogens include rhinovirus, coronavirus, respiratory syncytial virus (RSV), and adenovirus.

Antibiotics are not indicated for the treatment of uncomplicated upper respiratory tract infections. The most effective treatment for the common cold is symptomatic treatment. Many scientific studies emphasize this fact. In one study looking at over 2200 patients, no significant benefit was found to antibiotic use in patients with the common cold. Additionally, the use of antibiotics was associated with a three-fold increase in adverse effects. Although solid evidence exists against the use of antibiotics in this situation, almost 50% of patients receive antibiotics for the common cold in national surveys.

Since the common cold is a clinical diagnosis, caregivers need to be vigilant and recognize symptoms that may be associated with other respiratory conditions that require antibiotic treatment or closer monitoring. Some of these symptoms include shortness of breath, fever greater than 102°F (38.9°C), persistent symptoms >7 days, difficulty controlling salivation, and severe headache.

Sinusitis (Rhinosinusitis)

Only a very small percentage of colds (0.5-2%) are complicated by acute sinusitis. The exact factors that lead a cold to develop into sinusitis are unknown. However, thick secretions accumulating in the sinuses and increased dispersion of nasal bacteria and viruses into the sinuses from nose blowing may be factors. Some important predisposing conditions include poor dental hygiene, history of swimming or diving, or persistent nasal obstruction.

The most common causes of sinusitis are viruses, including rhinovirus, as well as parainfluenza and influenza viruses. The most common bacterial causes of sinusitis include the normal nasopharyngeal occupants *Streptococcus pneumoniae, Haemophilus influenzae,* and *Moraxella catarrhalis.* The differentiation of viral from bacterial sinusitis is a challenge to clinicians.

Studies have shown that the following symptoms are more likely to be associated with a bacterial etiology: maxillary toothache, transillumination, lack of response to decongestants or antihistamines, and purulent discharge seen on exam or reported by the patient. Other useful indicators include symptoms for >7 days and facial pain or swelling.

Effective methods to diagnose bacterial sinusitis include sinus aspiration or CT, although these are neither practical nor necessary to make the diagnosis of uncomplicated sinusitis.

Viral sinusitis should be treated symptomatically. Studies have shown that in immunocompetent patients, mild bacterial sinusitis is also self-limited. Patients with moderate to severe bacterial sinusitis should receive antibiotic treatment. Some controversy exists over appropriate treatment for bacterial sinusitis, but all agree that the most narrow spectrum agent effective against the likely pathogens should be used. First line agents include amoxicillin (Amoxil™), doxycycline (Vibramycin™), or trimethoprim–sulfamethoxazole (Septra™, Bactrim™).

Pneumonia

Pneumonia is the 6th leading cause of death in the USA. The most common bacterial cause of community-acquired pneumonia is *Streptococcus pneumoniae.* The emergence of antibiotic resistance among *S. pneumoniae* has further complicated treatment.

It is important to differentiate pneumonia from other causes of acute respiratory symptoms. Pneumonia can present with a variety of clinical findings including fever, cough, dyspnea, myalgias, tachycardia, and crackles on lung exam. Studies have shown that no individual clinical finding or group of findings can definitely make the diagnosis of pneumonia. There is some suggestion that a normal lung exam and normal vital signs make pneumonia a less likely diagnosis. The chest x-ray (CXR) is the standard for diagnosing pneumonia. A CXR should therefore be obtained whenever pneumonia is suspected in vulnerable individuals, including those with COPD or asthma, chronic diseases such as congestive heart failure (CHF) or diabetes mellitus (DM), and those who are immunocompromised.

The choice of antibiotic for presumed pneumonia is determined by whether the person can be treated as an outpatient or requires admission to the hospital. Clinical guidelines called the PORT criteria are very helpful in determining a patient's level of risk and need for hospitalization. (Please see table in the chapter on Pneumonia.)

The most common pathogens should be considered when choosing an antibiotic for the outpatient treatment of uncomplicated CAP, particularly *Streptococcus pneumoniae,* Mycoplasma, and viral etiologies. The most likely pathogens can vary based on patient co-morbidities. For example, in patients who use alcohol, consider covering anaerobes and Klebsiella. In smokers, consider *Moraxella catarrhalis* and *H. influenzae.* The possibility of *Pneumocystis carinii* pneumonia (PCP) should be considered in immunocompromised patients.

The first line of empiric treatment of uncomplicated CAP in those who do not require hospitalization should be doxycycline (Vibramycin™) or an advanced generation macrolide such as clarithromycin (Biaxin™) or azithromycin (Zithromax™).

Cellulitis

Cellulitis is a common skin condition. The diagnosis is mostly clinical, and the common findings include tenderness, warmth, swelling, or erythema. The most common pathogens include group A beta hemolytic Streptococcus and *Staphylococcus aureus.* Empiric treatment should focus on agents that cover these common pathogens.

Uncomplicated cellulitis can be treated with cephalexin (Keflex™) or dicloxacillin (Dynapen™). Patients with penicillin allergies can be treated with clindamycin (Cleocin™) or erythromycin (Eryc™, E-mycin™). For those persons with a history of intolerance to erythromycin, azithromycin (Zithromax™) or clarithromycin (Biaxin™) can be prescribed. Clindamycin (Cleocin™) should not be given to patients with a history of *Clostridium difficile.* Patients at risk for cellulitis from Gram negative pathogens, such as diabetics, should be treated with an agent that includes gram negative coverage, such at levofloxacin (Levaquin™) or amoxicillin/clavulanate (Augmentin™). Early uncomplicated cellulitis should be initially treated with a narrow spectrum antibiotic, and the more expensive fluroquinolones, such levofloxacin (Levaquin™), should be reserved for resistant or severe cases.

Diarrhea

Most cases of acute diarrhea are self-limited, whether the etiology is bacterial or viral. The treatment of acute diarrhea is supportive in most cases. However, antibiotic treatment should be considered in certain situations. Some bacterial causes of diarrhea include *Staphylococcus aureus,* Yersinia, Shigella, Salmonella, and *Escherichia coli.* Empiric antibiotic therapy should be considered in patients with fever, bloody diarrhea, or the presence of occult blood or fecal leukocytes on stool exam. Immunocompromised persons, the frail elderly, and other patients with chronic diseases may be considered for early empiric treatment for acute diarrhea.

Since most cases of acute diarrhea are self-limited, it is not necessary to obtain labs and stool studies. In more complicated cases, stool cultures and/or ova and parasite studies can be sent. The optimal time to utilize these more expensive cultures remains controversial.

Clinicians should remember that most cases of acute diarrhea resolve spontaneously without treatment. Fluroquinolones are the first line agents in most cases of acute diarrhea. Overuse of the fluroquinolones has already led to quinolone-resistant strains in many parts of the world. Consider the use of fluroquinolones when obtaining stool studies is impractical and the patient has prolonged symptoms or cannot be followed or monitored for several days. Patients who are immunocompromised should have further workup done if symptoms persist. Also, consider if patient is at risk for *Clostridium difficile,* which is treated with metronidazole (Flagyl™).

Summary

Antibiotic resistance continues to increase and will continue to limit our drug choices. When providing empiric treatment for infections, two considerations can facilitate appropriate use of antibiotics. First, consider if the signs and symptoms warrant antibiotic use in addition to symptomatic treatment. Second, consider the most common pathogens based on the patient's history and presentation, and choose the drug with the narrowest spectrum that will cover the pathogens involved. We urge all clinicians to be judicious in the use of antibiotics and resist the tendency to rely on broad spectrum and expensive antibiotics that are not necessary. As we all improve our choices of antibiotics, we will be engaging in cost effect practice that leads to fewer side effects and less antibiotic resistance. ▓

Antibiotics Medication List

Generic	Brand Name	Cost
amoxicillin	Amoxil	$
amoxicillin-clavulanate	Augmentin	$$$
azithromycin	Zithromax	$$
cephalexin	Keflex	$
clarithromycin	Biaxin	$$$
clindamycin	Cleocin	$$
doxycycline	Vibramycin	$
erythromycin	Eryc, E-mycin	$
levofloxacin	Levaquin	$$$
metronidazole	Flagyl	$
trimethoprim-sulfamethoxazole	Bactrim, Septra	$

References

Arroll B, Kenealy T. Antibiotics for the common cold. *Cochrane Database of Systematic Reviews.* 2002(3): CD000247.

Gilbert DN, Moellering RC, Sande MA. *The Sanford Guide to Antimicrobial Therapy.* Hyde Park, VT: Antimicrobial Therapy Inc.; 2000.

Gonzales R, et al. Principles of appropriate antibiotics use for treatment of respiratory tract infections in adults. *Annal of Internal Medicine* 2001;134(6):490-494.

Ilnyckyj A. Clinical evaluation and management of acute infectious diarrhea in adults. *Gastroenterology Clinics of North America* 2001;30(3):599-609.

Metlay JP, Kapoor WN, Fine M. Does this patient have community-acquired pneumonia? *Journal of the American Medical Association* 1997;278(17):1440-1445.

Park SI, Giannella RA. Approach to the adult patient with acute diarrhea. *Gastroenterology Clinics of North America* 1993;22(3):483-497.

Steinman MA, Landefeld CS, et al. Predictors for broad spectrum antibiotic prescribing for respiratory tract infections in adult primary care. *Journal of the American Medical Association* 2003;289(6):719-725.

Stulberg DL, Penrod MA, Blatny RA. Common bacterial skin infections. *American Family Physician* 2002;66(1): 119-124.

Williams JW, Aguilar C, Makela M, et al. Antibiotics for acute maxillary sinusitis. *Cochrane Database Systems Review.* 2003(2):CD000243.

Williams JW, Simel DL. Does this patient have sinusitis? Diagnosing acute sinusitis by history and physical examination. *Journal of the American Medical Association* 1993;270(10):1242-1246.

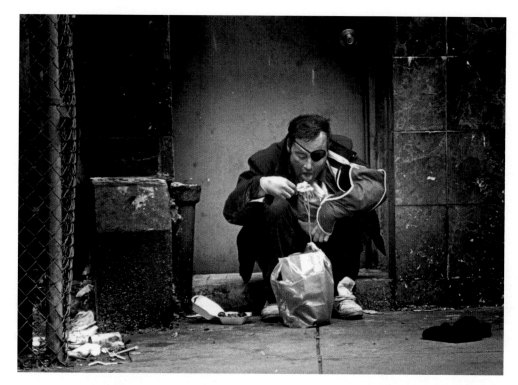

Nutritional Issues

Stefan G. Kertesz, MD, MSc

omeless persons in the USA experience a variety of nutritional problems that may affect health and quality of life. Significant numbers of homeless adults and children are hungry and report problems obtaining sufficient food when asked about their recent dietary history. Paradoxically, homeless individuals are at least as likely as the overall US population to be obese, and obesity carries a wide range of health consequences.

In addition to problems resulting from too few or too many calories, homeless persons are susceptible to specific vitamin and nutrient deficiencies. Nutritional deficiency diseases are uncommon in the USA, and clinicians frequently have difficulty recognizing these often subtle problems. Clinicians, counselors, and social workers seeking to help homeless persons obtain adequate nutrition face numerous challenges, especially for those with diabetes, hypercholesterolemia, and other chronic diseases that require specialized diets. This chapter reviews the common nutritional problems faced by homeless persons and recommends responses for their caregivers.

Prevalence and Distribution

We will consider the nutritional problems of hunger, overweight and obesity, and specific nutritional deficiency disorders. Some problems that are not specifically related to homelessness, such as excessive or harmful intake of particular vitamins or nutrients, will not be considered in this chapter.

Hunger

Homeless persons across the USA report significant problems obtaining food. Among 2938 currently homeless persons interviewed across the country in the 1996 National Survey of Homeless Assistance Providers and Clients, 19% reported going one or more days in the preceding week without anything at all to eat, and 40% went a whole day in the preceding month without anything to eat. Less than half the persons interviewed reported eating three times a day.

Although such problems were less common among homeless children living with their mothers, the findings in this national survey were troubling. Seven percent of mothers reported that at least once in the preceding month their children were hungry because they could not get enough food, and 1% indicated their children had gone a whole day without eating during the previous month.

While hunger is a serious problem among homeless persons, physical evidence of malnutrition due to lack of calories has not been consistently

Homelessness and Hunger.
Many people are forced to find food that has been discarded by others. In Boston and other cities, Salmonella food poisoning is seen frequently in homeless persons.
Photo by Robert T. Souther, www.geocities.com/ bob_souther

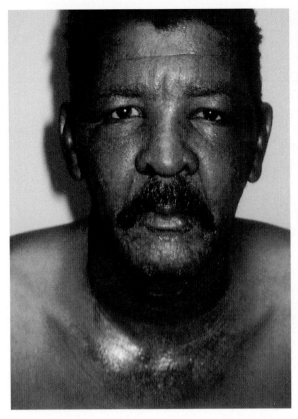 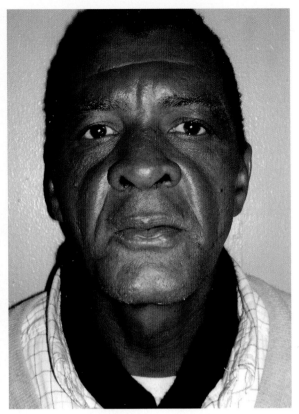

(left)
Pellagra.
This man at Long Island Shelter in Boston had been eating only corn chips each day for several weeks. His face shows cutaneous weeping, edema, erythema, fissuring, and scaling over the ears, face, and collar area.

(right)
Pellagra, One Year Later. The rash and other skin findings have resolved with adequate nutritional intake.
Photos reprinted with permission from Kertesz SG. Pellagra in 2 homeless men. Mayo Clinic Proceedings 2001;76:315-318.

documented in published studies. The results of these studies have varied because different cities and regions have different availability and accessibility of food resources, and the sub-groups of the homeless population studied have been inconsistent (e. g., those who use shelters and those who live on the streets). One New York study suggested that approximately 1/3 of homeless shelter-users had obtained less than 2/3 the recommended number of calories during the previous 24 hours. In contrast, studies of homeless persons in Alabama and Florida found that over 1/3 had evidence of either fat-wasting or muscle-wasting, problems related to excessive food intake. A study of 87 long-term outdoor-dwellers found that they averaged 500 calories less per day than was recommended and that among men, alcohol accounted for 44% of caloric intake.

Hunger is thus a serious problem among homeless persons, and evidence of malnutrition can be found in some but not all persons who are homeless. Such problems may be most common among chronically homeless individuals, particularly those with alcohol abuse. Even in the absence of measurable malnutrition, however, hunger is likely to affect a person's capacity to perform productive activity and remains inconsistent with the values of a humane society.

Overweight and Obesity

Despite the high frequency of hunger, homeless persons are at least as likely as other Americans to be overweight. Overweight is defined as a body-mass index of 25.0 to 29.9, which can be calculated after measuring height and weight. Obesity is indicated when the body mass index is 30 or greater. Together, these problems affect 61% of Americans, with 27% of Americans qualifying as obese. Homeless persons are equally if not more likely to have evidence of obesity, with approximately one-third of homeless adults qualifying as obese in two separate studies.

Obesity carries a broad range of long- and short-term health risks, including high blood pressure, diabetes, heart disease, stroke, arthritis, sleep apnea, depression, and asthma. Such problems can be especially difficult for homeless people. Not only are homeless individuals subject to increased risk of major illness (e.g. heart attack or stroke), but complications such as arthritis can also interfere with getting to and from work, appointments, or shelters. Additionally, obese individuals can face special barriers to shelter and/or rehabilitation because some facilities are unable to offer special accommodations, such as a lower bunk bed or night-time respiratory equipment for persons with sleep apnea.

Nutritional deficiency disorders

Several homeless studies based on detailed dietary questionnaires have described insufficient intake for a range of vitamins and minerals, including thiamine (vitamin B1), riboflavin (B2), pyridoxine (B6), folate, calcium, magnesium, iron, and vitamin A, among others. Deficient intake does not always lead to a classic vitamin deficiency disease, however. Most homeless persons are unlikely to develop a nutritional deficiency disease for the following reasons: (a) classic vitamin deficiency diseases take a long time to develop; (b) shelter-based meal programs most typically offer nutritionally appropriate meals; and (c) most American flour is enriched with B vitamins.

Certain homeless persons, however, are at special risk. In particular, homeless persons who do not make use of soup kitchens and those who are extremely heavy drinkers may be more likely to develop nutritional deficiency diseases. Homeless persons who chronically sleep outdoors ("rough sleepers") are at especially high risk for such problems. Those coping with diabetes and other special medical conditions face serious challenges in maintaining a medically appropriate diet. Finally, pregnant women are expected to maintain especially high intake of nutrients such as folic acid, calcium, and iron, and this can be a very difficult challenge for pregnant women who are homeless.

Symptoms and Diagnoses

For clinicians working in shelter clinics and on the streets, it is more important to recognize when medical evaluation and/or vitamin supplementation are required than to be able to recognize the signs and symptoms of specific nutritional deficiency diseases. Most nutritional deficiency disorders can present in ways that do not resemble textbook descriptions, and very often more than one nutritional deficiency can be present in the same person. For these reasons, it can be difficult to make a particular diagnosis. The most important consideration for a shelter-

Table 1: Manifestations of Major Vitamin Deficiency Disorders

Nutrient	Deficiency Disorder	Symptoms of Deficiency	Factors associated with deficiency
Thiamine (B1)	Beriberi	Heart failure, (with or without coexistent Wernicke's encephalepathy)	Alcohol, heart failure with loop diuretic therapy
	Peripheral neuropathy	Motor, sensory and/or reflex loss in hands & feet	
	Wernicke's Encephalopathy	Acute confusional state, eye movement abnormalities, fever, confusion, coma	
	Korsakoff Syndrome	Amnesia, impaired ability to learn (patient appears alert)	
Pyridoxine (B6)	B6 Deficiency	Dermatitis, glossitis, cheilosis, nausea, weakness	Phenytoin, isoniazid, oral contraceptives, pregnancy
Cyanocobalamin (B12)	B12 Deficiency	Macrocytosis, anemia, memory loss, irritability, numbness or paresthesias in hands & feet	Gastric atrophy, gastritis, or gastric resection; phenytoin, omeprazole, metformin; strict vegetarianism
Niacin	Pellagra	Dermatitis in sun-exposed areas (collar, forearms, face), mental status changes (depression, confusion, dementia, peripheral neuropathy), gastrointestinal disruption (diarrhea, abdominal discomfort, vomiting)	Alcoholism
Riboflavin (B2)	Riboflavin deficiency	Sore throat, irritation of oral mucous membranes, glossitis, anemia	Phenobarbital treatment, long-term avoidance of dairy products, malabsorption
Vitamin C	Scurvy	Hemorrhages and hyperkeratotic papules around hair follicles, bruising, bleeding into muscles or joints, gum breakdown, tooth loss, depression, neruopathy	Pregnancy, lactation, thyrotoxicosis, drug and alcohol abuse

based clinician is to recognize potential nutritional problems and quickly facilitate further evaluation and nutritional support by an expert.

Situations in which nutrition may be inadequate and require urgent attention:

- a person returns to the shelter or other care facility after a period of sleeping outdoors, with or without high levels of alcohol intake during that time. Such a person may be visibly ill with signs or symptoms of one of the classic diseases described below, or they may simply report fatigue;
- a homeless person has been unable to maintain good nutritional intake due to sustained problems of the digestive tract, such as diarrhea or vomiting, or because of lack of regular access to any source of food;
- a homeless person reports "eating normally" and appears well but is pregnant, has diabetes, or other medical conditions that require special dietary attention.

Some classic nutritional deficiency diseases are mentioned below, but clinicians should be prepared to refer patients for evaluation and to offer vitamins and additional nutritional support even if these diseases are not clearly evident.

Specific nutritional deficiency disorders

Some major nutrient deficiency disorders are reviewed in Table 1. More detailed information is available from conventional texts like those cited in the suggested references for this chapter. Definitive diagnosis often requires laboratory testing and consideration of other diseases that may have similar presentations.

Homeless persons who maintain a moderately balanced diet through regular use of shelter-based meal programs or other planned meal sources rarely develop any of the following disorders unless a coexisting medical condition predisposes to deficiency (such as alcoholism, isoniazid therapy, malabsorption, or pregnancy). Whenever regular nutritional and vitamin intake may have been seriously disturbed, shelter-based clinicians should consider the disorders listed below and have a low threshold to consult a clinician with nutritional expertise.

Treatment and Complications

Treatment of vitamin deficiency generally requires restoration of normal nutritional support. Supplementation with therapeutic doses of the missing vitamin constitutes appropriate treatment.

Isolated replacement of a single vitamin, however, is often inappropriate. Restoration of a single lacking vitamin may induce demand for other vitamins that participate in the same metabolic process. In some instances, treatment for one vitamin deficiency can cause symptoms due to the relative lack of another vitamin. Therefore, when a full nutritional deficiency disorder is manifest, shelter-based clinicians should seek consultative support and consider initiating treatment in a monitored hospital setting.

Prevention and Control
Dietary Counsel

Although soup kitchens offer relatively balanced meals, such meals are not always accessible to all homeless persons. Homelessness poses many challenges to a person attempting to adhere to recommendations concerning a well-balanced diet. Clinicians can take several actions to help. First, assess the available food sources in the community and advocate for appropriately funded food programs within shelters, soup kitchens, and food pantries. Second, have a dialogue with patients about how they obtain food and when and how they eat. In all instances, the patient's understanding, competing needs, resources, and comfort with the specific clinician will determine exactly how the dialogue on food and nutrition should evolve.

Traditional medical issues and more complex psychosocial considerations will influence how the discussion of food proceeds. As a practical matter, clinicians should attempt to identify issues that will require care, such as diabetes, alcohol abuse, diseases of the digestive system, and pregnancy. In the example of pregnancy, the most appropriate interventions will be to assure that the woman is taking prenatal vitamins, has access to sufficient calories through shelter meals and food stamps, and has decent and safe shelter each night.

Complex social and psychic issues will also influence the discussion of food between homeless patients and clinicians. As one example, consider the discussion of sugar intake by a homeless diabetic individual who also abuses alcohol. Some practical suggestions typically made to diabetics are useful for those living in shelters and on the streets, including the use of dilute juices, diet soda, eating bread instead of cake, and attempting to maintain regular meal intake. Clinicians must be mindful that these recommendations could have limited value for patients with limited capacity to understand them or limited choices in their environment. A casual recommendation to a diabetic patient with alcoholism ("eat less concentrated sweets") has potential to be helpful or harmful. The clinician wishing to be helpful must ground the dialogue in a well-informed relationship characterized by trust. Sometimes it is important to wait for such a relationship to develop before offering too much advice.

Food Stamps

The federal government assures access to food stamps to citizens and some non-citizens who meet specific income and asset requirements. Food stamps can be used to purchase food in grocery stores, although ready-to-eat items (such as a sandwich prepared and packaged at a grocery store) are generally not covered by food stamps, and this limits the utility of food stamps for homeless individuals. Items such as bread, fruit, and milk, however, do not require access to a kitchen and can be obtained with food stamps.

A person does not generally need to meet criteria for disability in order to receive this benefit. Since only 37% of homeless individuals reported receiving food stamps in the 1996 National Survey of Homeless Assistance Providers and Clients, it is likely that many homeless persons could qualify for this benefit but do not receive it. A person's particular situation, including household size and disability status, influences eligibility for food stamps. As a rough example, a single homeless person with assets less than $2,000 and income below $960 per month could qualify for food stamps up to $139 per month as of January, 2003 (See www.fns.usda.gov/fsp/default.htm for detailed information on this benefit). Some non-citizens also qualify for food stamps. Application procedures for this federally supported program vary from state to state and are generally obtained through a state benefits office or hotline.

Multiple Vitamins

Standard recommendations support the use of prenatal multiple vitamins among pregnant women. No consensus exists to support routine administration of multiple vitamins to homeless persons, but such a practice should be considered in any patient where dietary intake is irregular or where medical conditions like pregnancy or alcoholism raise special concerns.

Special Clinical Situations
Rough Sleepers

Of special note, when homeless "rough sleepers," particularly those who are alcoholic and

intoxicated, appear for medical care, the potentially life-threatening nutritional risks of thiamine deficiency and/or pellagra (niacin deficiency) must be anticipated and treated presumptively. In hospital emergency departments this is accomplished by offering intravenous fluids with both thiamine and a multivitamin containing niacin. Unfortunately, rapid intravenous nutritional support is not available when a "rough sleeper" is found acutely ill on the street or seeks care at a shelter, rescue mission, mobile services van, or outpatient clinic.

In these situations clinicians should refer patients to the hospital emergency department if any of the following conditions are present:
- the patient appears acutely ill;
- the patient is acutely intoxicated and the facility is not equipped to closely monitor the patient's mental status;
- signs or symptoms of intoxication fail to resolve over the expected time course.

Alcohol Withdrawal

Standard guidelines mandate administration of thiamine to all patients being treated for alcohol withdrawal. In the setting of alcohol withdrawal, the addition of a multiple vitamin can be justified on grounds that it is not harmful and could prevent emergence of a secondary vitamin deficiency.

Summary

Homeless persons are susceptible to both problems of overweight and nutritional deficiency. Vulnerability to either problem may predate the experience of homelessness itself and will vary depending on the current living conditions. The counsel and material assistance we offer patients must be grounded in a well-informed and trusting relationship. ⏹

Acknowledgement
The author is indebted to Marianne Feliciano, RN, for her advice concerning this manuscript.

Nutrition Medication List

Generic	Brand Name	Cost
isoniazid	INH	$
metformin	Glucophage	$$$
omeprazole	Prilosec	$$$$
phenytoin	Dilantin	$

References

Austin CK, Goodman CE, VanHalderan LL. Absence of malnutrition in a population of homeless veterans. *Journal of the American Dietetic Association* 1996;96(12):1283-1285.

Burt MR, Aron LY, Douglas T, et al. Homelessness: Programs and the People They Serve. Technical Report of Finding of the National Survey of Homeless Assistance Providers and Clients. The Urban Institute. 1999.

Carillo TE, Gilbride JA, Chan MM. Soup kitchen meals: an observation and nutrient analysis. *Journal of the American Dietetic Association* 1990;90(7):989-991.

Darnton-Hill I, Truswell AS. Thiamine status of a sample of homeless clinic attenders in Sydney. *Medical Journal of Australia* 1990;152(1):5-9.

Kertesz S. Pellagra in two homeless men. *Mayo Clinic Proceedings* 2001;76:315-318.

Wiecha JL, Dwyer JT, Jacques PF, et al. Nutritional and economic advantages for homeless families in shelters providing kitchen facilities and food. *Journal of the American Dietetic Association* 1993;93(7):777-783.

Wolgemuth JC, Myers-Williams C, Johnson P, et al. Wasting malnutrition and inadequate nutrient intakes identified in a multiethnic homeless population. *Journal of the American Dietetic Association* 1992;92(7):834-839.

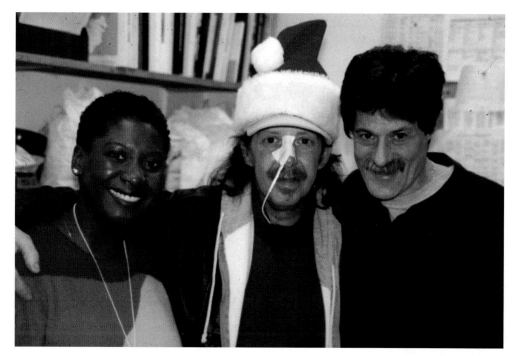

Pain Management

Daniel P. Alford, MD, MPH
Carol A. Waldmann, MD

Chronic pain is an extremely common and particularly challenging problem in the homeless population. Co-morbid psychiatric, behavioral, and addictive disorders are prevalent and complicate the management of pain in this population. Homeless individuals are less able to safeguard their medications and more vulnerable to theft and accompanying assault from others. Mutual mistrust between homeless persons and medical providers is widespread. Finally, acute and chronic pain is common among homeless persons due to the frequency of trauma and injuries in this group. Health professionals who care for homeless persons should develop expertise and comfort with the treatment of pain.

Pathogenic mechanisms of pain can be either nociceptive or neuropathic. Nociceptive pain is due to potential or actual tissue damage. Nociceptive pain is protective and elicits a coordinated reflex and behavioral response to keep injuries to a minimum. On the other hand, neuropathic pain is abnormal, persistent, and maladaptive pain with no obvious biological advantage.

Pain is often divided into three categories: acute pain, cancer pain, and chronic non-malignant pain. In the pain treatment community and the medical field as a whole, a general consensus has evolved on the treatment of acute and cancer pain. The US Department of Health and Human Services has disseminated Clinical Practice Guidelines for the management of acute and cancer pain. In addition, the World Health Organization (WHO) has developed an analgesic ladder for the management of cancer pain. While these guidelines are not universally followed, it is accepted that addiction should not interfere with the adequate treatment of pain in the acute or cancer setting.

The treatment of chronic pain is somewhat more complex for a variety of reasons. Chronic pain is subjective, often with no obvious organic lesion on examination or imaging studies. Myriad conditions can result in "chronic pain", and no single treatment modality fits all of them. By definition, chronic pain continues beyond the usual recovery period for an injury or illness, and therefore often without an ongoing nocioceptive injury. Considerable controversy exists regarding the effectiveness of long-term opioid medication for the treatment of chronic pain.

Epidemiology
Acute Pain
All people experience some acute pain during

Cancer Pain. This 50 year old man has squamous cell carcinoma of the head and neck. During the two years from diagnosis to death, he underwent two major surgeries, chemotherapy, and radiation therapy. Photo by James O'Connell MD

APPROACH TO CHRONIC PAIN

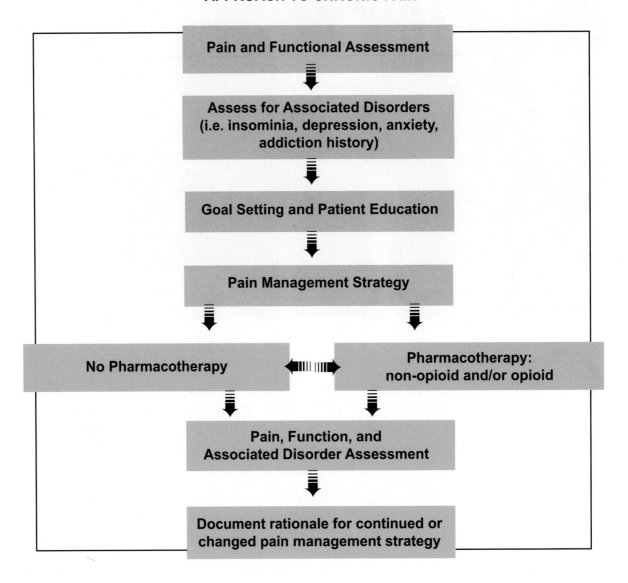

their lifetime. Acute pain is triggered by tissue damage, and the type of pain that generally accompanies injury, surgery, or illness. Muscle pain affects 53% of Americans. Lower back pain is the most common form of acute pain and the fifth most common reason for all physician visits. Low back pain is responsible for direct health care expenditures of more than $20 billion annually.

Cancer Pain

Most cancer pain is the result of tissue damage caused directly by the cancer or by complications, such as infections or blood clots. Approximately 30-40% of people diagnosed with any form of cancer experience moderate to severe pain. Cancer patients are more likely to downplay the severity of pain to their doctors because they fear it means worsening of the cancer or because they fear being seen as a burden or a "complainer".

Chronic Pain

The American Chronic Pain Association (ACPA) estimates one in three Americans (50 million people) suffer from some type of chronic pain. The cost to the American public is approximately $100 billion each year in health care, compensation, and litigation. Common causes include lower back problems, arthritis, reflex sympathetic dystrophy syndrome, repetitive motion injuries, shingles, headaches, and fibromyalgia. Diabetic neuropathy, phantom limb sensation, and other neurologic conditions can also cause chronic pain. Chronic pain is associated with physical, emotional, psychological, and social (including financial) disability. Over half of patients with chronic pain experience symptoms of depression or anxiety.

A subset of chronic pain patients have a syndrome that results in marked restrictions in daily activities and severe alterations in behavior and affect. These patients tend to rely excessively on medications and medical services and undergo multiple non-productive tests, treatments, and surgeries.

Approach to Chronic Pain

The approach to patients with chronic pain begins with a complete pain and functional assessment, followed by goal setting and a treatment plan. Both pain and functional status should be assessed and documented on initial and subsequent evaluations. Therapy should be evaluated based on pain relief and functional improvement. A variety of pain scales can be used, including numeric and visual analog intensity scales. One quick approach is to ask: "On a scale of 0 (no pain) to 10 (most severe pain), what is the level of pain at the present time? What is the level of the best and worst pain experienced in the past 24 hours?" Functional assessments should inquire how pain interferes with daily activities. Setting goals is a critical part of managing chronic pain. Health care providers and patients should discuss realistic expectations regarding pain control and functional improvement prior to initiating therapies. Improvement of both quality of life and functionality are as important as pain relief. In order to reach that goal, treatment of chronic pain must address all aspects of the pain syndrome, including issues of self-esteem, depression, anxiety, sleep, strength and mobility, financial and social support issues, and the experience of pain itself. Finally, the avoidance of the adverse effects of medication, including addiction, is another important goal.

Management of Chronic Pain

Management of chronic pain is most successful when a multidisciplinary treatment plan is employed that utilizes both pharmacologic and non-pharmacologic approaches. Functional rehabilitation may require physical, occupational, psychological, and stress management therapy. Cognitive behavioral therapy has been noted to be particularly useful in treating chronic pain. Treatment of co-morbid conditions such as obesity, addiction, mood disorders, and cardiopulmonary conditions should be aggressive.

While treatment of acute and cancer pain has improved significantly in the last several years, barriers still exist to the adequate treatment of chronic pain. The physiological mechanism of chronic pain is complex, and we do not fully understand why some episodes of acute pain in some people result in chronic pain while others do not. Evidence suggests the under-treatment of acute pain may play a role in long term changes in the brain that affect the ongoing perception of pain. Inflammation, injury, and disease can all cause neurological changes (neuronal plasticity) that result in increased or persistent pain.

New discoveries have been made in our understanding of the physiology of pain. Some common features of chronic pain include hyperalgesia (lowered pain threshold), allodynia (perception of pain caused by non-painful stimuli, such as touch or vibration), and the spread of pain to areas other than those involved with the initial tissue damage. In animal models, central nervous system plasticity can be clearly demonstrated by permanent changes in the brain after a temporary injury of a peripheral nerve. Hyperalgesia is a result of increased sensitivity of neurons or amplification of the pain signal in the dorsal horn, the section of the spinal cord that conveys pain. Allodynia results from the redistribution of neurons so that receptors that usually respond to touch stimulation (mechanoreceptors) now communicate with pain sensing areas of the dorsal horn.

Chronic pain does not have a single cause and has diverse manifestations and characteristics. The treatment of chronic pain must therefore be individualized. For example, low back pain is improved by intensive (>100 hrs) bio-psychosocial rehabilitation that includes physical therapy. On the other hand, corticosteroid injection improves the painful shoulder significantly more than physiotherapy. Unfortunately, access to intensive multidisciplinary pain treatment is not available to many people. Concurrent addiction, psychiatric illness, and unstable living situations such as homelessness may preclude chronic pain patients from the pain clinics that do exist. Homeless patients also often have fewer family and social supports. The limited access to appropriate specialty clinics and the lack of adequate social supports complicate the care of chronic pain for homeless individuals and place a heavy burden on their primary care clinicians. Evidence indicates that primary supports play an important role in the improvement of functional status of patients with chronic pain. Patients without the support of family or friends are likely to benefit from a close trusting relationship with caregivers.

Narcotic Analgesic Dosage Conversion Chart
(Each row contains identical dosages)

How to use this chart: First determine the patient's previous 24 hour regimen for any of the agents listed below. All dosages in the same row are therapeutically equivalent. Example: Patient is receiving Oxycodone 5-10mg po q4h = 30-60 mg/day . Using the table below, the equivalent dose of Fentanyl patch would be 25 mcg.

Codeine		Fentanyl Patch	Hydromorphone		Meperidine		Methadone		Morphine		Oxycodone	
Oral	IV	(Patch)	Oral	IV	Oral	IV	Oral	IV	Oral	IV	Oral	IV
150-447	104-286	25 mcg	5.6-17	1.2-3.4	-	60-165	15-44	8-22	45-134	8-22	22.5-67	12-33
448-747	287-481	50 mcg	17.1-28	3.5-5.6	-	166-278	45-74	23-37	135-224	23-37	67.5-112	33.1-56
748-1047	482-676	75 mcg	28.1-39	5.7-7.9	-	279-390	75-104	38-52	225-314	38-52	112.5-157	56.1-78
1048-1347	677-871	100 mcg	39.1-51	8-10	-	391-503	105-134	53-67	315-404	53-67	157.5-202	78.1-101
1348-1647	872-1066	125 mcg	51.1-62	10.1-12	-	504-615	135-164	68-82	405-494	68-82	202.5-247	101.1-123
1648-1947	1067-1261	150 mcg	62.1-73	12.1-15	-	616-728	165-194	83-97	495-584	83-97	247.5-292	123.1-147
1948-2247	1262-1456	175 mcg	73.1-84	15.1-17	-	729-840	195-224	98-112	585-674	98-112	292.5-337	147.1-168
2248-2547	1457-1651	200 mcg	84.1-96	17.1-19	-	841-953	225-254	113-127	675-764	113-127	337.5-382	168.1-191
2548-2847	1652-1846	225 mcg	96.1-107	19.1-21	-	954-1065	255-284	128-142	765-854	128-142	382.5-427	191.1-213
2848-3147	1847-2041	250 mcg	107.1-118	21.1-24	-	1066-1178	285-314	143-157	855-944	143-157	427.5-472	213.1-236
3148-3447	2042-2236	275 mcg	118.1-129	24.1-26	-	1179-1290	315-344	158-172	945-1034	158-172	472.5-517	236.1-258
3448-3747	2237-2431	300 mcg	129.1-141	26.1-28	-	1291-1403	345-374	173-187	1035-1124	173-187	517.5-562	258.1-281

Narcotic Conversion Chart. This chart provides equianalgesic dosage conversion guidelines for the common opiates. Courtesy of GlobalRPh.com

Pharmacotherapy for Chronic Pain

Not all chronic pain is the same, and different medication choices are made for different types of pain. Analgesics used for the treatment of chronic pain will be discussed in this section. The treatment of neuropathic pain will be discussed separately. Many conditions, such as migraine headache, have treatments specific to that diagnosis.

Non-Steroidal Anti-inflamatory Drugs (NSAIDs) inhibit the cyclooxygenase 2 (COX 2) enzyme. First generation NSAIDs are nonselective inhibitors of cyclooxygenase enzymes and also block cycloxoyenase 1 (COX-1), which is thought to play a role in the protection of the gastric lining. The nonselective NSAIDs include aspirin (Ecotrin™, ASA™, Bayer™, Anacin™), ibuprofen (Motrin™, Advil™), naproxen (Naprosyn™, Aleve™), ketoprofen (Orudis™), and many more. Taken in low doses, these NSAIDs offer mild to moderate analgesia. In larger doses, these NSAIDs have an anti-inflammatory effect. This is particularly beneficial when inflammation contributes to pain, such as musculoskeletal conditions including arthritis. NSAIDs taken on a long-term basis may have dangerous side effects, including gastrointestinal bleeding and renal failure. The newer COX-2 selective NSAIDs, celecoxib (Celebrex™) and rofecoxib (Vioxx™), are known as COX-2 inhibitors. With similar analgesic and anti-inflammatory effects as the nonselective NSAIDs, these COX-2 inhibitors may also marginally reduce some of the gastric side effects caused by other NSAIDs. COX-2 inhibitors have no effect on platelet aggregation but have the same nephrotoxic potential as nonselective NSAIDs. COX-2 inhibitors are very expensive, and the use of these medications should be reserved for persons with peptic ulcer disease or at risk for GI bleeding, such as individuals on chronic anticoagulation and the elderly. In general, lack of clinical response to one NSAID does not reliably predict response or lack of response to other NSAIDs.

Acetaminophen (Tylenol™) is a mild to moderate analgesic that can be used on a long-term basis and is as effective as NSAIDs. When used in doses higher than the recommended daily dose (greater than 4000mg/day) severe liver damage can result. In fact, patients with known liver disease should not take daily doses that exceed 3000mg/day. Acetaminophen does not reduce inflammation.

Tramadol (Ultram™) is a synthetic opioid analogue of codeine that has low affinity for the opioid receptors in the brain. The most active metabolite has an affinity for these receptors that is 6000 times lower than morphine. This analgesic effect is complemented by a separate effect, the blockade of painful impulses at the spinal level via inhibition of serotonin and norepinephrine re-uptake. This enhancement of the inhibitory pathway is similar to the action of tricyclic anti-depressants such as amitriptyline (Elavil™). This may be particularly beneficial in the treatment of neuropathic pain. The addiction potential of tramadol remains controversial. Early studies showed a very low addiction potential, but some later studies have challenged those findings. All agree that the addiction potential with tramadol is lower than with the other more potent opioids.

Opioids remain highly controversial in the treatment of chronic pain. The most common opioids used are morphine, oxycodone, hydrocodone, fentanyl, and methadone. Opioids primarily bind to mu receptors in the brain, spinal cord, and in the periphery, and decrease the transmission of painful stimuli and diminish the perception of pain by the brain. In the latter, the pain is not removed but experienced as less aversive. The effects of opioids include analgesia, euphoria, constipation, and respiratory depression. Used at appropriate doses, the physiologic side effects are minimal and can be easily controlled. As opposed to NSAIDs and acetaminophen, opioids have no analgesic ceiling. Analgesic doses are only limited by respiratory and central nervous system depression.

In general, opioid analgesics should be started at low dose and titrated slowly using the following broad guidelines: titrate to efficacy (pain relief and functional improvement) and minimize side effects; titrate initially with short-acting preparations and convert to long-acting preparations. The fentanyl (Duragesic™) patch is a convenient long-acting preparation. The patch is applied every 72 hours and will take approximately 8 hours after the first application to achieve peak serum levels. The lowest dose patch is 25 mcg, which is equivalent to 90 mg of morphine or 9-10 Percocet™ or Percodan™ per day. Unfortunately, patients who are stable on lower doses of short-acting opioids will not be able to tolerate the smallest fentanyl patch. A major concern with the use of long-term opioids is the potential for addiction and diversion. See our separate section on the treatment of chronic pain with opioids.

Adjuvant analgesics are used to treat pain, even though analgesia is not the primary indication for the use of these medications. Antidepressants and anticonvulsants are good examples. Antidepressants, including tricyclic antidepressants (TCAs) such as amitriptyline (Elavil™) and imipramine (Tofranil™), have been used successfully in some patients to treat both peripheral and central neuropathic pain. They are believed to potentiate the body's own pain relieving systems by affecting neurotransmitters such as norepinephrine. Studies evaluating selective serotonin reuptake inhibitors (SSRIs), such as fluoxetine (Prozac™) and paroxetine (Paxil™), have shown them to have inconsistent effectiveness in treating neuropathic pain compared to placebo. A meta-analysis found SSRI's to be less effective than TCA's, but with 50% fewer side effects. Pain relief usually requires lower doses than those used for treating depression. Therefore doses should balance pain relief and side effects. Such a balance is usually reached at a dosage of 75-150 mg of amitriptyline (Elavil™).

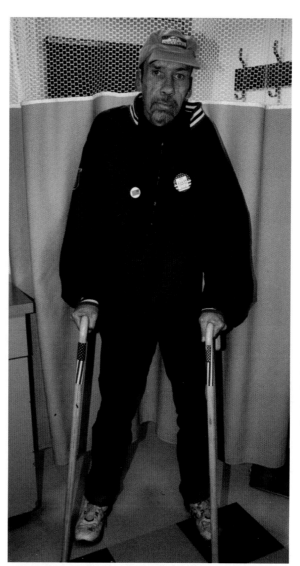

Compression Fractures of the Spine. This man with osteoporosis suffers from severe pain as a result of compression fractures in his back. Lung cancer was later diagnosed, with metastases to the T9 and T10 vertebral bodies. Photo by James O'Connell MD

Anticonvulsants such as carbamazapine (Tegretol™) and phenytoin (Dilantin™) have been commonly used at anti-epileptic doses with some success. Gabapentin (Neurontin™) is a second generation anticonvulsant that has shown great promise in the treatment of painful neuropathies. Studies have shown the efficacy of gabapentin (Neurontin™) to be equal to that of amitriptyline (Elavil™) but with fewer side effects. Anticonvulsants seem most effective with neuropathic pain described as lancinating or electric shock-like. The mechanism of action is unclear but presumed secondary to suppression of the spread of aberrant discharges through neuronal sodium channels.

Topical analgesic agents include lidocaine and capsaicin. Lidocaine is a local anesthetic agent available as a patch (Lidoderm™) as well as an injection for mononeuropathies. An oral antiarrhythmic lidocaine analogue, mexiletine (Mexitil™), has been used at doses of 200-400 mg three times a day with mixed results. Capsaicin (Zostrix™), an active ingredient in hot chili peppers, has been used with some success in patients with hyperalgesia and allodynia. This cream must be applied 3-4 times a day to be effective and often causes a burning sensation followed by anesthesia. Pain relief is usually modest and can take several weeks to take effect. A topical anesthetic like lidocaine gel can be used prior to application for the first several days to avoid the initial burning sensation.

Treatment of Chronic Pain with Opioids

Opioids are indicated for moderate to severe pain that has a significant impact on functionality and quality of life or when non-opioid pharmacotherapy has failed. Opioid therapy for chronic pain remains highly controversial. No controlled trials have evaluated the effectiveness of long-term opioids for the treatment of chronic pain. Some clinical evidence suggests that opioids are less effective with neuropathic types of chronic pain, a finding consistent with the known decrease in opioid receptors in the spinal cord dorsal horn after peripheral nerve damage. Other studies have found that patients with painful neuropathies may be relatively insensitive to opioids, but larger doses of opioids provide relief in double-blind, placebo-controlled trials. Many medications are useful in the treatment of chronic pain, but specific concerns have arisen around the use of opioids.

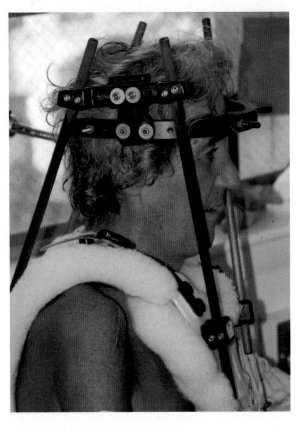

Neck Fracture. This man sustained a fracture of several vertebrae in the cervical spine when he collided with a bus while riding his bicycle. Photo by James O'Connell MD

The use of opioids raises concerns about tolerance, addiction, misuse, respiratory depression and other side effects, risk of diversion for non-medical uses, and regulatory issues. For these reasons, opioids are often underutilized, and their use is associated with tension and controversy. These concerns must be addressed in order to achieve the best treatment of chronic pain syndrome.

In 1997 the American Academy of Pain Medicine and the American Pain Society issued a joint statement on the treatment of chronic pain with opioids. This document, available on the website of either of these organizations, addresses many of the key concerns in detail and outlines suggested principles of practice for the use of opioids. These principles, an extension of the principles of good medical practice, should include a thorough evaluation of the patient, the development of a treatment plan, the determination whether specialty consultation is needed, the periodic review of treatment efficacy, and good documentation. The joint statement challenges many commonly held assumptions about opioid use and abuse:

- the *de novo* development of addiction when opioids are used for pain is low;
- respiratory depression induced by opioids is usually short lived, occurs in the treatment naïve, and is antagonized by pain;
- tolerance to analgesia has not proven to be a prevalent limitation to long-term opioid use;
- the risk of diversion can be reduced by paying attention to patterns of prescribing requests.

State laws and policies are evolving to recognize explicitly that the use of opioids in the treatment of chronic pain is appropriate in many cases.

Addiction, physical dependence, and tolerance are three discrete entities that are often confused. Treating clinicians and persons living with chronic pain should understand the definitions of these terms and their differences. In 2001 the American Academy of Pain Medicine, the American Pain Society, and the American Society of Addiction Medicine wrote a consensus statement that recognized the following definitions of these terms and recommended their use.

Physical dependence is a state of adaptation manifested by a drug class-specific withdrawal syndrome that can be produced by abrupt cessation, rapid dose reduction, decreasing blood level of the drug, and/or administration of an antagonist.

Tolerance is a state of adaptation in which

exposure to a drug induces changes that result in a diminution of one or more of the drugs effects over time.

Addiction is a primary, chronic, neurobiological disease with genetic, psychosocial and environmental factors influencing its manifestations. Addiction is characterized by behaviors that include one or more of the following: impaired control over drug use; compulsive use; continued use despite harm; and craving. Providers should not confuse addiction with pseudo-addiction. Pseudo-addiction is a behavior, seen in patients who have severe unrelieved pain, that mimics aspects of addiction. These patients are intensely focused on obtaining more opioids in order to achieve acceptable pain relief rather than trying to obtain more drugs. This behavior should resolve when adequate pain relief is provided.

Treatment Contracts

Much of the tension between health providers and patients arises when no explicit agreement has been reached on a treatment plan. Uncertainty about receiving adequate pain relief provokes much anxiety in patients with significant pain. Similarly, health providers can become very uncomfortable without clear behavioral expectations about the use of the prescribed medication. Controlled Substance Medication Consent and Agreement Forms delineate the possible side effects of opioids and are very useful for both patient and clinician. Treatment contracts codify the expected use of medication by the patient and the expected response to prescribing requests by the health provider. Examples of these forms can be found on the AAPM website.

Special Considerations for Homeless Populations

Many issues surrounding chronic pain are exaggerated in the homeless population. Homeless persons lack a full range of social supports. They often must be outside for most of the day and are unable to follow advice about physical activity and protection from weather. Adequate rest and sleep are often difficult for homeless persons. While *de novo* addiction after the use of opioid medication for pain is rare, substance abuse and addiction are common in the homeless population. Homeless people have less control of their possessions, rarely have access to a location where medications can be locked and stored, and are thus vulnerable to assault and theft. Such challenges must be acknowledged, and plans to avoid such complications should be a shared responsibility between patient and caregiver. Brainstorming with patients about strategies to avoid complications before troubles arise can help to form an alliance rather than an antagonistic relationship between the health provider and the patient. From the onset of treatment each patient should understand the prescribing limits that the provider will follow. Discussing these general rules beforehand assures that they are not "taken personally" or viewed as evidence of prejudicial treatment by the patient. Caregivers should empathize with their patients and recognize that homeless persons have minimal supports and will need considerable support from their primary care clinicians.

Opioid Treatment and Methadone Maintenance

People with addiction may require the use of opioids when they experience acute pain or cancer pain. Other chronic pain syndromes may also require the use of opioids. In such situations, explicit treatment agreements between patient and prescribing clinician are imperative. Multidisciplinary treatment, including substance abuse treatment, is critically important. The risk of addiction can be ameliorated slightly with the use of long-acting opioids, such as sustained release morphine (MS Contin™) and oxycodone (Oxycontin™) preparations, methadone (Dolophine™, Methadose™), or fentanyl patches (Duragesic™). This reduces the repeated pain/reward cycle that is characteristic of the rapidly acting, short duration medications such as oxycodone (Percocet™, Percodan™), hydrocodone (Vicodan™), and meperidine (Demerol™).

Studies confirm that patients with a history of opioid dependency are more pain sensitive than controls. Daily methadone maintenance treatment may confer some analgesia at peak plasma levels (2-3 hours after the dose), but these patients remain more pain sensitive (hyperalgesic) compared to controls. In addition, the daily methadone dose may cause cross-tolerance to the effects of administered opioid analgesics. Because methadone maintenance doses do not provide analgesia and may cause tolerance to opioids, the management of pain in these patients will often require higher doses and more frequent dosing intervals. Patients on methadone maintenance should continue with their regular daily dose in addition to the opioid being prescribed for pain management. Avoid using mixed agonist/antagonist opioid analgesics such as pentazocine (Talwin™) in methadone-maintained patients, as they may precipitate opioid withdrawal.

Summary

Chronic pain is common in the homeless population, and homeless persons experience significant barriers and obstacles to treatment for chronic pain. Trauma, mental illness, and addiction are common problems that contribute both to the incidence of chronic pain and the complications in caring for homeless persons with chronic pain. Barriers to care include poor understanding of chronic pain in the general medical community, inadequate access to multidisciplinary pain clinics, minimal social supports, inadequate shelter, and difficulty in storing medications. Chronic pain affects all aspects of life, including physical and mental health. The causes of chronic pain are complex and include brain plasticity and pain perception that is effected by mood, anxiety, and duration of painful stimuli. Each patient requires an individualized treatment plan. Many general strategies can be used to increase the success of treatment in most cases. Communication and empathy are critical in caring for homeless persons in pain. Clear expectations help reduce anxiety and tension between caregivers and patients. A caring and involved clinician can help reduce suffering, even when some physical pain persists. ■

Pain Management Medication List

Generic	Brand	Cost
aspirin	Anacin, ASA, Bayer, Ecotrin	$
ibuprofen	Advil, Motrin	$
naproxen	Aleve, Naprosyn	$$$
ketoprofen	Orudis	$
celecoxib	Celebrex	$$$
rofecoxib	Vioxx	$$$
acetaminophen	Tylenol	$
tramadol	Ultram	$$$
morphine sustained release	MS Contin	$$$$$
oxycodone sustained release	OxyContin	$$$
oxycodone	Percocet, Percodan	$$$
methadone	Dolophine, Methadose	$
hydrocodone	Vicodin	$
meperidine	Demerol	$$$
fentanyl patch	Duragesic	$$$$$
amitriptyline	Elavil	$
imipramine	Tofranil	$
carbamazepine	Tegretol	$
phenytoin	Dilantin	$
gabapentin	Neurontin	$$$$
lidocaine patch	Lidoderm, Xylocaine	$$$$
mexiletine	Mexitil	$$$
capsaicin	Zostrix	$
pentazocine	Talwin	$$$

References

American Pain Society. The Use of Opioids for the Treatment of Chronic Pain: A consensus statement from American Academy of Pain Medicine and American Pain Society. 1996.

Ashburn MA, Staats PS. Pain: management of chronic pain. *Lancet* 1999;353(9167):1865-1869.

Ballantyne JC, Mao J. Opioid therapy for chronic pain. *New England Journal of Medicine* 2003;349(20):1943-1953.

Besson JM. Pain: The neurobiology of pain. *Lancet* 1999;353(9164):1610-1615.

Gallagher RM. Treatment planning in pain medicine: integrating medical, physical, and behavioral therapies. *Medical Clinics of North America* 1999;83(3):823-849.

Katz WA. Approach to the management of nonmalignant pain. *American Journal of Medicine* 1996;101(1A):54S-63S.

Lipsky PE. Introduction. The role of COX-2-specific inhibitors in clinical practice. *American Journal of Medicine* 2001;110(Supplement 3A):1S-2S.

Marcus D. Treatment of nonmalignant chronic pain. *American Family Physician* 2000;61:1331-1346.

McQuay H. Pain: Opioids in pain management. *Lancet* 1999;353(9171):2229-2232.

Portenoy RK. Opioid therapy for chronic nonmalignant pain: clinician's perspective. *Journal of Law, Medicine and Ethics* 1996;24(4):296-309.

Savage SR. Opioid use in the management of chronic pain. *Medical Clinics of North America* 1999;83(3):761-786.

Stimmel B. Pain, analgesia, and addiction: an approach to the pharmacologic management of pain. *The Clinical Journal of Pain* 1985;1(1):14-22.

Woolf CJ, Mannion RJ. Pain: Neuropathic pain: aetiology, symptoms, mechanisms, and management. *Lancet* 1999;353(9168):1959-1964.

Drugs for pain. *The Medical Letter on Drugs and Therapeutics* 2000;1085:73-78.

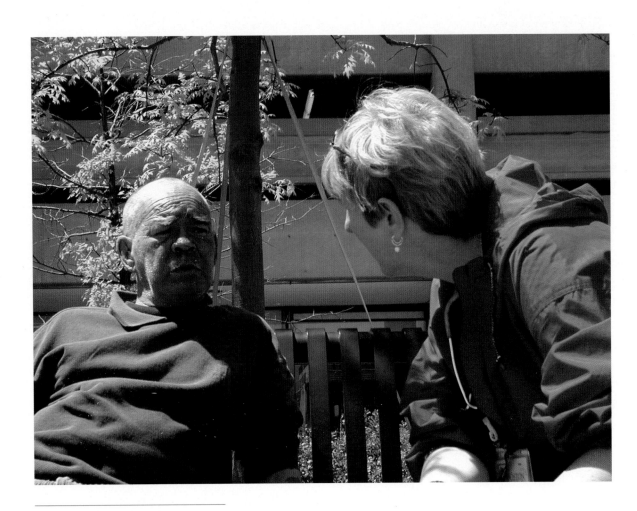

Street Team RN Cheryl Kane shares a few
quiet moments with this elderly man on his
bench near the Boston Aquarium.
Photo by Stan Grossfeld

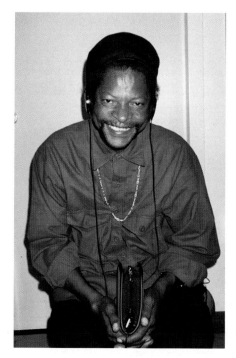
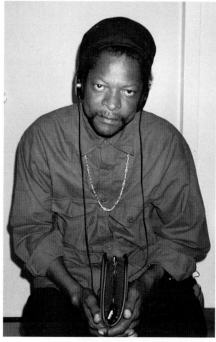

Traumatic Brain Injury (TBI)

Carol A. Waldmann, MD

Traumatic brain injury (TBI), caused either by blunt force or acceleration/deceleration forces, is common in the general population. Homeless persons are at particularly high risk of head trauma and adverse outcomes to TBI. Even mild traumatic brain injury can lead to persistent symptoms including cognitive, physical, and behavioral problems. It is important to understand brain injury in the homeless population so that appropriate referrals to specialists and supportive services can be made. Understanding the symptoms and syndromes caused by brain injury sheds light on some of the difficult behavior observed in some homeless persons. This understanding can help clinicians facilitate and guide the care of these individuals.

Prevalence and Distribution

Every year in the USA, approximately 1.5 million people sustain traumatic brain injury (TBI), 230,000 people are hospitalized due to TBI and survive, over 50,000 people die from TBI, and more than 1 million people are treated in emergency rooms for TBI. In persons under the age of 45 years, TBI is the leading cause of death. Health costs from TBI are estimated to be in the range of $35 billion per year. Eighty to ninety thousand Americans experience the onset of long-term disability as a result of a TBI. TBI is classified into categories of severe, moderate, and mild. Mild traumatic brain injury (MTBI), often referred to interchangeably as a concussion, can cause persistent disabling problems such as headache, confusion, memory and cognitive problems, mood changes, changes in sleep pattern, or sensory problems. In most cases of MTBI patients

recover fully, but up to 15% of patients diagnosed with MTBI by a physician experience persistent disabling problems. Up to 75% of brain injuries are classified as MTBI. These injuries cost the US almost $17 billion per year. The groups most at risk for TBI are those aged 15-24 years and those aged 65 years and older. Men are twice as likely to sustain TBI as women.

Causes

TBI occurs either with blunt force trauma to the head or as a result of rapid acceleration/deceleration. Diffuse brain injury can occur when the brain moves back and forth within the skull. The greatest amount of damage is often in the temporal and frontal lobes where the brain comes into contact with bony structures. Localized injury can also occur with penetrating head injuries. The leading

TBI and Mood Swings.
This man suffered a gunshot wound to the head and many subsequent traumatic brain injuries while homeless. These photographs show the rapid mood swings often seen after TBI.

Photos by Carol Waldmann MD

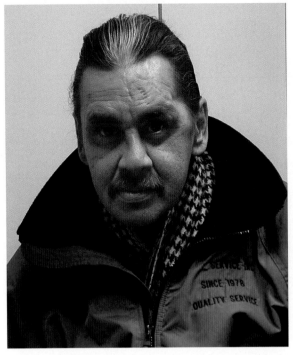

Brain Injury. This long time patient of BHCHP had a resection of a subdural hematoma in 1995. Note the visible change in the shape of his skull from brain surgery, which included partial resection of the temporal lobe.

studies, but the most frequent delineation of these categories is based on the Glasgow Coma Scale. Combined with the existence/duration of post-traumatic amnesia (PTA) and/or loss of consciousness (LOC), the following definitions are most useful:

- *severe brain injury* - GCS 8 or less, LOC >24 hrs, and/or PTA >24 hr;
- *moderate brain injury* - GCS 9-12, LOC 1/2-24hr, and/or PTA 1-24hr;
- *mild brain injury* - GCS of 13-15, LOC< 30 min, and PTA < 1hr

The Centers for Disease Control and Prevention (CDC) MTBI Working Group defined MTBI as "the occurrence of an injury to the head arising from blunt trauma or acceleration/deceleration forces" with one or more of the following conditions attributable to the head injury:

1. any period of observed or self reported:
   - transient confusion, disorientation, or impaired consciousness;
   - dysfunction of memory around the time of injury;
   - loss of consciousness lasting less than 30 minutes;
2. observed signs of other neurological or neuropsychological dysfunction, such as:
   - seizures acutely following injury to the head;
   - irritability, lethargy, or vomiting follow ing head injury, especially among infants and very young children or;
   - headache, dizziness, irritability, fatigue, or poor concentration, especially among older children and adults.

Diagnostic tests and imaging can be useful, particularly in the case of sports-related injuries. Neuropsychological testing is appropriate when

causes of TBI in the general population include motor vehicle accidents (MVAs), falls, firearm accidents, and sports/recreational injuries. Although no controlled studies have been done, homeless persons appear to be at high risk for TBI given that substance abuse, MVAs, and violence are common in this population. Substance abuse leads to a large number of falls. When a person passes out or "takes a header", it is equivalent to being dropped on the head from their height. Half of all TBI is associated with alcohol use, either in the injured or the person causing the injury. Alcohol use is also shown to result in a higher level of post trauma disability.

Diagnosis

The definition of mild, moderate, and severe traumatic brain injury has varied slightly in different

Based on Luerssen TG. Acute traumatic cerebral injuries. In: Cheek WR (ed). Pediatric Neurosurgery. 3rd ed. Philadelphia: WB Saunders; 1994.

Table 1: Glasgow Coma Scale

Score	Eye-opening	Motor	Verbal	Verbal (young)
6		Obeys		
5		Localizes	Appropriate and oriented	Appropriate
4	Spontaneous	Withdraws	Confused conversation	Not consolable
3	Verbal	Flexion (decorticate)	Inappropriate words	Persistently irritable
2	Pain	Extension (decerebrate)	Incomprehensible	Restless, agitated
1	None	None	None	None

Mild	13-15
Moderate	9-12
Severe (coma)	≤ 8

Grades of Concussion

Grade 1:
1. Transient confusion (inattention, inability to maintain a coherent stream of thought and carry out goal-directed movements)
2. No loss of consciousness
3. Concussion symptoms or mental status abnormalities on examination resolve in **less than 15 minutes**

Grade 2:
1. Transient confusion
2. No loss of consciousness
3. Concussion symptoms or mental status abnormalities (including amnesia) on examination last **more than 15 minutes**

Grade 3:
1. Any loss of consciousness
   a) Brief (seconds)
   b) Prolonged (minutes)

Features of Concussion Frequently Observed

1. Vacant stare (befuddled facial expression)
2. Delayed verbal and motor responses (slow to answer questions or follow instructions)
3. Confusion and inability to focus attention (easily distracted and unable to follow through with normal activities)
4. Disorientation (walking in the wrong direction; unaware of time, date and place)
5. Slurred or incoherent speech (making disjointed or incomprehensible statements)
6. Gross observable incoordination (stumbling, inability to walk tandem/straight line)
7. Emotions out of proportion to circumstances (distraught, crying for no apparent reason)
8. Memory deficits (exhibited by the athlete repeatedly asking the same question that has already been answered, or inability to memorize and recall 3 of 3 words or 3 of 3 objects in 5 minutes)
9. Any period of loss of consciousness (paralytic coma, unresponsiveness to arousal)

emotional or cognitive symptoms may be present. The primary tool for diagnosis remains careful history. All patients should be asked about injuries or accidents, as many patients do not spontaneously mention head injuries to their doctors. If they have had an injury a detailed history of signs and symptoms of head injury should be taken.

Neuropsychiatric Sequelae of TBI

MTBI (with or without LOC or PTA) can result in long term sequelae including somatic, mood, anxiety, cognitive, and behavioral disorders. Psychosis also occurs in some cases. The major risk factors for neuropsychiatric disturbances after brain injury include age, atherosclerosis, and alcoholism. Premorbid personality, social stressors, and lack of social supports also play significant roles in the level and type of disturbance. One study of 100 subjects revealed post injury personality disorders in 66%, with a pre-TBI personality disorder diagnosis in 24% of the sample. Cognitive disturbances after head injury include dementia, delirium, amnestic disorder, and intellectual impairment. Mood

disorders are common, including major depression in 25% and mania in 9% of patients. Anxiety disorders range in frequency from 11-70%, depending on the study cited. 10% of patients have apathy without depression. Schizophrenia-like psychosis occurs in 0.7-9.8%; most of these patients did not have a family history of schizophrenia. Diffuse brain damage with predominance in the frontal and temporal lobes (at times caused by MTBI) is thought to cause behavioral dyscontrol disorders. Symptoms include: mood problems, such as irritability, rage, and anger; cognitive deficits, including impaired memory, attention, and judgment; and behavioral dysfunction, including impulsivity, aggressivity, hyperactivity, hyperphagia, and pica. A wide range of somatic symptoms with a neurological basis also occur.

Management

The sequelae of TBI are diverse, and the management must be tailored to the individual. If individuals are seen soon after an injury, referral to a physician should be made as soon as possible. Baseline neurological, emotional, and cognitive findings should be carefully recorded. Patients at any stage should be evaluated for the ability to resume risky activity, such as operating machinery, driving motor vehicles, or participating in sports. Most research in this area has been around returning to sports activities and may be applied to other settings.

When cognitive or emotional symptoms interfere with normal relationships and functioning, as is often the case in the homeless population, patients should be referred to a neurologist and/or a psychiatrist. Referral to specialized multidisciplinary cognitive therapy programs should be considered. Patients should be educated about their condition, treatment plan, and prognosis. It is often a relief to patients and their support systems to understand the probable relationship of a head injury to changes in functional level, memory, concentration, personality, and emotions. Support is often available at the local chapter of the Brain Injury Association, but homeless patients often need significant additional support and assistance in accessing such services. Patients may also be eligible for disability benefits and should be assisted in obtaining these benefits, which may enable them to access services and housing. MTBI results in diminished reaction time, and those with recent concussions are at high risk for secondary injury. Individuals should be educated about this risk. Assistance in getting into a safe environment for recovery and secondary prevention should be provided if appropriate. Patients should be given written instructions about what activities may be dangerous and when certain of these activities can be resumed.

Summary

Brain injury is common in both the general population and specifically in the homeless population. Many homeless people are at risk of brain injury due to the high prevalence of accidents, substance abuse, and violence in this population. Persons with brain injury tend to decline in socioeconomic status due to neuropsychiatric disturbances following head injury. They are frequently unable to hold jobs or maintain interpersonal relationships, and are at increased risk of being involved in the criminal justice system. This increases the risk of becoming or remaining homeless. Alcoholism decreases the brain's ability to heal and increases the risk of neuropsychiatric and physical sequelae of brain injury. All head injuries in the homeless population, including MTBI, should be taken seriously. Referral to a health care clinician should be made as soon as possible after a head injury, and every effort should be made to find a safe environment for the injured person to recover. Physicians and mid-levels should routinely screen for past head injury and sequelae of TBI. Patients with evidence of ongoing symptoms should be referred to the appropriate services and counseled about secondary prevention, possible complications, and prognosis for recovery. ▪▪

Table 2: Signs and Symtoms of TBI

Behavior	Mood	Cognition	Somatic Symtoms
Impulsivity	Irritability	Impaired memory	Headache
Aggressivity	Depression	Decreased attention	Nausea
Hyperactivity	Mania	Poor concentration	Dizziness
Hyperphagia	Rage/ Anger	Poor executive	Vertigo
Pica	Anxiety	function	Diplopia
Loss of initiative		Impaired judgment	Insomnia
		Impaired judgment	Deafness
		Distractibility	Tinnitus
		Conceptual	Light sensitivity
		disorganization	Noise sensitivity
			Fatigue
			Dyscoordination
			Sleep disturbances
			Blurred vision
			Seizures

References

American Academy of Neurology. Report of the Quality Standards Subcommittee, Practice Parameter: The Management of Concussion in Sports (summary statement), 1997. http://www.aan.com/professionals/practice/guidelines.cfm

Centers for Disease Control and Prevention/National Center for Injury Prevention and Control Publication. *Heads Up: Brain Injury in Your Practice.* Traumatic Brain Injury Tool Kit. Jan 20, 2003. http://www.cdc.gov/ncipc/pub-res/tbi_toolkit/physicians/index.htm

Glascow Coma Scale (Adapted from Womack Army Medical Center, Internet Version). http://www.cdc.gov/ncipc/pub-res/tbi_toolkit/physicians/gcs.htm

Hibbard MR, Bogdany J, Uysal S, et al. Axis II psychopathology in individuals with tramautic brain injury. *Brain Injury* 2000;14(1):45-61.

McCrea M, Kelly JP, Randolph C, et al. Immediate Neurocognitive Effects of Concussion. 2002. http://www.cdc.gov/ncipc/pub-res/tbi_toolkit/mccrae/title.htm

National Institutes of Health Consensus Development Conference Statement: Rehabilitation of Persons with Traumatic Brain Injury. 1998. http://consensus.nih.gov/cons/109/109_intro.htm

Rao V, Lyketsos C. Neuropsychiatric sequelae of traumatic brain injury. *Psychosomatics* 2000;41(2):95-103.

Tate PS, Freed DM, Bombardier CH, et al. Traumatic brain injury: influence of blood alcohol on post-acute cognitive function. *Brain Injury* 1999;13(10):767-784.

Thurman DJ, et al. Traumatic Brain Injury in the United States: A Report to Congress: Centers for Disease Control and Prevention; 1999. http://www.cdc.gov/ncipc/pub-res/tbi_congress/tbi_congress.htm

Part Four:

The Management of
Chronic Diseases

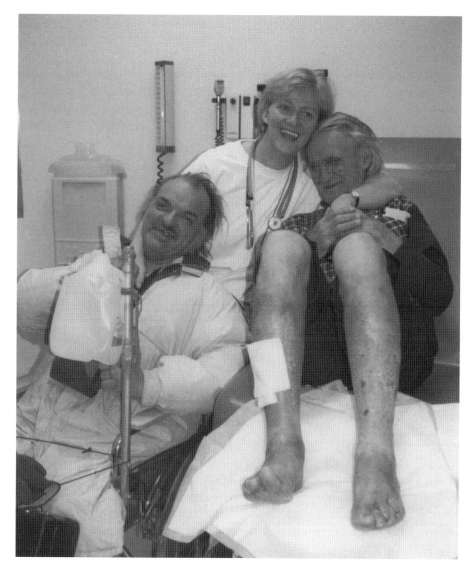

Chronic Medical Diseases in Homeless Populations

Gregory A. Wagoner, MD, MBA

Health care for homeless persons has long been rooted in caring for the emergent and episodic needs of a people whose daily lives are punctuated by uncertainty and vulnerability. Accident, injury, exposure to the extremes of heat and cold, and a range of communicable diseases facilitated by crowding repeatedly compromise the health and well being of people who are homeless. With the pressure to assure that each new event in their lives is cared for in the best way possible, the many other chronic conditions that are a part of their lives often do not get our full attention as clinicians.

Ellen Hoey, RN, embraces this wheelchair-bound man and his uncle. The uncle had several admissions to the hospital for recurrent cellulitis until Ellen taught his nephew how to change his uncle's daily dressings. Photo by James O'Connell MD

Readily accessible, consistent, and continuous care from a known and trusted clinician is not always available for many people experiencing homelessness. Likewise, the systems that support our care frequently do not give us adequate information to understand the nature of each chronic condition and what parts of a care plan are yet to be completed.

Convergent with the rise in awareness of the burden of chronic illness borne by homeless populations has been the quality improvement movement in health care and other industries and systems over the past 15 years. The conversation about the definition of quality of care and the method of examining issues of quality has been going on for decades. The 1970's were marked by peer review;

the 1980's by quality assurance; and since the 1990's, quality of care has been discussed in terms of quality improvement. Not surprisingly, individual clinicians, patients, health care organizations, and insurance providers may have contrasting perspectives on what constitutes quality of care.

Most homeless people have at least one, and often several, chronic diseases, yet often our delivery systems are focused on the episodic treatment of chief complaints at a given moment in time. Since the early 1990's, a slow shift in emphasis has occurred from this sporadic-type care focusing on individual and immediate issues to an emphasis on treatment of chronic disease in a revolutionary way. Instead of focusing on anecdotal evidence of best treatments for a given symptom complex, the emphasis has shifted. Now more resources are devoted to treatment based on clinical evidence, centered on the whole patient, and resulting in specific key improvements that are measurable and directly related to overall health, including morbidity, mortality, and quality of life. All around us is a push to close the gap between what we know – that extensive amount of evidence-based research that relates actions to outcomes – and what we actually do when we see a patient.

Studies consistently show that homeless people have a higher prevalence of chronic disease than the population as a whole, and the ability of someone who is homeless to manage disease optimally is severely impaired by a lack of control over living conditions and limited opportunities to consistently follow an optimal treatment plan. Given these factors, it is even more important to consider just how population-based, chronic disease management, in conjunction with measurable outcomes, affects care and quality of life. Moving from a dependent, provider-driven model to one in which the patient is empowered to set goals and determine priorities results in the inclusion of the patient in decisions. Since in reality patients do provide most of their own care through direct self-care and decision-making about how a recommended treatment plan will be followed, it appears natural to shift to a model in which the patient and the caregivers make decisions together. Whereas the clinician may define the main problem in a visit as non-adherence, the patient may define the main problem as loneliness – a priority that should result in a revised and markedly different treatment plan developed by both patient and provider.

As the quality improvement movement has resulted in measurable outcomes, such initiatives have fit well into the treatment of chronic disease in this collaborative fashion. In decades past there was little effort and even less success in measuring the level of quality in health care. Today this science has developed significantly, partly as a natural offspring of evidence-based medicine and partly as a result of initiatives sponsored by managed care systems in response to regulatory requirements. In measuring what we do, choosing outcomes that will truly make a difference is step one. Medical literature searches in a given chronic disease can result in a short and focused list of key quality outcomes to measure and improve. In the case of diabetes, even small reductions in HgbA1C levels result in significantly fewer future cardiovascular events, such as strokes or heart attacks. Measuring this value should be a part of every on-going treatment plan for diabetic patients, and collaborative goal setting around this measurement should be considered as one goal to be followed and improved.

Such goal setting highlights the need to build awareness of a disease through an education program that assures the patient is an informed partner in the design of a treatment plan. Only then can our homeless patients truly direct their care in a manner that understands and respects the reality of life in the shelters and on the streets. This awareness and education rests not only with the primary care provider during a clinic visit. Ideally this is a responsibility of a multidisciplinary team of professionals who tailor the education and treatment to the patient's readiness, willingness, knowledge level, and capacity to learn. This may include written literature, group visits, and nurse and other educator sessions, such as dietary discussion. All of this needs to be framed in the overall context of each homeless person, respecting their activities of daily living, resource availability, and personal desires and priorities. The priority for our patients is rarely improved control of their chronic diseases; rather, the basic priorities of safety, food, or shelter absorb their time and energy. Self-management goals must be set by the patient, with help from the providers and overall delivery system.

We are approaching an era of increasing opportunities to improve the care of our patients, even as resources remain stretched for most of us. As new models of integrated care emerge and new information systems become more available, clinicians will have more tools at the time of care to assist in joint decision-making with our patients. The weight of clinical evidence available in primary care is overwhelming, and none of us can know and remember all of the information that might improve our ability to care for our patients. As point-of-care knowledge and assistance increases, our ability to provide the best care possible at each visit will improve. We seek the skills, time, and knowledge to respond to new symptoms and new life situations facing our patients with chronic diseases. The next few years will yield dramatic changes in outcomes and better quality of life for us all. ▦

Reference

Chassin, MR. Quality of health care, Part 3: improving the quality of care. *New England Journal of Medicine 1996;* 335(14): 1060-1063.

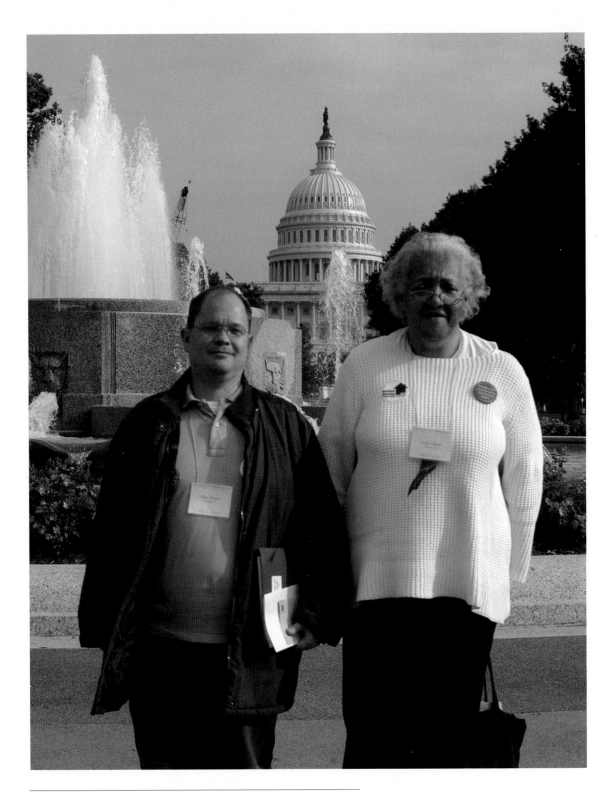

John Hatton and Ellen Dailey of BHCHP's Consumer Advisory Board at the Annual Health Care for the Homeless Program Meeting in Washington in May, 2003.   Photo by James O'Connell MD

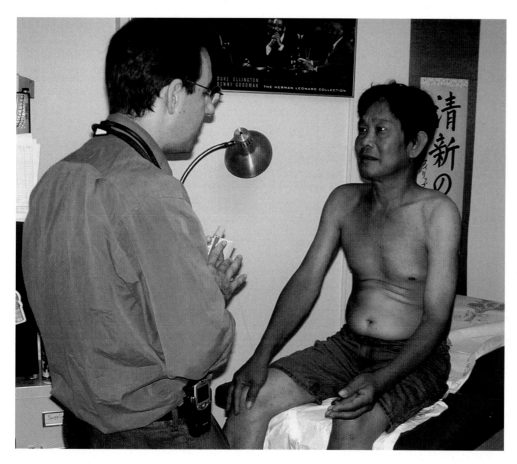

The Health Disparities Collaborative

Laura M. Gillis, MS, RN

A major goal of the US Public Health Service and the Bureau of Primary Health Care is the elimination of health disparities, particularly for minority populations, people living in poverty, and, in some cases, women. These health disparities refer to differences in deaths from the four top "killers" (heart disease, cancer, stroke, and diabetes), as well as other chronic illnesses.

- African Americans have the highest mortality rate from breast cancer, are twice as likely as white Americans to die from prostate cancer, and are at greater risk for end-stage renal disease secondary to co-morbid diabetes and hypertension.
- Hispanics and Native Americans are 2-3 times more likely than the general population to develop diabetes.
- Asian Americans are 3-5 times more likely to suffer liver cancer associated with untreated hepatitis.
- Inner city children and youth living in poverty have a higher incidence of asthma than those residing in less populated areas.

Health disparities are explained by four primary factors: limited access to appropriate health care; insufficient or ineffective treatment of mental health problems; exposure to higher levels of environmental pollutants; and lifestyle factors such as use of addictive substances, poor diet, and physical inactivity.

Scientific research and clinical practice have produced strong evidence concerning the successful management of chronic diseases such as diabetes. However, the implementation of this knowledge remains a challenge for all clinicians, and closing this gap between scientific knowledge and clinical practice is a primary objective of the Health Disparities Collaboratives. To eliminate health disparities and improve functional and clinical outcomes, health care organizations must be willing to change the way care is delivered. The Health Disparities Collaboratives thus call for a fundamental transformation in the service delivery model of care in the USA. This transformation affects not only how clinicians, such

Dr. Stefan Kertesz of BHCHP examines a patient at the BHCHP clinic at Saint Francis House. Photo by Jessie McCary MD

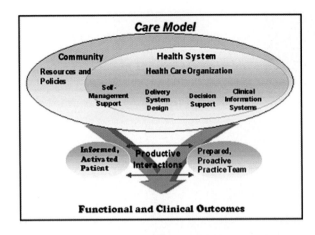

as doctors, nurse practitioners, physician assistants, dentists, nurses, and social workers deliver care, but also how patients participate in their own care and how communities learn to strengthen the provider-patient partnership.

The Health Disparities Collaboratives strive to achieve excellence in practice and improve the health of all Americans through the following goals:

- generate and document improved health outcomes for underserved populations;
- transform clinical practice through models of care, improvement, and learning;
- develop infrastructure, expertise, and multi-disciplinary leadership to support and drive improved health status; and
- build strategic partnerships.

The Health Disparities Collaboratives were developed by the Bureau of Primary Health Care (BPHC) in order to improve the health care provided to everyone and to eliminate health disparities. BPHC, a part of the U.S. Department of Health and Human Services, is responsible for funding programs to expand access to high quality, culturally and linguistically competent, primary and preventive care for underserved, uninsured, and underinsured Americans. To achieve this mission, BPHC funds community, migrant, homeless, and public housing health centers that care for over 3,500 communities and 12 million people, including 7 million minority individuals.

In 1998 BPHC funded one state Primary Care Association and one regional Clinical Network in each of five regional clusters to begin the first Collaborative. In addition, National Clinical Networks, created to focus on oral health, migrant farm worker health care, and homeless health care, began to work with the Institute for Healthcare Improvement (IHI) to develop the infrastructure to support the Health Disparities Collaboratives.

The first Collaborative in 1998 focused on

diabetes, with 88 health centers selected to participate. Additional Collaboratives have since been initiated, concentrating on asthma, depression, cardiovascular disease, HIV, and cancer, with plans for prevention, diabetes prevention, finance, and office redesign. As of December 2003, over 500 health centers have participated in at least one of these Collaboratives, including almost 30% of the over 160 Health Care for the Homeless Projects. All BPHC-supported health centers are expected to take part in the Health Disparities Collaboratives.

How can participation in a Collaborative make dramatic improvements in health outcomes possible, even for homeless patients? Three factors are essential for this to occur: 1) commitment of the health center's administration and providers; 2) support from the regional infrastructure comprised of primary care associations and clinical networks; and 3) adherence to three models of change promoted by the Health Disparities Collaboratives. These three models of change are the Learning Model, the Care Model, and the Improvement Model.

The Learning Model involves 12 months of intensive learning during the implementation phase, called Phase I, of a Collaborative. The Learning Model is adapted from the IHI's Breakthrough Series. The following components comprise the Learning Model.

- Health center leadership selects the staff team to work on the Collaborative. The team does initial pre-work to gain an understanding of the Collaborative and the issue being studied (diabetes, asthma, cardiovascular disease, or depression).
- The team participates in three Learning Sessions with teams from other centers and with expert advisors. At these sessions, change ideas and results are shared among all teams.
- Each Learning Session is followed by an Action Period, during which each center develops, tests, and implements trial runs for their change ideas, using the PDSA model (described below under Improvement Model).
- After the final Learning Session, each health center works on ways to move the new model into other clinical areas or other sites.

The Care Model is a population-based model predicated upon knowing which patients have the target illness, assuring that care is based upon scientific evidence, and actively aiding each patient to participate in all aspects of care. This model was developed by a national program of the Robert Wood Johnson Foundation, called Improving Chronic Illness Care, at the MacColl Institute in Seattle, Washington. It is recommended that a sub-group of the entire patient population be the focus of change for the duration of the Collaborative.

The Care Model has six components:
- the health care organization;
- community resources and policies;
- self-management support;
- decision support;
- delivery system design;
- clinical information systems.

The change concepts associated with each of the six components of the Care Model are described below.

Health Care Organization
- Goals to improve chronic care are part of the organization's business plan.
- Senior leaders visibly support improvement in chronic illness care.
- Benefit packages designed by the health care organization promote good chronic illness care.
- Provider incentives encourage better chronic illness care.
- Improvement strategies that are known to be effective are used to achieve comprehensive system change.

Community Resources and Policies
- Effective programs are identified and patients are encouraged to participate.
- Partnerships with community organizations are formed to develop evidence-based programs and health policies that support chronic care.
- Health care organizations coordinate chronic illness guidelines, measures, and care resources throughout the community.

Self-Management Support
- Providers emphasize the patient's active and central role in managing chronic illness.
- Standardized patient assessments include self-management knowledge, skills, confidence, supports, and barriers.
- Effective behavior change interventions and ongoing support with peers or professionals are provided.

- The care team assures care planning and assistance with problem solving.

Decision Support
- Evidence-based guidelines are embedded into daily clinical practice.
- Specialist expertise is integrated into primary care.
- Provider education modalities proven to change practice behavior are utilized.
- Patients are informed of guidelines pertinent to their care.

Delivery System Design
- Team roles are defined and tasks delegated.
- Planned visits are used to provide care.
- The primary care team assures continuity.
- Regular follow-up is assured.

Clinical Information Systems
- A registry contains clinically useful and timely information.
- Care reminders and feedback for providers and patients are built into the information system.
- Relevant patient subgroups can be identified for proactive care.
- Individual patient care planning is facilitated by the information system.

In addition to the Care Model, the Collaboratives use an Improvement Model developed by the Associates in Process Improvement and tested and used in many IHI-sponsored Collaboratives. When used with the Care Model, the Improvement Model provides a process to improve the quality of care at an accelerated pace. The Improvement Model is based on the following three fundamental questions.

What are we trying to accomplish?
This question is meant to establish an "aim statement" that focuses the organization's effort for improvement. This aim statement helps focus on specific actions or elements of the Care Model and defines which patients and providers will participate. The aim statement should be time-specific, measurable, and as concise as possible. A few trials that test an aim statement may be required before it becomes truly focused.

How will we know that a change is an improvement?
Measures and definitions are necessary to

answer this question. Data is needed to assess and understand the impact of changes designed to meet an aim statement. When shared aim statements and data are used, learning is further enhanced in sharing with other organizations in the Collaborative. Superior performances and best practices are more quickly identified and disseminated through benchmarking.

What changes can we make that will result in any improvement?

Testing and re-testing are necessary to conclude that a result is an improvement. The PDSA ("Plan, Do, Study, Act") Cycle is a trial-and-learning method to discover effective and efficient ways to change a process. The "study" part of the cycle is the key to learning which changes lead to improvement. "Study" compels the team to learn from the data collected and to assess the effects of any changes on other parts of the system, as well as on patients and staff. Changes can also have varying effects under different conditions, such as different practice teams or different sites. Most importantly, the "study" phase is an ideal time to think through how the Care Model can help generate new ideas and new approaches to positive change. PDSA cycles should be short and quick, requiring only hours, days, or a few weeks to complete.

Measurement is essential to ensure that changes made in clinical practice lead to desired improvements. All teams use national measures determined by a panel of clinical experts. In addition, each team selects at least one additional measure to use in assessing clinical outcomes. An electronic registry is used to collect data, schedule office visits, labs, and educational sessions, and generate reminders and guidance for patient care. Health centers are expected to track and provide monthly reports on the core measures used by all Collaborative participants as well as the additional measure(s) they have selected. The Bureau of Primary Health Care provides free software for the electronic registry to all health centers that participate in a Health Disparities Collaborative. The latest version, released in July 2002, is called the Patient Electronic Care System (PECS).

The Health Care for the Homeless Clinicians' Network is one of three national clinical networks that provide support and technical assistance to teams in the Health Disparities Collaborative. The Network's role in the Collaboratives is to increase the understanding of the special needs of homeless people, partner with Collaboratives' staff at the national and regional levels, serve as a resource and mentor to health center teams, and participate as faculty at Learning Sessions.

The Health Care for the Homeless Clinicians' Network, founded in 1994, is a national professional association of clinicians from many disciplines who are dedicated to the prevention of homelessness and strive to improve the health and quality of life of homeless people. Organized to provide peer support to clinicians from various disciplines, the Network has many goals and objectives, including: actively sharing information and experience to enhance clinical practice; promoting clinical research; educating clinicians, communities, homeless people, and policymakers on the interrelationship between homelessness, health, and public policy issues; and collaborating with other clinical networks, professional associations, and groups who work with our homeless neighbors. ■

Reference

Sam, C. Eliminating US health care disparities among racial and ethnic groups. Presentation at the Society of General Internal Medicine 24th Annual Meeting, May 2001.

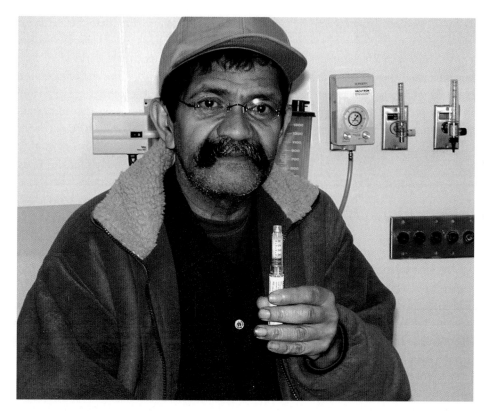

Diabetes

Gregory A. Wagoner, MD, MBA

Diabetes mellitus is commonplace and touches the lives of most Americans, either directly or by affecting friends, family members, or colleagues. About 18 million people are reported to suffer from diabetes in the USA, about 6.3% of the entire population. Over one-third (40%) of Americans with diabetes are over the age of 65. And diabetes is on the rise in the USA. From 1980 to 1996 the prevalence of diabetes rose 18.4%, while in the brief period between 1997 and 2000 this rate increased another 12%.

Diabetes is more common in black and Hispanic people than in white people. Among those younger than 75 years of age, African-American women had the highest prevalence. In other poor populations, the percentages are higher than the general population. Most observers and clinicians fear that the prevalence of this chronic and debilitating disease is reaching epidemic proportions among many vulnerable populations.

Persons with diabetes can develop many complications as a result of damage to organs, such as the kidneys, eyes, heart, blood vessels, and skin. Treatment of the disease and prevention of these complications require a significant commitment on the part of both the patient and the care provider. For many people, life-style changes may alleviate the need for medication in the early stages of the disease. These changes primarily involve diet and exercise, neither of which is easy to control for persons who

sleep in shelters and eat in soup kitchens. Walking is often the only practical exercise, as exercise facilities are not generally accessible to homeless people.

Jane L is a 48 year old diabetic diagnosed six months previously at the local homeless clinic after complaining of fatigue and frequent urination. She reported that her mother had diabetes and died of a stroke at age 55. Her primary care clinician has given her abundant written information about her disease, but Jane does not comprehend the complications of her illness and is confused about how the treatment works. The fatigue and the frequent urination continue unabated, and Jane now feels depressed and anxious about her new diagnosis of diabetes.

Jane lives at a shelter for women, eats daytime meals at a nearby women's center or downtown soup kitchen, and walks about 4 miles each day as she completes her daily routine. Wary of medication, she

A diabetic patient simplifies the process of injecting insulin by using an automatic injection device, an "insulin pen".
Photo by Jessie McCary MD

manages to take pills for blood pressure and thyroid problems. She has been told that she will need to start a new pill for her diabetes but may require insulin via a needle if her blood sugars do not respond to the pills or her changes in diet and activity. Despite good intentions, she has little control of her diet and must accept the meals offered. With the pressure of finding a bed for the night and the next meal, finding the time and place to exercise is virtually impossible.

Her blood sugar and glycosylated hemoglobin (hemoglobin A1C) tests remain high, and after a month her doctor prescribes two injections of insulin daily. Jane has no insurance and is unable to fill the prescription for insulin, syringes, and needles for several weeks. She needs education and training in the use and administration of insulin, a place to refrigerate her medication as well as a safe place to keep her needles, and assistance with monitoring her progress once she begins the injections. All of these present complex barriers that need to be overcome during her daily search for housing, food, and safety.

Suffice it to say, she will need to make the care and treatment of her diabetes an integral part of her daily needs – a day already filled with so many survival issues that such a burden is extremely difficult to bear. She continues to see her primary care clinician regularly but becomes depressed by the number of appointments she needs to remember, including the eye doctor, the nutritionist, the podiatrist, and the dentist. Sometimes, in the midst of her poverty and homelessness, it simply doesn't feel worth the effort. She believes that she will probably "get by" as long as she just keeps doing what she did before. Her sugars improve a little, but the fatigue and her depression are overwhelming and she just wants to sleep.

This story is not unusual and typifies the challenges faced by homeless persons who have been diagnosed with diabetes. Coordination of care and adherence to the treatment plan can be daunting to both patient and provider. The necessary education and support often require more time and resources than are available, and important components of the prevention and treatment of diabetes are deferred or forgotten in our current clinical settings.

The alternative is evidence-based decision-making and a supportive system of care in which decisions are made by both patient and provider. Jane needs a health care delivery system that emphasizes collaborative, team-based care that will support the major behavioral changes necessary to control the diabetes and reduce the risk of devastating complications.

Solid clinical evidence provides the basis of current treatment guidelines for diabetes, which should be an integral component of the care that each homeless person receives. The majority of the data come from a few key studies that are available in the literature. These guidelines help eliminate "doing the wrong things" and emphasize activities that yield the greatest rewards in the form of quality of life and risk prevention. By adopting the Care Model, practitioners have a heightened chance of eliminating the gap between what we know and what we do.

The Care Model, as used and developed through the Bureau of Primary Health Care's Health Disparities Collaboratives, incorporates key measurements and activities that have been shown in the literature to be clearly beneficial for populations with diabetes. Several key studies form the majority of this evidence. The HOPE study demonstrated the benefit of the use of ACE-inhibitors for persons with diabetes over the age of 55. In another study sponsored by the Medical Research Council and the British Heart Association, the use of statins resulted in 33% reduction in heart attacks and strokes. The benefits of blood pressure control were studied in a large clinical trial called the UK Prospective Diabetes Study. A total of 1148 patients with diabetes showed dramatic reductions in strokes, microvascular complications, and diabetes-related deaths. Every reduction of 1% in the HgbA1C resulted in reductions of 17% in mortality, 18% in myocardial infarctions, 15% in strokes, and a 35% in cardiovascular endpoints.

Lowering blood glucose has been definitively shown to slow the onset of complications of diabetes in one of the largest and most comprehensive studies to date. The Diabetes Control and Complications Trial (DCCT), conducted by the National Institute of Diabetes and Digestive and Kidney Diseases, compared standard and intensive therapy of type 1 diabetes through glucose control measurements. The findings were dramatic. Eye disease was reduced by 76%, neurological pathology was reduced by 60%, and kidney disease was cut in half.

Based on a list of key measurements on diabetes furnished by the Health Disparities Collaborative on diabetes, the Boston Health Care for the Homeless Program chose several indicators to be followed on a monthly basis among the diabetic patients included in the collaborative:

- two HgbA1C's annually (at least 3 months apart);

- blood pressure control (under 130/80);
- annual dental exam;
- documented self-management goals;
- ACE inhibitors used in patients over 55 years of age;
- HgbA1C under 7.0%;
- population of focus size.

Components of Care

As discussed in a previous chapter, the Care Model has six components of care, which are explained in detail. The remainder of this chapter will use one example from each component to illustrate current testing or complete implementation of change within the diabetic collaborative patient population.

Health Care Organization

The organization has begun integrating the Care Model into the business plan in several ways. The spread of this effort through additional parts of the organization is part of the Annual Plan for the upcoming year. Participation in the model of care is a part of performance evaluations for all clinicians. The Board receives regular informational updates, including monthly reports.

Clinical Information Systems

Through the use of the software and registry system provided by the Health Disparities Collaborative, reports are now generated for the diabetic population of focus that indicate areas where further actions are likely indicated. For instance, we can generate a report of all those diabetics in our population who have not had dental exams in the past year. This report can then be used to generate reminders or inform the clinician so that these services will be scheduled at the next visit.

Decision Support

The organization now has deployed portable HbgA1C devices at selected sites. These devices provide a way to measure this number accurately and have results within minutes, so that feedback to the patient occurs during the same visit. The devices also need no electric supply, and are useful on the street or in other locations without power.

Delivery System Design

A team has been created which is multidisciplinary and allows for better coordination of access for our diabetic patients and more complete exchange of information. Other areas of change

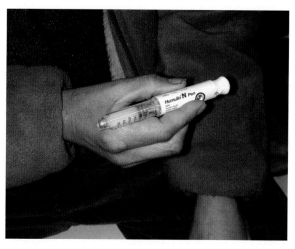

The patient dials in the desired number of units of insulin instead of manually filling a syringe. Photo by Jessie McCary MD

have included the use of an eye specialist referral form which patients take to the eye doctor and then return with the necessary information. This form has improved greatly our ability to obtain feedback from specialty visits.

Community Resources

Using qualified volunteers, diabetes education classes have been instituted at our 92-bed respite care facility and one large shelter in our system. These classes have allowed for more detailed and individualized information exchange in a place where access for our patients is easy and the setting familiar. These classes have been extremely successful, both as measured by participant enthusiasm and overall attendance.

Self-Management Support

An easy-to-use handout has been used to work with diabetic clients to choose a self-management goal that they want to work on. Clinicians in the collaborative have established standardized ways to document and follow these goals in the electronic medical record.

Summary

The delivery of care based on the Care Model has been shown to be effective and realistic. The Boston Health Care for the Homeless Program can document wonderful examples that serve as proof that this model of care works. Although we have only been involved in this initiative for less than a year at the time of this writing, staff members involved in this initial phase have enthusiastically supported its use and endorsed its spread to all areas of the organization. Comparison of the care delivered through this approach versus the traditional model reveals gaps that must be eliminated in order to assure high quality care for all of our diabetic clients. Diabetes management is difficult even under the best of situations, and for the homeless diabetic, broad support and access to appropriate services is extremely difficult. This model of care results in an evidence-based prioritization of actions by both the patient and the clinician. Care moves from an approach characterized by more episodic, reactive visits with little patient involvement to a model that includes the patient and results in improvements that will hopefully reduce morbidity and mortality in the future. ▇

References

American Diabetes Association. Insulin administration. *Diabetes Care* 2002;25:S112-115.

Brehove T, Bloominger MJ, Gillis L, et al. *Adapting Your Practice: Treatment and Recommendations for Homeless People with Diabetes Mellitus.* Nashville: Health Care for the Homeless Clinicians' Network; 2002.

Ridolfo AJ, Proffitt BJ. *Diabetes and Homeless: Overcoming Barriers to Care.* Nashville: Health Care for the Homeless Clinicians' Network; 2002.

Uphold CR, Graham MV. *Diabetes Mellitus: Clinical Guidelines in Family Practice.* Gainesville, Fla.: Barmarrae Books; 2002:140-155.

Web sites:
American Diabetes Association   www.diabetes.org
Health Disparities Collaboratives   www.healthdisparities.net
National Guidelines Clearinghouse   www.guideline.gov

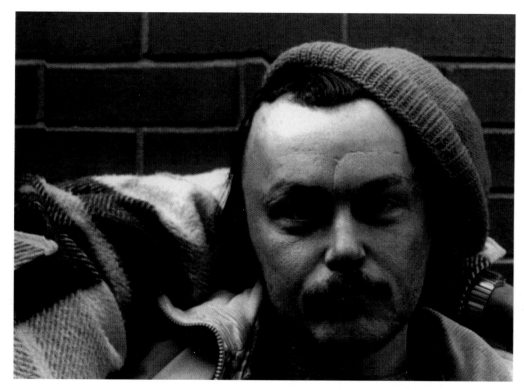

Depression

Lawrence E. Gottlieb, MPA, MSW

Today we have far greater knowledge and awareness of the prevalence of mental illness, including depression, in primary care settings than ever before. As many as 25% of primary care patients have a significant mental health disorder (most often anxiety or depression). All too often, mental health conditions are neither diagnosed nor adequately treated in primary care settings. The costs associated with untreated mental disorders in primary care are considerable. For example, the annual health care cost for untreated patients with depression is nearly twice that for patients who do not have depression. According to a study supported by the Agency for Healthcare Research and Quality (HS09397), the proper diagnosis and timely treatment of these mental health disorders can prevent many costly acute care hospitalizations and save significant health care dollars.

Depressed patients in primary care settings commonly present with somatic symptoms rather than complaints of depressed mood. Therefore clinicians must be proficient in the assessment and management of depression. However, the diagnosis and treatment of depression in the adult homeless population can be very challenging for primary care practitioners. This is generally due to the complex set of bio-psycho-social factors experienced by homeless adults. These factors may include chronic alcohol and substance abuse, various forms of physical and emotional trauma (e.g., PTSD), persistent poverty with limited access to affordable housing, lack of access to and continuity of medical and mental health services, and the formidable task

of survival on the streets or in the emergency shelter system.

In the *Homeless Survey of 2000 in Hartford, Connecticut,* 27 of 66 (41%) homeless individuals who completed the survey reported having depression as a medical issue. Only drug abuse (other than alcohol) was reported higher (42%) by homeless respondents to the survey. The National Institute of Mental Health and the Federal Task Force on the Homeless also estimate that roughly one-third of homeless persons suffers from mental illness. Various studies have estimated the prevalence of co-occurring disease (both mental illness and substance abuse) in the adult homeless population to be from 30% to 60%.

This man suffered from lifelong and untreated depression. His depression improved with medication prescribed by a psychiatrist who had observed him in the shelter and on the streets. Photo by Norma Laurenzi

Signs and Symptoms of Depression

Clinical depression can be very difficult to diagnose in the homeless population. Depression is often viewed as a normal response to the situation of living in a "state of homelessness", and the typical manifestations are considered the result of trying to survive life on the streets or the turmoil of the emergency shelter system. Depressive symptoms in the adult homeless population may also accompany chronic substance abuse, and clinicians should be cautioned about making a diagnosis of clinical depression when patients are impaired. A diagnosis of depression should be made cautiously during short-term periods of sobriety, as "rebound" sadness and other depressive symptoms can occur during withdrawal periods in persons who suffer from chronic substance abuse.

Clinical depression is a syndrome with biological changes characterized by a specific cluster of signs and symptoms. Three common forms should be recognized by primary care clinicians: major depression, chronic depression, and minor depression. According to the *Diagnostic and Statistical Manual of Mental Disorders IV* (DSM-IV), chronic depression is also known as "dysthymia". Minor depression is classified as "adjustment disorder with depressed mood" or "depressive disorder not otherwise specified (NOS)."

Major Depression

DSM-IV identifies nine signs and symptoms of major depression that can be categorized into four groups:
- *depressed mood*: subjective feelings of sadness or emptiness most of the day, nearly every day;
- *anhedonia*: markedly diminished interest or pleasure in all or almost all activities;
- *physical symptoms*: fatigue, significant change in appetite or weight, sleep disturbances, and psychomotor retardation or agitation;
- *psychological symptoms*: feelings of worthlessness, inappropriate guilt, inability to concentrate, and recurrent thoughts of death or suicidal ideation.

For a diagnosis of depression, the patient must exhibit either a depressed mood or anhedonia, as well as four of the physical or psychological symptoms noted above. If both depressed mood and anhedonia are present, then only three other symptoms are necessary to make the diagnosis. These symptoms must be present for at least two weeks and occur nearly every day for most of the day.

Chronic Depression

Chronic depression, or dysthymia, is characterized by a persistently depressed mood, present for more days than not, for at least a two-year period of time. Depressed mood must be accompanied by two other depressive symptoms (see above list). These symptoms must be present for at least two years with no major depressive episode.

Dysthymic disorder is not a major depressive episode in partial remission. Many patients have suffered with dysthymia for their entire adult lives, and some may have come to accept depressed mood as a part of life. A large majority of individuals with dysthymia, however, will develop major depressive episodes.

Minor Depression

Sadness is an appropriate response to stressful life events, such as job loss, death of a family member, loss of a close friend, health impairment, marital difficulties, or financial hardship. When the reaction appears excessive or continues for longer than two months, these patients are considered to have an adjustment reaction with depressed mood. Other patients may have mixed depressed mood and anxiety symptoms, some of which recur on an intermittent basis.

Patients suffering from one of these depressive disorders that do not fit well into any other category can be diagnosed with the syndrome of minor depression or, according to DSM-IV, "depressive disorder not otherwise specified (NOS)."

These minor forms of depression are distinguished from major depression by the absence of a full complement of five depressive symptoms and from chronic depression by their shorter duration. If at any time, however, the symptoms change, the diagnosis and management strategies should be adjusted accordingly.

The BPHC's Depression Collaborative and Worcester's HOAP

In July of 2002, the Bureau of Primary Health Care's (BPHC) Health Disparities Collaborative included depression in its list of chronic illnesses, along with diabetes, cardiovascular disease, and asthma. The goal of the Bureau's Health Disparities Collaboratives is to develop improvements in chronic disease management in underserved populations who receive primary care services across all health center programs. Teams focusing on one of the four chronic illnesses were selected through a competitive process based on their readiness to engage in a "redesign" of chronic illness care in their health centers. Among the health centers selected to engage in the process were a number of HCH programs. Depression care was adapted to the Care Model, and teams were assembled across the country by region and by disease to discuss the implementation of both the Care and Improvement Models in each setting.

Teams are required to report monthly and to maintain a confidential database or "registry" of patients participating in the Collaborative. These patients are described as a "population of focus" who belong to a designated team of providers and support staff (nurse educators, care managers, etc.). Teams of providers report patient progress compared to a set of national "key measures" on a monthly basis to the Bureau through 10 Regional Cluster coordinators. Sites can also select specific measures that are unique to their population of focus. Goals of the project include improving patient care and quality of life, reducing the overall cost of chronic illness care in primary care settings, helping patients become more active in managing their illness, and "redesigning" patient visits to better meet the needs of patients. The model supports the use of a wide spectrum of health center and community resources.

Community Healthlink (CHL) is a community-based mental health facility located in Worcester, Massachusetts, and is the site of a 330(h) HCH program. The HCH program at CHL, the Homeless Outreach and Advocacy Project (HOAP), has been operating since 1985. HOAP serves between 2300-2400 unduplicated homeless adults annually. HOAP provides a broad range of services to Worcester's adult homeless population, including: primary care; mental health and substance abuse services; transitional and permanent housing services; emergency case management; and a small respite program. The majority of HOAP's patients are single adult homeless males (65%) between the ages of 25 and 55, with the largest single group of male patients falling within the specific age range of 39-44.

The initial screening for depression takes place via a self-administered tool called the Patient Health Questionnaire (PHQ-9). In a multi-center study of 8 family practices and internal medicine sites with 3000 patients and 62 physicians, the instrument was found to have 73% sensitivity and 98% specificity for the diagnosis of major depression. The instru-

ment is easy to administer and can be scored quickly (1-2 minutes for 85% of patients). The PHQ-9 is administered on regular follow-up visits in order to monitor a patient's response to treatment.

The PHQ-9 provides screening, diagnostic, and outcome data for patients with depression through a series of questions (11 in total) that measure the signs and symptoms of clinical depression. Recording the number of overall symptoms and a severity score correlates to a specific diagnosis of depression. The greater the frequency of depressive symptoms reported by the patient, the higher the severity score. Patients with a severity score of 10 or greater are classified as having a "Clinically Significant Depression" (CSD) and are engaged in the program.

The original national key reporting measures required for all depression teams are listed below. These key measures have been discussed at length with current depression teams at several of the National Learning Sessions, and modifications are frequently made. The measures are:
- number of patients with a diagnosis of depression;
- number of patients with a CSD;
- CSD patients with PHQ score less <5;
- CSD patients with documented follow-up within 2 weeks of initial assessment;
- CSD patients with 2nd PHQ within 6 weeks of initial assessment;
- patients with self-management goal within 12 months;
- number of patients with documented PHQ score at six months.

New homeless patients seen at the HOAP main clinic site in Worcester were given the PHQ-9 questionnaire beginning in July 2002. The HOAP primary care team is relatively small and includes one physician (0.6 FTE) and two nurse practitioners (2.0 FTEs). As of May 2003, the collaborative patient database was capped with 73 patients entered into the registry. Of these 73 initial patients, 48(66%) were male and 25(34%) were female. Sixty-one patients (84%) had a PHQ severity score of 10 or greater, indicating a Clinically Significant Depression (CSD). One of the national key measures being tracked is follow-up after the initial or index assessment. There is a two-week standard for the first follow-up appointment. Despite often high rates of no-shows in homeless populations, HOAP found that 73% of patients were seen within 2 weeks of the initial assessment.

Components of Change

Treating depression in the homeless adult population presents many challenges. Clinical depression has often gone untreated for many years or may have been treated only episodically in emergency settings. More often than not, homeless individuals receive only emergent or acute treatment for a variety of mental illnesses and then return to the community with incomplete follow-up care.

HOAP has a significant mental health and substance abuse treatment component as a part of its core services. Depression was often relegated to a "low level" priority in comparison to other mental illnesses among HOAP's homeless patients, such as schizophrenia, bi-polar disorder, schizo-affective disorder, and psychotic disorders. HOAP primary care providers often prescribe anti-depressant medications but are much more comfortable referring patients to the HOAP psychiatrist and mental health team for medication and ongoing psychotherapy. The collaborative did raise the "visability" of depression in our population, and patients participating in the collaborative were referred for mental health treatment much more quickly. Also, substance abuse disorders were present in a significant number of patients, making the diagnosis of clinical depression more difficult.

Self-Management Issues

One of the major goals of the collaborative process is the active involvement of patients in the overall management of their illness. For illnesses such as diabetes, CVD, and asthma, patients can often participate by making changes in life-style, exercise, or choices about reducing the consumption of foods high in fat or salt content. Depressed individuals in most settings have opportunities to make changes such as practicing stress reduction techniques, going for walks, or talking to a sympathetic friend. Homelessness limits such choices and opportunities, and therefore self-management goals must be adapted to other than "ideal" circumstances. For example, patient adherence with medication regimens is often a goal for providers working with homeless patients. Although 100% adherence is usually the target, this may be an unrealistic expectation for many homeless individuals who may not have a place to store or refrigerate medicines and who may have great difficultly remembering to take medicines at prescribed times throughout the day. As a direct result of our provider team conferences, we have decided that a "harm reduction" philosophy is more realistic for homeless individuals. Patients are reminded that their use of substances such as alcohol or drugs directly contributes to overall feelings of depression. For patients who are depressed and continue to use substances, a self-management goal might be to commit to using less alcohol or heroin or to use less frequently. We have found that self-management goals tailored to each individual work more effectively in the homeless population.

References

Cole S, Raju M, Barrett J. Assessment and management of depression in primary care practice. *Annals of General Hospital Psychiatry* 2000 (Reprinted in the Participant's Monograph, Health Disparities Collaborative, Learning Session I.)

O'Keefe E, Maljanian R, McCormack K. (Hartford Community Health Partnership). Hartford Homeless Health Survey 2000. March, 2000.

Part Five:
Immunizations

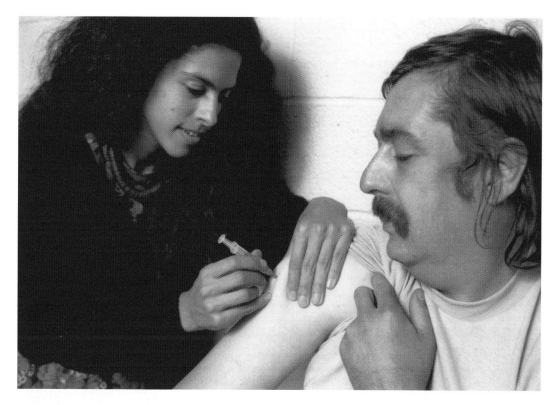

Adult
Immunizations

*Pat Petrosky Tormey,
RN, MPH
Michelle Canning,
RN, BSN*

Routine vaccination has dramatically reduced the prevalence of diphtheria, tetanus, pertussis, polio, measles, mumps, rubella, and *Haemophilus influenza* type b (Hib) in the USA. Nonetheless, with the exception of polio, these diseases still occur in the USA, and polio continues to occur in other parts of the world. With international travel now commonplace, the fact that these vaccine-preventable diseases occur anywhere in the world means that outbreaks can occur in the USA if our immunization rates fall.

This section reviews the less commonly seen vaccine-preventable diseases, the immunizations to prevent these diseases, and the immunization schedules recommended in the USA, as of 2004.

"Uncommon" Vaccine-Preventable Diseases

Diphtheria, mumps, rubella, polio, and tetanus, illnesses once epidemic in the USA, are now relatively rare because of widespread immunization programs. However, aggressive immunization programs and prompt reporting of suspect cases are critical to prevent the recurrence of large outbreaks of diseases in this group. In Massachusetts and many other states, the law requires that documented or suspected cases of these diseases be promptly reported to the local board of health or the appropriate health agency.

Diphtheria

Widespread immunization has made diphtheria

very rare in the USA. From 1980 through 2000, an average of 2-3 cases were reported each year. However, diphtheria continues to occur in other parts of the world. A major epidemic of diphtheria occurred in countries of the former Soviet Union beginning in 1990. By 1994, more than 157,000 cases and more than 5000 deaths were reported in all of the 15 newly independent states. One cause of the outbreak was the lack of routine immunizations of adults in these countries.

A person with diphtheria is infectious as long as the bacteria are present, usually about 2 weeks but as long as 4 weeks. A person is usually not infectious 48 hours after receiving the appropriate antibiotics; however, elimination of the bacteria needs to be documented by two consecutive negative cultures after the antibiotics are completed. Once a person has been exposed to diphtheria, symptoms can occur 1-10 days later.

Diphtheria, a bacterial infection that most

BHCHP nurse practitioner Maya Mundkur Greer administers a tetanus shot to a guest at St. Francis House. Photo by David Comb

Recommended Adult Immunization Schedule UNITED STATES • 2002-2003

| | For all persons in this group | Catch-up on childhood vaccinations | For persons with medical/exposure indications |

VACCINE / AGE	19-49 YEARS	50-64 YEARS	65 YEARS & OLDER
Tetanus, Diphtheria (Td)*	1 dose booster every 10 years		
Influenza	1 dose annually for persons with medical or occupational indications, or household contacts of persons with indications	1 annual dose	
Pneumococcal (polysaccharide)	1 dose for persons with medical or other indications. (1 dose revaccination for immunosuppressive conditions)		1 dose for unvaccinated persons / 1 dose revaccination
Hepatitis B*	3 doses (0, 1–2, 4–6 months) for persons with medical, behavioral, occupational, or other indications		
Hepatitis A	2 doses (0, 6–12 months) for persons with medical, behavioral, occupational, or other indications		
Measles, Mumps, Rubella (MMR)*	1 dose if measles, mumps or rubella vaccination history is unreliable; 2 doses for persons with occupational or other indications		
Varicella*	2 doses (0, 4–8 weeks) for persons who are susceptible		
Meningococcal (polysaccharide)	1 dose for persons with medical or other indications		

Recommended Immunizations for Adults with Medical Conditions
UNITED STATES • 2002-2003

| | For all persons in this group | Catch-up on childhood vaccinations | For persons with medical/exposure indications | Contraindicated |

Medical Conditions ▼ / Vaccine ▶	Tetanus-Diphtheria (Td)*	Influenza	Pneumococcal (polysaccharide)	Hepatitis B*	Hepatitis A	Measles, Mumps, Rubella (MMR)*	Varicella*
Pregnancy		A					
Diabetes, Heart Disease, Chronic Pulmonary Disease, Chronic Liver Disease, including Chronic Alcoholism		B	C		D		
Congenital Immunodeficiency, Leukemia, Lymphoma, Generalized Malignancy, Therapy with Alkylating Agents, Antimetabolites, Radiation or Large Amounts of Corticosteroids			E				F
Renal Failure/End Stage Renal Disease, Recipients of Hemodialysis or Clotting Factor Concentrates			E	G			
Asplenia, including Elective Splenectomy and Terminal Complement Component Deficiencies			E, H, I				
HIV Infection			E, J			K	

* Covered by the Vaccine Injury Compensation Program.

A. If pregnancy is at second or third trimester during influenza season.

B. Although chronic liver disease and alcoholism are not indicator conditions for influenza vaccination, give one dose annually if the patient is 50 years or older, has other indications for influenza vaccine, or if patient requests vaccination.

C. Asthma is an indicator condition for influenza but not for pneumococcal vaccination.

D. For all persons with chronic liver disease.

E. Revaccinate once after five years or more have elapsed since initial vaccination.

F. Persons with impaired humoral but not cellular immunity may be vaccinated. *MMWR* 1999;48 (RR-06):1-5.

G. Hemodialysis patients: Use special formulation of vaccine (40 ug/mL) or two 1.0 mL 20 ug doses given at one site. Vaccinate early in the course of renal disease. Assess antibody titers to hep B surface antigen (anti-HBs) levels annually. Administer additional doses if anti-HBs levels decline to <10 milli international units (mIU)/mL.

H. Also administer meningococcal vaccine.

I. Elective splenectomy: vaccinate at least two weeks before surgery.

J. Vaccinate as close to diagnosis as possible when CD4 cell counts are highest.

K. Withhold MMR or other measles-containing vaccines from HIV-infected persons with evidence of severe immunosuppression. *MMWR* 1996;45:603-606, *MMWR* 1992;41 (RR-17):1-19

often involves the upper respiratory passages, causes a sore throat, a slight fever, chills, and often a thick covering (membrane) that forms in the back of the throat. The membrane, which varies in color from bluish-green to grayish-green or black if there has been bleeding, can impair breathing and swallowing. If diphtheria is not properly diagnosed and treated, it can also produce a powerful toxin (poison) that spreads throughout the body causing

serious complications, such as paralysis or heart failure. About 1 person in every 10 who contract diphtheria will die from this infection.

Diphtheria vaccine protects people by creating immunity to the toxin that causes symptoms of illness, rather than immunity to the diphtheria bacteria itself. The vaccine acts on the toxin and not the bacteria, and is thus called a toxoid. Diphtheria toxoid is made from inactivated toxins and cannot cause disease. Since diphtheria disease may not give the person immunity, persons recovering from diphtheria should be evaluated for immunization with diphtheria toxoid.

Children under 7 years of age normally receive 5 doses of diphtheria toxoid in early childhood. Doses begin as early as 6 weeks of age. To assure continued immunity, booster injections of diphtheria toxoid (given with tetanus toxoid as Td) are recommended every 10 years following the primary series. The first booster dose may be given at 11-12 years of age if at least 5 years have elapsed since the last dose of DTaP, DTP, DT or Td.

Diphtheria toxoid comes in several forms:
- **DTaP** (diphtheria and tetanus toxoids and acellular pertussis vaccine) is the vaccine of choice for children 6 weeks through 6 years of age;
- **DT** (diphtheria and tetanus toxoids) is for children under the age of 7 for whom pertussis immunization is contraindicated; and
- **Td** (tetanus and diphtheria toxoids) is the vaccine of choice for children 7 years old and older and for adults. Td contains a lower dose of diphtheria toxoid than does DTaP or DT, diminishing the risk of adverse reaction in this older age group.

Adults working in shelters should show evidence of immunity to diphtheria. To prove immunity, they should have one of the following:
- documentation of a primary series with Td within the past 10 years; or
- documentation of a primary series in childhood and a booster within the preceding 10 years.

Those without proof of immunity are candidates for immunization with the appropriate diphtheria vaccine preparation (usually Td).

Mumps

Prior to mumps vaccine licensure in 1967, mumps was a common childhood disease. The number of reported cases in the USA has dropped from over 150,000 in 1968 to only 231 in 2001. Since 1990 in the USA, persons age 15 years and older have accounted for 30-40% of the cases. Cases of mumps are more common in the winter and spring; however, cases can occur at any time of the year.

Mumps spreads from an infected person to others who are susceptible (never had the disease mumps or have not had two doses of the mumps vaccine) through direct contact with infected respiratory secretions (sneezing, coughing, contact with mucous or saliva). A person is infectious from 3 days before until about 9 days after the onset of gland swelling. Once a susceptible person is exposed, symptoms usually appear within 14-25 days of exposure.

Mumps is a viral infection that causes the salivary glands to become inflamed, resulting in swollen cheeks and jaw, the classic symptom of the disease. The swelling of the cheek and jaw may occur on both sides of the face or only on one side and may be first noted as earache and jaw tenderness. Symptoms that may occur 1-2 days before the swelling of the cheek and jaw include fever, headache, tiredness, muscle aches, and decreased appetite. Mumps is usually a mild disease with symptoms resolving after 10 days. However, mumps can cause serious complications such as deafness, meningitis (infection of the brain and spinal cord coverings), painful swelling of the testicles or ovaries, and rarely, death.

The mumps vaccine used today is made from a live, attenuated (weakened) mumps virus. In the USA mumps virus is usually given together with measles and rubella vaccine, in an immunization called MMR vaccine.

Two doses of mumps vaccine are routinely recommended for all children, with the two doses separated by at least 4 weeks. In the USA the first dose is given on or after 12 months of age, and the second dose is given at age 4-6 years before the child enters kindergarten. Any mumps-containing vaccine given before 12 months of age does not count as a valid dose and needs to be repeated when the child is at least 12 months of age.

Adults working in shelters should show evidence of immunity to mumps by having one of the following:
- documentation of at least one dose of mumps vaccine given at or after 12 months of age; or
- a blood test result showing immunity to mumps virus; or
- documentation of birth in the USA before 1957 (probably had the disease mumps and now has immunity).

Rubella

The largest number of rubella cases in the USA occurred in 1969, when 57,686 cases were reported. The rubella vaccine was licensed in 1969, and the number of cases fell rapidly. By 1983, fewer than 1000 cases per year were reported. A moderate

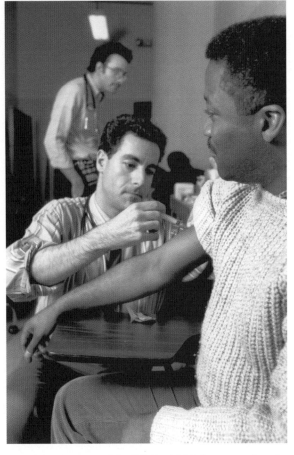

Late BHCHP physician Tom Bennett with a relieved guest at the shelter clinic in 1988 after administering a flu shot during the annual citywide immunization effort in November in Boston's shelters. Photo by David Comb

7 days before to about 7 days after the onset of the rash. A person who is infected with the rubella virus but has a very mild case or no rash (about 20-50% of all rubella infections) is still able to spread the virus. An infant born with CRS can shed the virus for a year or more.

Rubella, also called German measles, is a moderately contagious disease that is caused by a virus. In children, a rash is usually the first sign of illness. Older children and adults often have a low-grade fever, feel tired, have swollen lymph nodes (especially those behind the ears and at the back of the neck), and may have cold-like symptoms 1-5 days before the rash. The flat, pink rash of rubella usually begins on the face and then spreads over the entire body within 24 hours. The rash lasts about 3 days and is sometimes itchy. Some adults, especially women, will also have swollen and painful joints for as long as one month.

Rubella is often a mild disease, and 20-50% of cases may not have a rash. Complications of rubella are rare but can include encephalitis (swelling of the brain) and thrombocytopenia (a decrease in platelets, which are cells in the blood which help clot formation). Rubella that occurs during pregnancy, especially in the first trimester, can cause miscarriage or lead to very severe problems in the unborn child called congenital rubella syndrome (CRS).

Rubella vaccine was first licensed in the USA in 1969, and the vaccine we use today was licensed in 1979 and is a live, attenuated (weakened) vaccine. While rubella vaccine can be given by itself, in the USA it is usually given together with measles and mumps vaccine in an immunization called MMR. Two doses of rubella vaccine, as combined MMR vaccine, separated by at least 4 weeks, are routinely recommended for all children in the USA. The first dose is given at or after 12 months of age and the second dose upon entering kindergarten at 4-6 years of age.

Adults working in shelters should show evidence of immunity to rubella by having one of the following:
- documentation of at least one dose of rubella vaccine given at or after 12 months of age; or
- a blood test result showing immunity to the rubella virus; or
- documentation of birth in the USA before 1957; however, birth before 1957 is not accepted evidence of rubella immunity for women who might become pregnant.

resurgence occurred in 1990 - 1991 due to outbreaks in California and within the Amish community in Pennsylvania. Since the mid-1990's, most reported rubella cases in the USA have occurred among Hispanic adults who were born in other countries where rubella vaccine is not routinely given. Recent outbreaks have occurred in workplaces in which many employees were born outside the USA.

Congenital rubella syndrome (CRS) surveillance is maintained through the National Congenital Rubella Registry. Infants with CRS are born to mothers who contracted rubella disease during the pregnancy; CRS includes defects of the eyes, ears, heart, brain, and bones. The largest yearly number of reported CRS cases to the registry was 67 cases in 1970. Two cases were reported in 2001. Rubella outbreaks are almost always followed by an increase in CRS.

The rubella virus lives in the nose and throat of an infected person and is sprayed into the air when the person sneezes, coughs, or talks. Having direct contact to the infected droplets or articles that are contaminated with infected droplets (such as cups, utensils, mouthed toys, or tissues) can expose others to the virus. It takes about 12-23 days from the time of exposure for people to start showing signs of the disease. A person with the disease is contagious

Polio

Following widespread use of the polio virus vaccine in the mid-1950's, the number of polio cases declined rapidly in many industrialized countries. In the USA the annual number of reported cases of paralytic polio decreased from more than 20,000 in 1952 to less than 100 in the mid-1960's. The last case of paralytic polio caused by a person being exposed in the USA to the wild polio virus was in 1979. However, from 1980 through 1999, an average of 8 cases of paralytic polio were reported annually in the USA. Six of these cases were acquired outside this country, but the vast majority (95%) were vaccine associated paralytic polio (VAPP) caused by the live oral polio vaccine (OPV). After being vaccinated with OPV, people can excrete virus for 2 weeks in the throat and for as long as 2 months in the feces. In order to eliminate VAPP from the USA, the recommended vaccine for polio since 2000 has been the inactivated polio vaccine (IPV).

The polio virus lives in the throat and intestinal tract of an infected person. This virus is spread by direct contact with the feces of an infected person (changing a diaper) or by indirect contact (eating foods/drinks prepared by an infected person who did not wash their hands well after using the toilet or after coughing). The infected person is contagious 7-10 days before the symptoms start until about 6 weeks afterwards. Infected persons without symptoms (asymptomatic group) shed the virus in their stool and are able to spread the virus to others. Once exposed, a person develops symptoms in 3-35 days, usually in 1-3 weeks.

Polio (poliomyelitis) is a very contagious disease caused by three types of enteroviruses. Polio infection may present in one of the following four forms:

- *asymptomatic infection*: up to 95% of all polio infections are asymptomatic. Estimates state that for every one case of paralytic illness there are 200 asymptomatic cases;
- *minor nonspecific illness*: about 4-8% of polio infections fall into this group. The person may have an upper respiratory infection (sore throat and fever), gastrointestinal symptoms (nausea, vomiting, abdominal pain, constipation, or diarrhea), or flu-like illness. The person recovers completely in less than 1 week;
- *aseptic meningitis*: in about 1-2% of polio infections, the person presents with symptoms of stiffness of the neck, back, and/or legs. Usually these patients report a history of symptoms similar to those listed in the minor nonspecific illness group and lasting several days before the stiffness appears. The stiffness may last 2-10 days, and the person completely recovers;
- *paralytic disease*: in less than 1% of all polio infections, the person becomes paralyzed. The paralysis usually follows a minor nonspecific illness of 1-10 days. Most often the paralysis affects the leg muscles but can affect other muscles, including those that control breathing. Some people with paralytic polio recover completely, some recover but have a permanent muscle weakness or paralysis, and some die.

There are 2 kinds of polio vaccine: inactivated polio vaccine (IPV) and live, oral polio vaccine (OPV). IPV, the first polio vaccine, was licensed in 1955 and was used extensively from that time until the early 1960's. OPV was then licensed and became the vaccine of choice in the USA and most other countries. Both IPV and OPV protect against polio. OPV is better at controlling polio disease in outbreaks; however, OPV can actually cause vaccine associated paralytic polio (VAPP) in a small number of those who receive this vaccine. Because the risk of getting polio in the USA is now extremely low, using OPV is no longer worth the risk and only IPV is now used in this country. In other parts of the world where outbreaks of polio still occur, OPV continues to be widely used. Aggressive efforts are being made to eradicate the poliovirus worldwide by 2005.

In the USA children usually receive 3 doses of IPV by 2 years of age and a fourth dose upon school entry. A fourth dose is not needed if the third dose was given on or after the child's fourth birthday. Routine vaccination of adults who live in the USA is not recommended unless they travel to countries where polio still occurs or work in selected laboratories.

Tetanus

Before tetanus toxoid vaccine became part of the routine childhood immunization schedule in the late 1940's, 500-600 tetanus cases were reported yearly in the USA. Since the mid-1970's, an average of 50-100 cases have been reported each year. A low of 27 cases were reported in 2001. Tetanus in newborns is very rare in the USA but common in some developing countries.

People with tetanus are not contagious. People get tetanus from the environment and not from other people. The bacteria enter the body through a major or minor wound or cut. Tetanus may follow severe burns, splinters, ear or dental infections, animal bites, abortion, surgery, deep puncture or crush wounds, frostbite, and self-performed body piercing and tattooing. Injection drug users are at particular risk for tetanus, especially those who inject drugs subcutaneously ("skin pop"). The elderly are also more susceptible because of declining immunity or because they never received a primary series of tetanus immunizations as children and/or boosters every 10 years as adults. Once the tetanus bacteria enter the body, symptoms of tetanus develop in 3-21 days.

Tetanus, also known as "lockjaw", is caused by a bacteria usually found in soil, dust, animal feces, and manure. Illness from tetanus happens when the bacteria enter the body through a wound or cut in the skin. Once inside the skin, the bacteria release a toxin that leads to a persistent contraction of muscles in one area or, more commonly, muscle contractions with a descending distribution pattern. With this descending pattern, the first contractions or spasms are with the jaw muscles, followed by stiffness of the neck, difficulty swallowing, and rigidity of the abdominal muscles. The spasms may occur frequently and last for several minutes. Spasms may continue for 3-4 weeks, while complete recovery may take months. Complications of tetanus include fractures of the spine or long bones, and death results in 11% of reported cases.

Tetanus vaccine is made from the toxins produced by the bacteria and is inactivated so it cannot cause disease. This vaccine protects people by creating immunity to the toxins produced by the tetanus bacteria. As with diphtheria vaccine, this is called a "toxoid" because it acts on the toxins rather than the bacteria. Tetanus toxoid is available as a single antigen preparation, combined with diphtheria as pediatric DT or adult Td, and with both diphtheria toxoid and acellular pertussis vaccine as DTaP. Pediatric formulations (DT and DTaP) contain a similar amount of tetanus toxoid to adult Td.

Primary tetanus immunization, usually combined with diphtheria toxoid and acellular pertussis vaccine (DTaP), is recommended for all children at least 6 weeks of age and less than 7 years of age. Four doses of DTaP are usually given by 24 months of age (2, 4, 6, and 15-18 months of age), with a fifth dose of DTaP at 4-6 years of age. If the fourth dose of DTaP is not given until on or after the fourth birthday, a fifth dose is not needed at 4-6 years of age. To assure continued immunity, booster injections of tetanus toxoid given with diphtheria toxoid as Td are recommended every 10 years following the primary series. The first booster dose may be given at 11-12 years of age if at least 5 years have elapsed since the last dose of DTaP, DTP, DT, or Td. Health care providers should always evaluate a person who had the disease tetanus for immunization against tetanus. Diseases caused by exotoxins do not always render a person immune.

Adults working in shelters should show evidence of immunity to tetanus. To prove immunity, they should have documentation of one of the following:

- a primary series with Td within the past 10 years; or
- a primary series in childhood and a booster within the preceding 10 years.

Those without proof of immunity are candidates for immunization with the appropriate tetanus vaccine preparation (usually Td).

All wounds should be thoroughly cleaned as soon as possible to prevent multiplication of the tetanus bacteria. The decision to give tetanus toxoid is dependent upon the person's vaccine history and the condition of the wound.

For clean, minor wounds:

- people with a history of receiving 3 or more immunizations, with the last dose given within the preceding 5 years, do not require a booster dose;
- those who received 3 or more immunizations, with the last dose more than 10 years ago, should be given a booster dose (Td); and
- persons with uncertain histories require a dose of tetanus toxoid (DTaP/DT if the person is less than 7 years; Td if the person is 7 years or older). Arrangements should be made for completion of the primary series of immunization.

For wounds that are neither clean nor minor:

- those with a history of 3 or more doses of tetanus toxoid need a booster dose only if the last dose was more than 5 years ago;
- those with an uncertain immunization history or those who have received less than 3 doses of tetanus toxoid require a booster dose of tetanus toxoid and tetanus immune globulin (TIG). TIG gives immediate, temporary immunity to tetanus.

Arrangements should be made as appropriate for completion of the primary series.

Special Considerations for Homeless Populations

As soon as a shelter learns of a guest or staff member having a communicable disease, the shelter should immediately contact the local health department. The local health department will work with shelter staff to institute appropriate control measures in order to minimize spread of the infection.

When a shelter guest or staff member contracts a vaccine preventable disease, a determination must be made as to who may have been exposed. The next step is then to identify those susceptible to the disease from among those who may have been exposed. A person is susceptible if they have no immunity to the disease. A person becomes immune by receiving the appropriate immunizations or, for some of the diseases, by having had the disease in the past.

A cornerstone of prevention of communicable diseases in shelters is the establishment of the immunization status of each staff member and, when possible, each guest. An immunization history should be taken at the time of hiring for each shelter employee, and any uncertainties may be resolved with past medical records or an appointment with a primary care provider. The vaccine history for shelter guests is often unknown or unclear. In family shelters, upon admittance, the available immunization histories and the children's primary health care providers should be documented. Participating in a state or local immunization registry can be another method for obtaining immunization histories. Even though obtaining immunization histories for staff and guests is a difficult task, when these diseases occur, it will be invaluable.

Immunization Schedules

The schedules in the beginning of this chapter are based on the 2003 recommendations of the Advisory Council on Immunization Practices (ACIP), the American Academy of Pediatrics, and the American Academy of Family Physicians (AAFP). ◼

References:

Pickering LK, Peter G, Baker CJ, et al., eds. *The 2003 Red Book: Report of the Committee on Infectious Disease.* Elk Grove Village, Illinois: American Academy of Pediatrics; 2003.

CDC National Immunization Program website. http://www.cdc.gov/nip

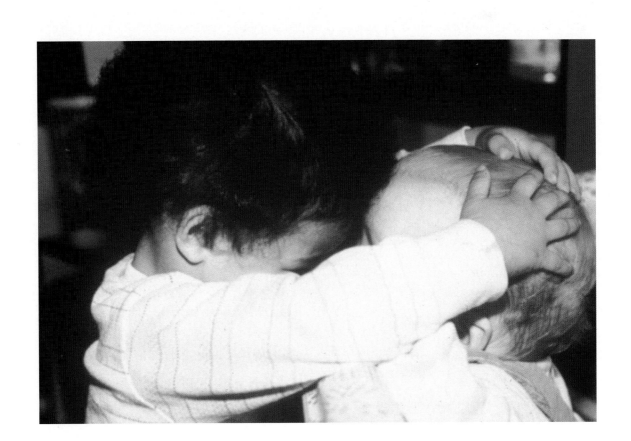

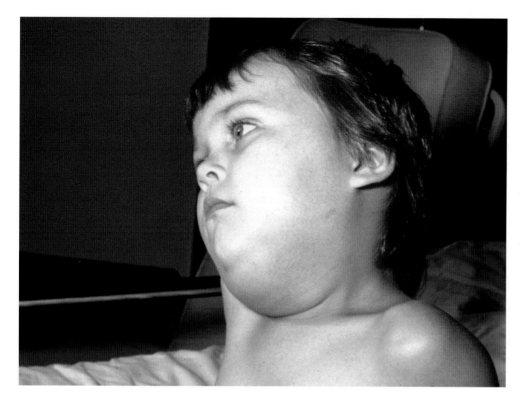

Childhood
Immunizations

Robert Gamble, FNP

The development of effective vaccination programs against childhood infectious diseases has been one of the most significant advancements in public health over the last century. Smallpox has been eradicated worldwide, and wild poliovirus has been eliminated in the Western Hemisphere. The prevalence of diseases such as measles, diphtheria, and *Haemophilus influenzae* type b invasive disease, which used to cause substantial mortality in children, has been dramatically reduced with the advent and refinement of routine vaccine administration programs. The addition of new childhood vaccines against pneumococcal disease and refinements in the scheduling of existing vaccines has made the management and administration of vaccines for children a complicated process. This chapter will focus on the management of childhood vaccinations as laid out in the 2002 Recommended Childhood Immunization Schedule from the Advisory Committee on Immunization Practices (ACIP) of the CDC. Many of the diseases mentioned in this chapter, such as hepatitis B, measles, and pertussis, are discussed in more detail in previous chapters.

Mumps. This child has the swollen cheeks typical of mumps. This virus infects the parotid gland in children, as well as the testicles in teenage and adult males. Photo courtesy of the CDC

Special Considerations for Homeless Pediatric Populations

A major problem often encountered when working with homeless families is missing or inadequate documentation of children's vaccinations. Families often become homeless under traumatic circumstances, such as after a devastating fire or fleeing from frightening domestic violence, and are unable to bring the vaccination records of their children with them. Many homeless families have been relocated repeatedly, have received vaccinations at different health care facilities, and possess incomplete or conflicting documentation of vaccinations. Health care providers should try to obtain the most complete records possible. Only written and dated records are acceptable as evidence of vaccination, with the single exception of the pneumococcal polysaccharide vaccine (PPV). If records cannot be obtained, the person must be considered susceptible and started on an age-appropriate schedule for the missing vaccines. Alternatively, serologic testing to confirm immunity for specific antigens (measles, mumps, rubella, varicella, tetanus, diphtheria, hepatitis A, hepatitis B, and poliovirus) can confirm immunity for children who, by history, have completed these vaccines.

Because homeless families live in close proximity in shelter settings, the determination of their immunization status is especially important, as unimmunized guests could precipitate an infectious disease outbreak in the shelter. An outbreak of varicella (chickenpox) could be extremely dangerous to other immunocompromised guests. A rubella outbreak could cause severe birth defects among pregnant mothers living at the shelter. In addition, health care providers and shelter staff should have documented immunity to varicella, rubella, and hepatitis B when working with homeless families.

Because it is often difficult for homeless families to obtain consistent routine health care for the children, the opportunity should be taken at every clinic visit to review a child's vaccination records. Any required or missing vaccine doses should be administered at that time, particularly if the provider feels that it will be difficult for the patient to make a return visit to receive further vaccines. Because of the complexity of the immunization schedule, this means that at certain age intervals a child could be facing up to five vaccinations at one visit. Extensive clinical evidence shows that simultaneous administration of vaccines during the same clinic visit greatly increases the probability that children will be immunized by the appropriate age. For homeless children, who can so easily slide through gaps in the health care system, this is particularly important. ACIP now states that all combinations of the live and inactivated vaccines in the Routine Childhood Immunization Schedule can be given safely and effectively at the same visit, with no decrease in the rate of seroconversion and no increase in adverse effects from the vaccines. The only exception is that the live vaccines (MMR and varicella) should be given at least 4 weeks apart. The MMR vaccine will also affect the sensitivity of PPD testing for tuberculosis; PPD may be planted at the same time as an MMR is given, but for 3 months after MMR vaccination, the PPD may be falsely negative.

When children are on a "catch-up" schedule of multidose vaccines, it may be necessary to immunize them at shorter than recommended intervals between doses, particularly if up-to-date immuniza-tions are required for entry into school or daycare programs. ACIP has developed guidelines for the minimum ages and intervals between vaccine doses, which are outlined in Table 1. Table 2 shows the overall "catch-up" schedule.

Pediatric Vaccines

This section will discuss particular considerations for each of the vaccines that appear in the ACIP Recommended Childhood Immunization Schedule (Table 1). Some vaccines immunize against individual diseases, while others (e.g. DTaP and MMR) are vaccines that combine several antigens in a single vaccine dose. Many of the diseases covered by this vaccine schedule are discussed in detail in other chapters. The more "uncommon" vaccine-preventable diseases will be described briefly here.

Hepatitis B

The disease process of hepatitis B is discussed in detail in a previous chapter.

The first Hep B vaccine dose is usually administered shortly after birth, before the infant and mother are discharged from the hospital. Infants born to hepatitis B surface antigen positive mothers should also receive a 0.5 ml dose of Hep B immunoglobulin (HBIG) within 12 hours of birth.

An infant's first postpartum clinic visit is a good teaching opportunity to discuss the importance of regularly scheduled vaccines with the infant's caregivers and to ensure that they have begun to fill out the infant's immunization record. Parents should be instructed to bring this record to all subsequent clinic appointments.

The Hep B vaccine is an inactivated vaccine. Hep B vaccines produced by different manufacturers may be used interchangeably to complete a three-dose Hep B series.

DTaP

DTaP is a combination vaccine, conferring immunity for diphtheria, tetanus, and pertussis. Diphtheria, one of the "uncommon" vaccine-preventable diseases, is a bacterial infection that usually affects the upper respiratory airways. Before the advent of universal vaccination measures, diphtheria was a common and frequently fatal disease. In 1920, almost 150,000 cases of diphtheria were reported in the USA, with over 13,000 fatalities. In contrast, from 1980 to 1989, only 24 cases of respiratory diphtheria were reported nationwide, resulting in 2 deaths.

Table 1: Routine Childhood Immunization Schedule

Recommended Age	Vaccine
At birth	HBV-1
2 months of age	DTaP-1 IPV-1 Hib-1 HBV-2 (HBV-1, if no documentation of birth dose) PCV7-1
4 months of age	DTaP-2 IPV-2 Hib-2 HBV-3 (if dose 2 at 2 months) PCV7-2
6 months of age	DtaP-3 IPV-3 (can be given between 6-8 months) Hib-3 HBV-3 (can be given between 6-18 months) PCV7-3
12 months of age	MMR-1 (can be given between 12-15 months, but after first birthday) Varivax (can be given between 12-18 months, but after first birthday) Hib-4 PCV7-4 (can be given between 12-15 months) DtaP-4 (can be given between 15-18 months)
4-6 years old	DTaP-5 IPV-4 MMR-2
11-12 years old	HBV series Td MMR-2 (if no history of 2nd dose) Varivax (if no history of chicken pox)
13-18 years old	Td MMR Varivax (will require two doses, if no documented history of disease or vaccination)

The disease process for tetanus is discussed elsewhere in this chapter, and pertussis is covered in a previous chapter. Pertussis, also known as whooping cough, is a common cause of chronic cough in adults but can be a fatal respiratory disease for children.

The DTaP vaccine is routinely given at 2, 4, 6, and 15 months of age, with a fifth booster dose given before entering kindergarten or elementary school. Unlike other vaccine series, the DTaP series has been demonstrated to have greater efficacy if the same brand of vaccine is given for all doses of the vaccination series, and children should be given the same brand when possible.

At age 11-12 years, a tetanus-diptheria combination (Td) booster should be given, with subsequent Td boosters every 10 years.

The pertussis component of the original DTP vaccine has been associated with rare instances of acute encephalopathy and prolonged convulsions in children. In 1998, most companies changed to an acellular form of the pertussis component of the vaccine, forming the DTaP vaccine (aP = acellular pertussis). Since the recommended vaccine schedule has been changed to use the acellular form of pertussis, no cases of encephalopathy have been reported. However, further vaccination with DTaP is still contraindicated for any child who developed encephalopathy within 7 days of a previous DTaP vaccination and had no other identifiable cause for the reaction. ACIP has also issued precautions for further vaccination with DTaP if a child had any of the following events after a previous DTaP vaccination:

- temperature greater than or equal to 40.5°C (105°F) within 48 hours of vaccination;
- collapse or shock-like state within 48 hours of previous vaccination;
- persistent, inconsolable crying for more than 3 hours, occurring within 48 hours of previous vaccination; and
- convulsions with or without fevers within 3 days of previous vaccination.

In these instances, a later schedule of pertussis vaccine can be considered after the child has completed a thorough neurological evaluation and the providers and parents have evaluated risks

Table 2: The Catch-up Schedule

Visit	Under 7 years old	7 years and older
First visit	HBV (2nd if birth dose documented) DtaP IPV MMR (if >12 months old*) Varicella (*) Hib (if no previous doses, or if one dose before 12 months old, recommend 2 doses) PCV-7 (without previous doses; 12-23 months, 2 doses 8 weeks apart; 24-59 months, 1 dose; 2 doses for "high risk")	HBV Td IPV MMR Varicella (if no history of disease)
Second visit	HBV (4 weeks between dose 1 and 2) DtaP (4 weeks) IPV (4 weeks) HiB (4 weeks) PCV7 (4 weeks)	HBV (8 weeks, dose 2 and 3; note: 16 weeks between dose 1 and 3) Td (4 weeks) IPV (4 weeks) MMR (4 weeks) Varicella (if >13 years old, 2 doses required)
Third visit	HBV (4 weeks between dose 1 and 2) DtaP (4 weeks) IPV (4 weeks)	HBV Td (6 months) IPV (4 weeks)
Fourth visit (now <11 years old)	DtaP (6 months) IPV (4 weeks) Hib (8 weeks) PCV7 (8 weeks)	Td booster at minimal interval of: (a) **6 months** if 1st dose at <12 months old and now <11 years old (b) **5 years** if 1st dose at >12 months old, 3rd dose at < 7 years old and patient is now 11 years old or older (c) **10 years** if 3rd dose given at age > 7 years old IPV Booster (with minimal intervals)

(*) indicates minimal intervals required.

and benefits of continuing a pertussis-containing vaccine series.

The DTaP vaccine is *not* contraindicated in the following circumstances: low-grade fever; current antimicrobial therapy; infant prematurity; or a family history of convulsions, sudden infant death syndrome (SIDS), or an adverse event following a DTP vaccination.

Hib

The disease process of meningitis from *Haemophilus influenzae* type b (Hib) is discussed in detail in a previous chapter.

Before the advent of an effective Hib vaccine, 1 in 200 children under the age of 5 in the USA developed invasive Hib, making it the leading pediatric invasive disease. 60% of these children developed meningitis; 3-5% of them died, while another 20-30% were left with permanent damage including hearing loss and mental retardation.

The Hib vaccine is routinely given at 2, 4, 6, and 12-15 months of age. Hib vaccines produced by different manufacturers may be used interchangeably to complete a four-dose Hib series. Children who have had invasive Hib disease and are less than 24 months old should be given a vaccine series, as they likely will not develop immunity from their invasive infection. For older healthy children who have not been previously immunized, a single Hib vaccine dose after 15 months of age will provide sufficient coverage. Vaccination is not needed if a child is over 7 years of age.

IPV

Polio was a serious childhood infectious disease until the advent of the polio vaccine. Polio is caused by a highly contagious enterovirus. The disease is generally either asymptomatic or a mild nonspecific febrile illness. In 1% of cases, the illness progresses to aseptic meningitis or paralytic disease. Since

Table 2: (cont.) Haemophilus Influenza Type B Vacine Catch-up Schedule

Age of Child	Vaccine History	Recommendations
7-11 months	0 doses	3 doses: dose number 2 one month after dose 1; dose 3 two months after dose 2 at 12-15 months old
	1 dose	1-2 doses at 7-11 months with booster at least two months later at 12-15 months
	2 doses	1 dose, then booster 2 months later at 12-15 months
12-14 months	0 doses	2 doses with 2 months minimum interval
	1 dose before 12 months	2 doses with 2 month interval
	2 doses before 12 months	1 dose
15-59 months	Any incomplete schedule	1 dose
60 months or older	Any incomplete schedule	1 or 2 doses if "high risk"

PCV7 Vaccine Catch-up Schedule

Age of Child	Vaccine History	Recommendations
7-11 months	0 doses	2 doses, 4 week interval with booster 8 weeks later at 12-15 months old
	1 dose	1 dose with booster 8 weeks later at 12-15 months
	2 doses	1 dose, then booster 8 weeks later at 12-15 months
12-23 months	0 doses	2 doses at 8 week intervals
	1 dose before 12 months	2 doses at 8 week intervals
	2 doses before 12 months	1 dose>8 weeks after most recent dose
24-59 months	Any incomplete schedule	1 dose
Children with underlying medical conditions (e.g. sickle cell disease, asplenia, HIV infection, AIDS, other immuno-suppressive conditions and treatments)	Any incomplete schedule	2 doses at 8 week intervals

polio vaccines were first introduced in the 1950s, wild poliovirus has been completely eradicated in the Western Hemisphere, with the last case detected in Peru in 1991.

There are two types of polio vaccine in use: inactivated polio vaccine (IPV) and oral polio vaccine (OPV), which is a live vaccine. Over the past five years ACIP has shifted from recommending a sequential IPV/OPV schedule to using an all-IPV series for polio immunization. The shift to IPV was made to reduce the risk for vaccine-associated paralytic poliomyelitis, a rare but serious consequence to vaccination with OPV (one case per 2.4 million OPV doses distributed). OPV is more effective against wild virus and is now reserved for use in regions in Africa and Asia where polio is still endemic, as well as for places where injectable polio vaccines are logistically difficult to provide.

IPV is routinely given at 2, 4, and 6 months, and then at 4-6 years of age. Children who began the polio vaccine series with OPV can complete their scheduled series with IPV.

MMR

MMR is a combination vaccine, conferring immunity for measles, mumps, and rubella. The disease process for measles is covered in a previous chapter. Measles remains a significant public health

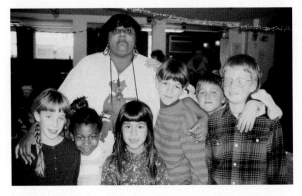

Marsha Adderly has worked in BHCHP's respite program since 1987. She is pictured here with several children from the nearby Neighborhood School, who volunteer to share in holiday festivities with the guests and patients.
Photo by James O'Connell MD

issue, with occasional outbreaks in the USA. In 1991, 100 children died from measles because of inadequate immunization.

Mumps is a viral infection, causing painful swelling of the salivary glands, giving a typical "chipmunk" appearance. Fever, headache, and stiff neck are usually present. Mumps generally has an incubation period of 2-3 weeks, followed by an acute phase which usually resolves within 7 days. Complications occur more frequently with older patients and can include encephalitis, meningitis, and inflammation of the testicles. A single attack of mumps will confer lifelong immunity from the disease.

The incidence of mumps dropped dramatically in the USA as a result of routine immunization against the disease, declining from 152,209 reported cases in 1968 to 1537 cases in 1994.

Rubella (German measles) is another viral infection, causing rash, fever, and lymphadenopathy. This cluster of symptoms is similar to measles and other viral exanthems. For most people, rubella is usually a mild and self-limiting disease. However, a mother who becomes infected during pregnancy can pass the rubella virus on to the fetus, causing severe fetal malformations known as congenital rubella syndrome. This syndrome can include defects in the eyes, ears, heart, brain, and bones.

The incidence of rubella has also been well controlled by routine immunization programs against the disease. Only 227 cases of rubella and 7 cases of congenital rubella syndrome were reported in the United States in 1994.

The first MMR dose is routinely given at 12-15 months, with a second dose given at 4-6 years, before a child enters school. MMR is a live virus that is given subcutaneously and needs to be administered within 8 hours of being reconstituted. MMR should not be administered within 4 weeks of a varicella vaccination, another live virus vaccine, for risk of interference in developing immunity to both live virus vaccines.

Varicella

The disease process of varicella is discussed in a previous chapter.

Varicella vaccine is routinely given once after 12 months of age. Varicella vaccination or serologic evidence of immunity is now required for children before entry into elementary school or child care facilities in all states. Children age 13 or older with no previous evidence of immunity should be given 2 vaccinations at least 4 weeks apart. Varicella is a live virus, given subcutaneously, and needs to be administered within one hour of reconstitution. Varicella vaccine is contraindicated for children with blood dyscrasias, leukemia, lymphoma, or other lymph and bone marrow cancers. Under certain guidelines, some HIV-infected children might be candidates for varicella vaccine and a specialist should be consulted. Varicella should not be administered within 4 weeks of vaccination with MMR.

PCV

The most recent addition to the Recommended Immunization Schedule is the pneumococcal conjugate vaccine (PCV), which provides immunity against *Streptococcus pneumoniae* bacteria, or pneumococcus. Pneumococcus is a leading cause of invasive bacterial disease in children, responsible for the majority of cases of pneumonia, bacteremia, and meningitis. Each year, pneumococcus causes approximately 700 cases of meningitis in children under the age of 5 in the USA, resulting in 200 deaths. Pneumococcus also causes the majority of cases of sinusitis and acute otitis media in children. The extensive use of antibiotics to treat these infections has been a major factor in the emergence of antimicrobial resistance among pneumococcal strains, increasing the risk for more virulent invasive pneumococcal disease.

ACIP now recommends all children under 23 months of age should receive a PCV vaccine series. The routine immunization schedule is 2, 4, 6, and 12-15 months of age. Immunization is also recommended for children age 2-6 who are in certain high-risk groups: (1) sickle cell disease, sickle hemoglobinopathies, or asplenia; (2) HIV infection; (3) renal failure; (4) immunodeficiency from immunospressive therapy, organ transplant, or malignant neoplasms; (5) chronic cardiac or pulmonary disease; or (6) diabetes mellitus. In addition, ACIP notes that a PCV series should be considered for children age 2-6 who attend group day care centers, as well as for children of African-American, Native Alaskan, or American Indian descent.

Influenza (for selected pediatric populations)

The disease process for influenza is discussed in a previous chapter.

ACIP recommends annual influenza vaccines for children over 6 months of age who have certain risk factors, including: asthma, cardiac disease, sickle-cell disease, HIV, and diabetes. These children should receive an age-adjusted dose: 0.25 ml for age 6-35 months, and 0.5 ml for age 3 and up. ∷

References

Centers for Disease Control. General recommendations on immunization. *MMWR* 2002; 51(RRD2);1-36.

Centers for Disease Control. Achievements in public health, 1900-1999: impact of vaccines universally recommended for children – United States, 1900-1998. *MMWR* 1999; 48(12); 243-248.

Centers for Disease Control. Preventing pneumococcal disease among infants and young children. *MMWR* 2000; 49(RR-9).

Centers for Disease Control. Prevention of varicella: updated recommendations of the Advisory Committee on Immunization Practices (ACIP). *MMWR* 1999; 48(RR06);1-5.

Centers for Disease Control. Haemophilus b conjugate vaccines for prevention of Haemophilus influenzae type b disease among infants and children two months of age and older recommendations of the ACIP. *MMWR* 1991; 40(RR01);1-7.

Centers for Disease Control. Diptheria, tetanus and pertussis: recommendations for vaccine use and other preventive measures recommendations of the Advisory Committee on Immunization Practices (ACIP). *MMWR* 1991; 40(RR10);1-28.

Centers for Disease Control. Pertussis vaccination: use of acellular pertussis vaccines among infants and young children. *MMWR* 1997; 46(RR-7);1-23.

Centers for Disease Control. Poliomyelitis prevention in the United States: updated recommendations of the Advisory Committee om Immunization Practices (ACIP). *MMWR* 2000; 49(RR-5);1-19.

Gershon, A. *Mumps.* In Fauci AS, Braunwald E, Isselbacher KJ, et al, eds. *Harrison's Principles of Internal Medicine.* 14th ed. New York: McGraw-Hill 1998: 1127-1128.

Gershon A. *Rubella (German Measles).* In Fauci AS, Braunwald E, Isselbacher KJ, et al, eds. *Harrison's Principles of Internal Medicine.* 14th ed. New York: McGraw-Hill 1998: 1125-1127.

Groth, J. Immunizations and the Vaccine-Preventable Diseases. In O'Connell JJ and Groth J, eds. *The Manual of Common Communicable Diseases in Shelters.* Boston: Boston Health Care for the Homeless Program; 1991: 203-218.

Holmes, RK. Diptheria, other Corynebacterial Infections, and Anthrax. In Fauci AS, Braunwald E, Isselbacher KJ, et al, eds. *Harrison's Principles of Internal Medicine.* 14th ed. New York: McGraw-Hill 1998: 892-899.

CDC's National Immunization Program (NIP): http://www.cdc.gov/nip

Part Six:

Food Management
in Shelters &
Soup Kitchens

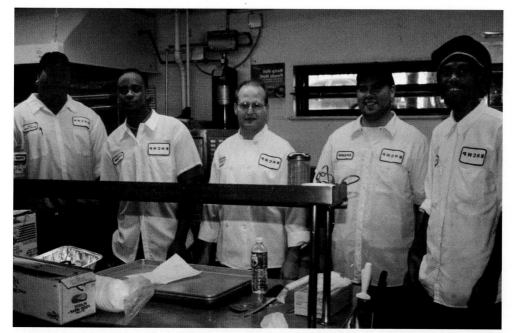

Food Management

Julia E. Gunn, RN, MPH
T. Scott Troppy, MPH
Andrew Ellington, BS

F ood-borne illness is a common problem. The Centers for Disease Control and Prevention estimates that approximately 76 million cases of food-borne illness occur each year in the USA. Although the majority of illnesses are mild, an estimated 325,000 persons are hospitalized. Food-borne illness is caused by a variety of bacteria, toxins, and viruses that do not necessarily make foods look, smell, or taste unusual.

A unique concern for homeless programs is the management of donated food. Maintaining the safety and quality of donated food is critical. Potentially hazardous foods require particular vigilance to prevent food-borne illness. These foods include meats, poultry, seafood, cooked rice, cooked beans, and dairy products such as cheese, eggs, and milk.

Food Donation

For homeless programs, food donations are a valued gift. However, care must be exercised to assure that the food does not become a health hazard for the guests of homeless programs and shelters. A few simple procedures can help prevent food-borne illness.

Evaluate the Suitability of Food Items
for Donation
Excellent for donation:
- canned foods such as beef stew, sauces, vegetables, or fruit;
- fresh or frozen vegetables or fruits that are purchased within 24 hours of donation;
- rice and pasta;

- coffee and tea;
- other dry staples.
Accept with extreme caution:
- uncooked meats and poultry, even if frozen or refrigerated and stored at the appropriate holding temperature;
- fish and shellfish, even if frozen or refrigerated and stored at the appropriate holding temperature.
Never accept:
- cooked or raw meats or poultry that have not been kept frozen or refrigerated;
- cooked or raw meats or poultry containing stuffing;
- food from public gatherings such as buffets, weddings, or tasting events;
- other potentially hazardous food that has been cooked and has not been stored at appropriate holding temperatures;
- unpasteurized juices;
- milk and eggs, including products made from milk or eggs such as cheese and sauces;

Chef Stephen Paquin (center) and his staff in the kitchen at Barbara McInnis House have taken great pride in meeting the varied dietary needs of guests with acute and chronic medical problems.
Photo by James O'Connell MD

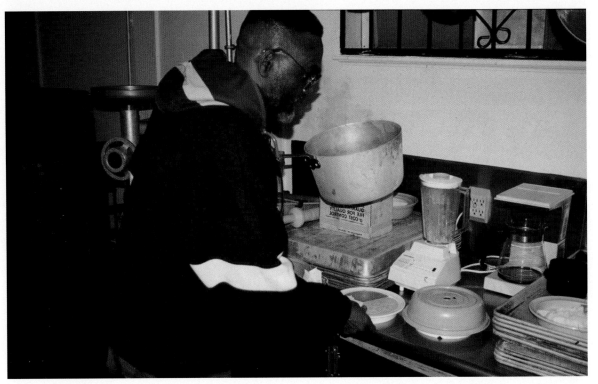

- cooked beans or rice;
- food with expiration dates that have passed.

Maintain Foods at Proper Holding Temperatures
- Cold foods should always be refrigerated at 45°F (7°C) or below. Hot foods should always be kept hot (140°F/60°C or higher) until served.
- Make sure all foods are securely wrapped or stored in containers with airtight lids.
- Do not accept cans with dents or damage to the seam or without the original label attached.
- Separate raw meat, poultry, and seafood from other items to avoid cross-contamination.
- Do not accept toxic items, such as soap powders, cleaners, detergents, or abrasives without an appropriate place to store them that is separate from food.
- Ask donors to call ahead to check on specific program needs and available resources to accept the food items, such as adequate storage capacity.

Reception of Donated Food
- Clean all surfaces that you will be using when the food arrives.
- Do not accept potentially hazardous food that has not been held at proper temperatures during storage or preparation.

- Use a food thermometer to check the temperature of donated food and reject any item in the danger zone.
- Always check frozen foods for large ice crystals that can be a sign of improper handling. Ice crystals may indicate that food was partially thawed and then refrozen.
- Check the packaging of donated food.
- Consider using the FIFO method: First In, First Out. Rotating food supplies decreases spoilage and waste.
- Do not re-use disposable containers. Aluminum pans food should be recycled but not re-used.
- WHEN IN DOUBT, THROW IT OUT!

Food Handlers (Employees and Volunteers)

Successful shelter food programs often use the services of volunteers in addition to employees. Volunteers often make it possible to feed hundreds of people each day. Food handling and preparation for large numbers of people requires adherence to food safety principles. In addition, homeless programs serve many persons who are at particular risk of food-borne illness because of underlying health problems.

Hands

All persons involved in food preparation must thoroughly wash their hands with soap and warm water. Critical times for handwashing include:

- prior to any food preparation;
- between different kitchen procedures;
- after handling the trash or taking out the garbage;
- after using the restroom or changing a diaper.
- WHEN IN DOUBT, WASH YOUR HANDS!

Recommended Way to Wash Your Hands
- wet hands with warm water;
- use soap;
- rub your hands briskly together to loosen dirt and germs for about 20 seconds;
- pay special attention to finger nails and areas around rings;
- rinse thoroughly under running water;
- dry hands with a paper towel or with an air dryer;
- use paper towel to shut off the water.
- alcohol-based hand gels are not currently approved for use in food service establishments. However, there may be unique circumstances, such as temporary limited access to hand washing facilities, when the use of alcohol-based hand gels may have some benefit.
- gloves are not a substitute for good hand washing. When they are used for a procedure such as slicing meat, remove and discard the gloves and wash your hands before starting a new task.

Hair
- All personnel working with food must use a baseball cap, scarf, hair net, or other hair restraint to keep hair out of food. These coverings minimize touching one's hair.

Illness in a Food Handler
- An ill food handler (employee or volunteer) should be excused from work. This includes persons with a cough or a cold, regardless of fever. Bacteria and viruses are easily spread through droplets when coughing or sneezing.
- Food handlers with diarrhea or vomiting pose a higher risk of food-borne illness and should refrain from working. Whenever close contacts or family members of a food handler are ill with gastrointestinal illness (vomiting or diarrhea), the employee or volunteer should not work directly with food.

Such illnesses spread easily within a family, and some family members may carry and spread germs even though they are without symptoms.
- Volunteers or employees with sores, open wounds, or infected skin on the hands or face should not prepare food. They should be assigned other functions for the program that do not involve direct contact with food. Open lesions should be covered with a bandage and changed as needed. Skin infections can contaminate food with bacteria (especially Staphylococcus), which can result in serious food-borne illnesses.

Preparation
Equipment and Environment
- Wash equipment and surfaces often.
- Use hot soapy water to wash cutting boards, dishes, utensils, and counter tops after preparing each food item and before starting the next item.
- To sanitize washed surfaces and utensils, put 1 teaspoon of bleach in 1 quart of water and use a spray bottle if necessary. This solution should be made fresh daily.
- Cutting boards:
  - always use a clean cutting board;
  - use one cutting board for produce and a separate one for raw meat, poultry, and seafood;
  - replace worn or deeply grooved cutting boards;
  - cutting boards used for meat or poultry must be washed and sanitized before cutting other foods, such as vegetables.
- Knives used for meat or poultry should be washed and sanitized before use with vegetables or other foods.
- Use utensils for mixing and stirring. Never use ungloved fingers or hands for food preparation.

Thawing Food
- Foods should be thawed in a refrigerator – never defrost at room temperature!
- In a microwave, follow the directions provided by the microwave manufacturer and cook the food immediately.
- In cold water (less than 70°F/21°C), but make sure the sink or container is clean before use. Immersion in cold water allows

the middle to thaw without exposing the edges to room temperatures:
– wrap food item airtight;
– submerge food item in cold water and change the water every 30 minutes; or completely submerge food item in constantly running cold water.
- Refrigerate or cook food immediately after thawing.

Marinating
- Always marinate in the refrigerator.
- Use food-grade plastic, stainless steel, or glass containers for marinating.
- Marinades used for raw meat, poultry, or seafood should not be used in cooked foods unless boiled before application.
- Never reuse marinades for other foods.

Produce
- Wash fruits and vegetables with cool tap water.
- Do not use soap.
- Consider using a brush for thick-skinned produce.

Tasting Food
- Food should be at a safe internal temperature before tasting.
- Use a clean utensil each time food is tasted. Never put a used utensil back into the food.

Cooking
- Use a food thermometer to check the internal temperature of food items. The internal temperature is the temperature of the food determined by a food thermometer, not the temperature of the oven.
- Check the temperature in several places to make sure that the food item is evenly heated.
- Wash and sanitize thermometers after each use.
- There are several styles and types of food thermometers. Additional information on food thermometers is available at http://www.fsis.usda.gov/oa/thermy/ktherms.htm.
- Placement of food thermometers:
– beef, pork, or lamb roasts - midway in the roast, avoiding the bone;
– hamburgers, steaks, or chops - thickest part, away from bone, fat, or gristle;
– whole poultry - thickest part of the thigh (avoiding the bone);
– stuffed poultry - the center of the stuffing should be checked after the thigh reads 180°F (82°C) (stuffing must reach 165°F (74°C);
– poultry parts - thickest area, avoiding the bone. The food thermometer may be inserted sideways if necessary;
– casseroles and other combination dishes - thickest portion of the food or the center of the dish.
- Heat all potentially hazardous hot foods to an internal temperature of at least 165°F (74°C).
- While guests are being served, maintain the internal temperature at 140°F (60°C).
- Never partially cook food (especially meat) for the purpose of completing the cooking at a later time.
- Stuffing should be placed in meat or poultry just prior to roasting.
- With frozen meat, lengthen the cooking time by 50% of that recommended for meat at room temperature. For example, if the recommended cooking time is 1 hour for a roast at room temperature, for a frozen roast the cooking time would be 1½ hours.
- Do not use recipes in which eggs remain raw or partially cooked. Pasteurized eggs should be used in place of raw eggs whenever possible.

Microwave Cooking
- Remove large bones before cooking meat. Bones prevent thorough cooking.
- Stir or rotate food half way through microwaving time for more even cooking.
- Partial cooking in a microwave may be done only if the food is to be completely cooked immediately.

Reheating Food
- Cooked, commercially vacuum-sealed, ready-to-eat foods, such as hams and roasts, are safe to reheat.
- Foods cooked ahead and cooled or leftovers should be reheated to 165°F (74°C).
- Reheat sauces, soups, and gravies to a boil.
- Slow cookers, steam tables, or chafing dishes are not recommended for reheating food.

Preparation of Baby's Milk

- When infant formulas are used, fully prepared formulas in individual bottles offer the least chance of contamination. Bottles with plastic inserts are a good alternative.
- Plastic or glass bottles can easily be cleaned with hot soapy water and then sanitized with a mild bleach and water solution.
- Contamination can happen not only when the bottle is prepared but also when open bottles of milk or cans of formula are handled by others in communal refrigerators.
- The ideal rule calls for a new bottle with each feeding. This is often impractical, and any bottle that will be used for more than one feeding should be refrigerated immediately after use.
- Discard unused formula or use the leftovers within a few hours.

Storage

- Cover food immediately after use with plastic or foil, or store in containers with tight-fitting lids. Do not over fill the containers.
- Refrigerate food immediately after use. Do not over fill the refrigerator.
- Cooked food does not need to cool before storage.
- Remove stuffing from meats prior to refrigerating. Label all foods including the preparation date.
- Leftover hot food that was not held at a temperature of 140°F (60°C) or above while being served should be discarded.
- Freeze food at 0°F (-17°C) or less. Articles to be frozen should be placed in freezer bags or wrapped in freezer paper or aluminum foil in order to avoid freezer burns. Freezer burns can destroy the taste and texture of the food.

Staples

- Store items such as uncooked pasta, rice, and flour in airtight containers and place them in cool, dry areas that are at least six inches off the floor.
- Close all boxes after use, and date and label all staples in your storage areas for easy identification by all staff.
- To avoid chemical or physical contamination, never store food near items such as soap, detergent, insect spray, abrasives, steel wool pads, or cleaners.

Dishwashing

- Dishes, pots, pans, and utensils should ideally be washed in a dishwasher with a rinse cycle set at 180°F (82°C).
- If this is not possible, soiled dishware and utensils should be washed and rinsed and then sanitized in a dilute bleach solution to prevent the growth of bacteria. A mixture of 1/4 cup of bleach (Clorox™) in one gallon of water is sufficient for this purpose.
- Allow dishes, pots, pans, and utensils to air dry. Dishtowels can spread bacteria and other germs.
- Sanitize towels with a mixture of a bleach and water (1/4 cup bleach to one gallon water) after you use them to wipe counters and cutting boards and before you use them for any other procedure. Outbreaks of food-borne illnesses can be traced to contaminated towels or cutting boards used in a facility.

Summary

Homeless shelters and programs can take many steps to reduce the risk of food-borne illness. If a cluster of illness (particularly gastrointestinal) is noted, be sure to contact the local health department. Prompt consultation with the health department is essential to evaluate the situation and institute appropriate control measures to ensure the health and well being of the guests, the staff, and the community. ∷

The authors of this chapter gratefully acknowledge the invaluable contribution of M. Kathleen Hennessy, who authored this chapter in the original Manual.

References
Helpful Food Safety Websites
- Food Safety and Inspection Service: www.fsis.usda.gov/
- Government Food Safety Information: www.foodsafety.gov/
- Centers for Disease Control and Prevention: www.cdc.gov/foodsafety

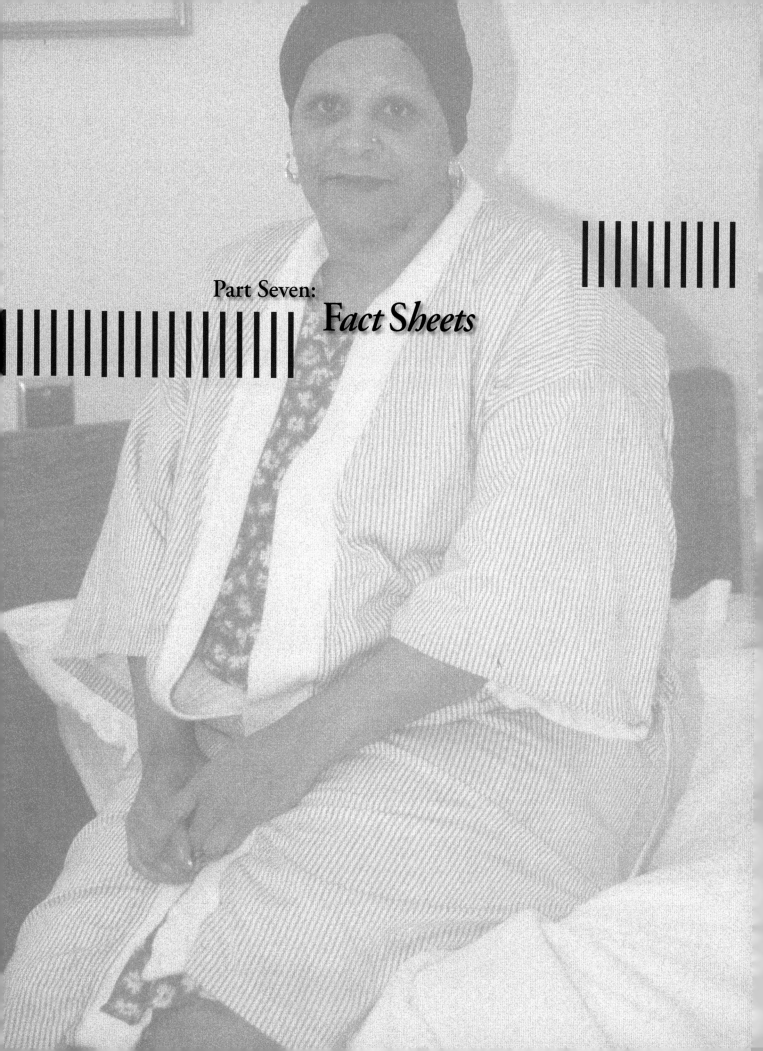

Part Seven:
Fact Sheets

English	Spanish
Chlamydia	Clamidia
Conjunctivitis (Red Eye)	Conjuntivitis (Ojos Colorados)
Diarrhea	Diarrea
Gonorrhea	Gonorrea
Hepatitis A	Hepatitis A
Hepatitis B	Hepatitis B
Hepatitis C	Hepatitis C
Herpes Simplex Virus (HSV)	Herpes Simplex Virus (HSV)
Herpes Zoster (Shingles)	Herpes Zoster (Culebrilla)
HIV/AIDS	VIH y SIDS
Impetigo	Impétigo
Influenza	Gripe
Lice	Piojos
Measles	Sarampión
Meningococcal Disease	Enfermedad Meningocócica
Pertussis (Whooping Cough)	Pertusis
Ringworm	Tiña
Scabies	Sarna
Streptococcal Pharyngitis (Strep Throat)	Faringitis
Syphilis	Sífilis
Tuberculosis (TB)	Tuberculosis (TB)
Upper Respiratory Infection (URI/Common Cold)	Infección Respiratoria Alta
Vaccinations	Vacunaciones
Varicella (Chickenpox)	Varicela
Viral Meningitis	Meningitis Viral

What is Chlamydia?

Chlamydia is a sexually transmitted disease (STD or VD). Although it is very common, many people have never heard of it.

What does Chlamydia look like?

Most women and many men who have Chlamydia don't know it because it doesn't appear to cause them any obvious problem. You may not know that you have the disease, but it can still cause many problems, especially in women. It can cause tubal pregnancy, chronic pain around the female organs, or prevent women from ever getting pregnant.

Many people who have Chlamydia also have gonorrhea. When people do get sick from Chlamydia, the symptoms are often the same as those caused by gonorrhea.

What happens when you get Chlamydia?

If you have Chlamydia, you may feel burning when you urinate. A watery or mucous-like fluid may come out of your penis or vagina, and your sex organs may itch.

If you are a woman and you have Chlamydia, you may feel pain below your stomach. It may hurt when you have sex, and sometimes you may bleed between your periods.

If you are pregnant and you have Chlamydia, you can pass the disease to your newborn at birth. Your baby may get infected eyes and lungs.

What do you do if you have Chlamydia?

Usually, it's easy to treat Chlamydia. You and your partner will have to take antibiotic pills for one or two weeks.

How do you keep from getting Chlamydia?

There are two ways to keep away from Chlamydia:
1) don't have sex;
2) if you do have sex, use a condom every time.

Make sure you and/or your partner use condoms from start to finish every time you have sex.

You cannot get Chlamydia from toilet seats, doorknobs, towels, or from lifting heavy objects and straining muscles.

Conjunctivitis (Red Eye)

What is conjunctivitis?
Conjunctivitis, sometimes called "red eye," is a very common eye problem.

What does it look like?
If you have conjunctivitis, one or both of your eyes are red. Your eyes and eyelids burn or itch. Your eyes may water and leave a crust which can make your eyelashes stick together, especially when you wake up in the morning.

How do you get conjunctivitis?
Germs get into your eyes all the time. Some germs can grow under your eyelids. When you rub or touch your eyes, the germs can infect the eyes very easily.

Sometimes, conjunctivitis isn't caused by germs. Chemicals, allergies, or other illnesses can also give you red eye.

What do you do if you have conjunctivitis caused by an infection?
A doctor or nurse will probably give you eye drops, an ointment, or pills. These are antibiotics.

Your eye will look better after 2 or 3 days of medicine. But the germs will still be alive. You need to take all of the medicine (usually it lasts for 7 to 10 days) to get rid of all the germs. Otherwise, you can get conjunctivitis again.

You don't need an eye patch if you have conjunctivitis.

If your eye stays red after treatment or you feel pain or your vision if fuzzy, see your doctor or nurse again.

How do you keep from getting eye infections?
Never share eyedrops or eye ointments, even with your family.

Do not share towels, washcloths, or makeup. In particular, never share these things with someone who has conjunctivitis.

If your child or your partner has an infected eye, wash your hands with lots of warm water and soap both before and after putting medicine in her or his infected eye.

If your partner, a friend, or someone in your family has conjunctivitis, you may also need to take medicine to keep from getting the disease.

What is diarrhea?

Diarrhea is usually a change in a normal bowel pattern, with abnormal amounts of stool or liquid stool. You can get diarrhea from viruses, bacteria, or parasites. You can also get diarrhea from other medical problems.

What happens when you have diarrhea?

If you have diarrhea, you have to go to the bathroom a lot. Your bowel movements are loose and mixed with liquid. Sometimes, you get cramps, you throw up, or you have a fever. You may see blood or mucous in your bowel movements.

When diarrhea lasts for more than three days, or if it seems severe, see a doctor or a nurse. They can take a sample of your bowel movement to see what kind of diarrhea you have.

What do you do if you or your child has diarrhea?

Whenever you have diarrhea, drink a lot of clear liquids to replace the fluids you have lost. If your baby has unusually loose stools or an increase in the usual number of bowel movements, contact your health provider. Diarrhea can quickly make babies very sick.

If your child has diarrhea, special liquids, such as Pedialyte™ or Enfalyte™, which can be bought at a drug store, can help prevent your child from becoming dehydrated. If the diarhhea is not severe and the child is not vomiting, you should allow the child to eat a normal diet in moderation. Keep in mind that starchy foods are better absorbed.

If your child's diarrhea is severe or won't stop, contact a doctor or nurse.

Take your child to a hospital or clinic if you see any of these signs:

- your child can't make tears;
- the mouth of your child is dry;
- the eyes of your child look sunken or have dark circles around them;
- your child is very sleepy;
- your child is less than 12 months of age and is having very large or very frequent stools;
- your child has not wet a diaper in 8 hours.

If your child has diarrhea, vomits, or has a fever over 101°F (38.4°C), see a doctor or nurse.

How do you keep from getting diarrhea?

Always wash your hands:

- before fixing any food or formula;
- before eating or feeding a child;
- after changing diapers or going to the bathroom.

Toilet-trained children should always wash their hands after they go to the bathroom. You or another adult should remind children to wash their hands and watch them in the bathroom. If children are putting toys in their mouths, try to keep them from sharing these toys with other children. This is especially important if one of the children is sick.

If you have diarrhea, do not fix or serve food to anyone outside of your family. You can serve and fix food when your symptoms go away or your doctor or nurse tells you it's OK.

Gonorrhea

What is gonorrhea?
Most people know gonorrhea as "the clap" or "the drip". Gonorrhea can infect your eyes, throat, vagina, rectum, joints, skin, penis, or urethra. Gonorrhea is very common.

How do you get gonorrhea?
It's an infection you can get by having sex with a person who has gonorrhea. If you're pregnant and you have gonorrhea, the germs can be passed to your baby at birth.

You are more likely to get gonorrhea if you have more than one sex partner than if you have only one partner. If you have sex with someone who has sex with different people, you have a good chance of getting gonorrhea.

If you are sexually active, go to a clinic for a gonorrhea exam regularly. Your health care provider can recommend how often you should visit.

What does gonorrhea do to you?
If you're a man and you have gonorrhea, your penis may hurt, burn, or itch when you urinate. Also, a yellow fluid may drip from your penis ("the drip").

If you're a woman and you have gonorrhea, most often you will not feel sick, even though you are infected. When gonorrhea does make you sick, you may feel pain, burning, and itching. You may also have a discharge. Sometimes the infection can spread to your tubes, ovaries, and pelvis. It is very important to get treatment as soon as possible to avoid long term problems.

Most women and some men with gonorrhea don't have any symptoms. People without symptoms can still spread the disease.

What do you do if you get gonorrhea?
Treatment for gonorrhea is usually simple. Often you get a single shot of antibiotics followed by a week or two of pills. Sometimes, an infection needs stronger antibiotics or an overnight stay in the hospital.

How do you prevent gonorrhea?
If you don't have sex, you won't get gonorrhea.

Condoms are the next best way to prevent gonorrhea.

USE CONDOMS FROM START TO FINISH EVERY TIME you have sex. It's the best way to prevent gonorrhea and other STDs (sexually transmitted diseases).

What is hepatitis A?

Hepatitis A is a virus that irritates your liver.

People with hepatitis A can feel very tired and have a fever, poor appetite, nausea, yellow eyes and skin, dark urine, and white bowel movements. Some people, especially children, don't have yellow skin or eyes. You usually feel sick from hepatitis A for about 2 weeks, although some people can get sick for several months and others never get sick at all.

How do you get hepatitis A?

Hepatitis A is spread through the stool of infected people. This can happen when an infected person goes to the bathroom, doesn't wash his hands, and then touches objects which others might put into their mouths. Hepatitis A can spread when you change diapers or when children put their hands into their diapers and then touch objects that go into the mouth.

You can't get hepatitis A when you talk to, touch, or sleep in the same room with a sick person.

How do you treat hepatitis A?

There is no treatment for hepatitis A. If you get sick, lots of rest and high calorie foods can make you feel better.

How can I keep from getting hepatitis A?

If you are at high risk for getting hepatitis A or may get seriously sick from hepatitis A, you can get a vaccination. This vaccination is for sexually active men who have sex with men, drug users (injection and non-injection drug users), persons with chronic liver disease, and children living where there are high rates of hepatitis A.

Whether or not you are vaccinated against hepatitis A, it is always important to wash your hands before you touch food, eat, feed your baby, change your baby's diapers, or go the bathroom. Always put soiled diapers in a wastebasket that children can't get into.

If your children get hepatitis A or the person you live with has hepatitis A, you can get a shot called immune globulin (IG) to make sure you don't get very sick. The shot has to be given within 2 weeks of exposure, so see a caregiver as soon as possible.

Can you get hepatitis A more than once?

After you get sick from hepatitis A, you can't get it again. But remember, you can still get other types of hepatitis.

Hepatitis B

What is hepatitis B?

Hepatitis B is a virus that affects your liver. The early symptoms are like the cold or flu. After about a month, your skin may turn yellow and begin to itch. Your urine looks like Coca-Cola, but the color of your bowel movements is light. You may not see any of these symptoms for 6 weeks to 6 months after you first get the disease.

These symptoms can last for 1 to 2 months. Usually, you are healthy again after the symptoms go away. Some people die from hepatitis B, and others have life-long liver problems.

What do you do if you have hepatitis B?

Rest and high calorie foods may help your fever and itching. Usually, food goes down better in the early part of the day.

Avoid drugs such as Tylenol™ that are broken down by the liver. Alcohol and drugs can also damage the liver.

How do you get hepatitis B?

The virus doesn't spread when you talk to, touch, or sleep in the same room with an infected person.

Having sex without a condom or sharing needles with an infected person can spread the virus very easily.

Some people can be infected and never feel or look sick. However, they can still spread the virus.

How do you keep from getting hepatitis B?

Vaccination can prevent you from getting hepatitis B. It is now recommended that all children and adolescents receive the hepatitis B vaccine. The vaccine is also recommended for adults who are high risk, which includes injection drug users.

If you inject drugs, you can also keep from getting hepatitis B by not sharing needles. If you share needles, use a watered down bleach solution to clean your works before and after you inject to kill the hepatitis B on the needle. Ask shelter staff about where to find bleach.

Use a condom every time you have sex. Often, shelter staff know where you can get condoms.

Don't share toothbrushes and razors.

Cover any cuts or sores with a bandage.

If you touch any of the fluids that come out of another person's body, especially blood and urine, you need to wash you hands very well.

Be careful when throwing away razors and other sharp things! The shelter staff can tell you where to put them.

Watch children to make sure they don't bite or scratch one another.

If you get exposed to hepatitis B, ask your doctor or nurse about vaccines.

What is hepatitis C?

Hepatitis C is a virus that causes liver disease. The hepatitis C virus is found in the blood and liver of people with hepatitis C infection.

How is hepatitis C spread?

The virus is spread primarily through blood. People most at risk are those who have had a blood transfusion or an organ transplant before 1992 or people who use or have used needles contaminated by blood (for example, the injection of drugs). Since July 1992, the blood supply has been carefully checked for this virus and the blood supply is considered to be safe.

The hepatitis C virus can be spread whenever blood (or fluids containing blood) come in contact with an opening on the skin or other tissues. This can occur even when these openings cannot be seen. Hepatitis C virus can also be transmitted by sexual contact, but this does not happen as easily as the spread of HIV, the virus that causes AIDS. Tattooing and body piercing are also risk factors.

The hepatitis C virus is not spread by casual contact like hugging, sneezing, coughing, or sharing food. As with all blood-borne infections, razors, toothbrushes, and drinks should not be shared. You cannot get hepatitis C by donating blood.

How serious is hepatitis C?

Hepatitis C infection can be very serious. Most people who become infected will carry the virus for the rest of their lives. Some of these people will develop liver damage and feel very sick. Other people may feel healthy for many years after being diagnosed with hepatitis C infection. This virus can eventually cause cirrhosis (scarring of the liver) and/or liver cancer in some infected people. While most people will not develop liver failure or cancer with hepatitis C, a significant number of people will. We cannot tell who will or will not have these problems. We do know that homeless and poor patients are at higher risk for infections and complications.

Who is at risk for getting hepatitis C?

People are at risk for developing hepatitis C infection if they:

- have used street drugs or shared needles, even just once;
- have received a blood transfusion, blood products, or an organ transplant before July 1992;
- have had many sexual partners, especially if they did not use condoms;
- are health care workers (like doctors or nurses) who may be exposed to blood or needles;
- are babies born to mothers who have hepatitis C;
- are homeless;
- suffer from alcoholism;
- are veterans of the Vietnam war;
- have tattoos or body piercing with infected needles or ink;
- have been on kidney dialysis.

Continued next page.

Is there a treatment for hepatitis C?

A drug called interferon, in combination with Ribavirin™, is used to treat hepatitis C infection. People diagnosed with hepatitis C infection should not drink any alcohol or take certain medicines that can cause liver damage. It is recommended that persons infected with hepatitis C be vaccinated for hepatitis A and hepatitis B, two other viruses which cause liver damage. Antibiotics (medicine to fight an infection from bacteria) do not work against the hepatitis C virus. Ask your doctor about treatment options and steps you can take to protect your liver.

How can hepatitis C be prevented?

There is no vaccine for hepatitis C. The best way to keep from getting the hepatitis C virus is to avoid any contact with blood. This includes not sharing needles, razors, or toothbrushes. Blood banks now screen donated blood for hepatitis C virus, so your risk of getting infected from a blood transfusion is extremely low. You can also get hepatitis C from sex with an infected partner; using a condom may reduce your risk of becoming infected.

To prevent the spread of hepatitis C:

- if you shoot drugs, never share works with anyone. Don't share cocaine or other snorting straws, since these can get blood on them too. Find out about treatment programs that can help you stop using drugs.
- use a latex condom every time you have sex.
- only get tattoos or body piercing from places using sterile equipment.
- health care workers and people who clean up in hospitals or places where needles or sharps are used should follow standard (universal) precautions for every patient.
- if you have hepatitis C, don't share razors or toothbrushes.
- if you have hepatitis C, don't donate blood, sperm, or organs.

Adapted from the MA Department of Public Health Fact Sheets.

What is herpes simplex?

Herpes simplex is a virus. It is not very dangerous for most people, but it can be very painful.

Once you get herpes, you have the germs for life. Most of the time, you don't notice you have herpes. Now and then, you get blisters that open up and become painful. Stress, sunlight, and sometimes getting sick with other things can bring the blisters out again.

What does herpes look like?

If you have herpes, you usually get groups of little blisters. A ring of skin around the blisters becomes bright red. The blisters will open up and become painful. Then, they'll get a scab over them and dry up.

You can get the blisters on your lips or the corners of your mouth. People call these cold sores or fever blisters. Doctors call them oral herpes.

You can get the blisters on your penis, on the inner lips of your vagina, or around your anus. The blisters can also spread to your buttocks, the small of your back, and your thighs. This is called genital herpes.

The blisters of both genital and oral herpes break open and then crust over. Cold sores on the lips take about a week to go away. Sores of genital herpes can take two weeks to go away.

If you have a rash that looks like herpes, see a doctor or nurse. They can show you how to take care of your rash.

How do you get herpes?

You get herpes by touching the sores of people with herpes.

You get oral herpes by kissing or nuzzling someone who has sores or is infected but does not have sores.

You get genital herpes by having sex with someone who has sores or who is infected but does not have sores.

Most people get herpes from people who are infected but do not have sores.

Newborn babies can get herpes from their mothers if their mothers have sores.

What do you do if you have herpes?

Wash your hands often with warm water and soap. Wash your hands every time you touch your sores.

Cover your sores with a cloth or bandage until they crust over.

Keep the rash clean and dry. When it's clean, the rash can't get infected.

No medicine gets rid of the virus completely. Some medicines can help heal the sores. There is no vaccine to prevent herpes.

If you have genital herpes, a nurse or a doctor can give you some medicine that may help.

See a doctor or nurse if you have herpes and:
- your rash spreads;
- you feel ill (headaches, fever, strange behavior);
- your rash spreads to your eye;
- you think you might be pregnant.

How do you keep from getting herpes?

Many people are already infected with herpes but do not know it because they have never had the blisters or sores.

Most people get herpes from infected people without sores.

Don't touch the sores or saliva of someone who has herpes.

Don't have sex or kiss your partner when he or she has sores.

Always use a condom every time you have sex with anyone, because even people without sores now or in the past may be infected and give you the infection.

Herpes Zoster (Shingles)

What is herpes zoster?

Herpes zoster is a rash known as shingles. Shingles comes from the same germ that causes chickenpox. After you have chickenpox, the virus "sleeps" for many years and can "wake up" at any time to cause painful blisters on your skin.

What does shingles look like?

The rash looks like chickenpox but is usually limited to one area. You get many little red bumps that can itch and ooze.

You can get shingles more than once, but you can't get chickenpox more than once.

How do you get shingles?

You have to get chickenpox before you can get shingles. If your immune system is healthy and you touch the blisters of someone with shingles, you don't get shingles. But you can get chickenpox if you have not had chickenpox before.

The drainage from the blisters of shingles can spread germs to other people who have not had chickenpox. You should cover open or wet blisters with a bandage or clean clothes.

If you have not had chickenpox and you have contact with someone with a shingles rash, see a doctor or a nurse.

What do you do if you have shingles?

Keep the shingles lesions clean with soap and water to prevent them from getting infected. You may need to take pain relievers.

See a nurse or a doctor often. They can help you with the pain. Also, they can make sure that your rash doesn't get worse.

See a caregiver immediately if any of these signs or symptoms appear:

- blisters spread to your eyes or other parts of your body;
- blisters are still appearing after one week;
- you get more sleepy, cranky, or confused.

What is HIV?

HIV is a virus that spreads through sexual contact and blood contact. The virus can also pass from a pregnant woman to her unborn baby or to a baby through breast milk.

What is AIDS?

AIDS stands for "acquired immune deficiency syndrome." AIDS results when the body's immune system is damaged by the human immunodeficiency virus (HIV). This can result in infections and certain kinds of cancer. AIDS can be prevented!

How is HIV transmitted?

HIV is a virus that is spread through person to person contact with body fluids – blood, semen, vaginal fluids, or mother's milk.

The virus is most often transmitted during sexual contact and through sharing needles and other drug works. It can also be passed to a baby during pregnancy or at birth.

Sexual contact can be between men and women or between partners of the same sex.

How do other sexually transmitted diseases affect HIV?

When a person has another STD like gonorrhea, Chlamydia, or herpes, he or she is at greater risk of getting HIV.

How can I tell if my partner has HIV?

There is no way to tell if a person is infected with HIV. He or she can look healthy and feel healthy.

How can I tell if I have been infected with HIV?

When a person is initially infected with HIV, he or she may have fevers, chills, swollen lymph nodes, and a rash. This usually resolves in several days. People with HIV may not know it. They may feel and look very healthy. They can still spread the virus. The only way to find out is to have HIV testing done either by a saliva sample or a blood sample.

Does a positive HIV test mean I have AIDS?

No. It means you have been infected with the virus. Treatment with medication may prevent the development of AIDS. If your HIV test is positive, you can spread the virus to sexual partners, needle use partners, or your unborn child.

What do I do if I am pregnant and may have HIV?

If you are pregnant or planning to become pregnant, consult your doctor about getting a test for HIV. If you are HIV positive, your doctor can help you and your baby if you get into care as soon as possible.

What do I do if I am HIV positive?

It is important to remember that HIV is now a treatable disease. Get medical care as soon as possible. If you do not need medications, it is important to stay as healthy as possible and to get regular check ups.

What do I do if someone I know is HIV positive?

People with HIV need support and understanding, as well as respect for their confidentiality. If someone tells you he or she has HIV, offer friendship but respect their privacy.

How can I keep from getting HIV?

You can become infected if you do not practice safer sex. Men should always wear a condom (rubber). Lubricate the condom with water-based substances such as K-Y Jelly™, For-Play™, PrePair™, or Probe™. Don't put any oil or Vaseline™ on the condom because it may break. Avoid nonoxynol 9 spermicide. Never use a condom more than once. Don't take chances. Use a condom from start to finish every time you have sex.

Oral sex on a man should also be done with a condom in place. For oral sex on a woman, use a dental dam. Don't let blood or sexual fluids enter your mouth or your partner's.

Continued next page.

Dry kissing, masturbation, hugging, and touching are safe. Deep (French) kissing has not been shown to pass on the virus but may be risky, especially if there are sores or blood in someone's mouth.

DON'T SHOOT DRUGS! The best protection from HIV is to get help through a drug program. When using drugs, NEVER SHARE NEEDLES, straws, or other works. Always clean your works with bleach before and after use.

Because HIV spreads through blood, don't share sharp objects like razors and toothbrushes that may have blood on them.

You cannot get the virus by being stung by insects, sitting on toilet seats, washing dishes, or being around someone with AIDS. Sharing bathrooms, dishes, and laundry cannot spread the virus. A person infected with HIV cannot transmit the virus when he or she hugs and touches you or sneezes towards you.

Where can I get information about HIV/AIDS?

Much information about HIV/AIDS is now available. The shelters have brochures and sometimes videos. There are now many magazines with information about HIV/AIDS. If you have access to the internet, the following websites can give you information that is easy to understand:
www.projinf.org
www.thebody.com
www.aegis.com

What is impetigo?
Impetigo is a very common skin infection that can spread very easily in places where people are close together, such as day care centers and shelters.

What does impetigo look like?
Red blisters that later become crusted can appear anywhere on the body but most often around your mouth, your nose, or on your arms and legs. It can also look like pus-filled blisters on any part of the body.

How do you get impetigo?
You can get impetigo when you have an open cut on your skin or when you scratch an insect bite. The sores can quickly spread to other parts of your body.

You can get impetigo if you touch the sores of someone else. If you have impetigo, you can spread it until all your sores get better.

What should you do if you have impetigo?
If you have impetigo, a doctor or a nurse will give you an antibiotic ointment or pills. You must complete the whole recommended treatment in order to keep the infection from coming back.

If you have impetigo, clean your sores with warm water and soap every day, then cover them with clothing or a bandage. Don't share towels or clothing with other people until all your sores go away.

If you have impetigo, wash your hands often with a lot of soap and clean water to keep from spreading the infection. Wash your hands every time you touch impetigo sores or change the bandages or clothing that covers the sores.

Make sure you carefully throw away soiled bandages and keep any clothing or linen that might have drainage on them away from others. Clothing and linen soiled with drainage can be disinfected by washing in a hot water wash cycle with chlorine bleach.

How can you keep from getting impetigo?
Try to avoid scratching insect bites and picking scabs.

Keep any insect bites or cuts clean with soap and water. If it looks like a bite or cut is draining or forming a crust, see a doctor or a nurse.

What is influenza?

Influenza is the flu, a virus that comes around once a year, usually in the late fall or winter months.

When you have the flu, you get a fever, chills, headaches, dry cough, and often a runny nose. You feel very tired and can feel achy all over for several days.

For most people, the flu comes and goes quickly. But the flu can make you very sick if you have problems with your heart or lungs. You can also get very sick from the flu if you are infected with HIV, the virus causing AIDS.

How do you get the flu?

The flu is easy to catch when many people live close together. You get the flu by breathing germs from someone who is coughing or sneezing or by staying in a shelter where many people are sick.

What should you do if you get the flu?

If you have the flu, you should take it easy and drink plenty of liquids. You can help a sore throat by gargling with warm water and some salt.

Use Tylenol™ (acetaminophen) to treat the fever or muscle aches.

You should see a doctor or nurse if you are getting worse, are not better after a few days, or if you have heart or lung problems.

How can you keep from getting the flu?

You can get a flu shot every year so you don't get the flu or give it to other people. Shelters usually give flu shots in November.

You can't get the flu from a flu shot. Most people don't have any side effects from the flu shot. However, sometimes the shot can make you feel achy and tired, or you may have a low fever and chills. This is not common and only lasts for about 2 days. Your arm may be sore for a couple of days from the shot.

If you are allergic to eggs, you should not get a flu shot.

If you are ill and have a fever, wait until you feel better before you have a flu shot.

You should wash your hands with warm water and soap after blowing your nose or your child's nose to prevent giving the flu to others.

What are lice?
Lice are tiny bugs that live on the human body.

There are three types of lice:
Head lice live on people's hair and make the scalp itch. The eggs often look like dandruff, but you can't pull them off your hair easily.

Head lice spread when a person with head lice comes into contact with another person's hair. They can also spread when people share hats, combs, and other things that touch the head or hair. Head lice are very common among children.

Body lice live on people's clothes, especially in the seams. They do not usually live on the skin. People usually find they have body lice when they get a rash from scratching.

Body lice spread when you touch or come into contact with a person with body lice. They can also spread by sharing things like clothing or bed sheets that have body lice on them.

Pubic lice is most commonly spread by close body contact or sexual contact. If you have pubic lice, you should ask a doctor or nurse to exam you for other sexually transmitted diseases.

How do you get rid of lice?
For head lice and pubic lice, ask a doctor or nurse about shampoos or cream rinses that will kill lice in your hair. Usually, you have to leave the shampoo on your hair for up to 10 minutes. You then rinse your hair well and dry it with a towel. Once your hair is dry, you may have to comb any remaining eggs out of your hair with a fine-toothed comb. This takes a lot of time. Some people prefer to cut or shave their hair instead of combing.

To keep the lice from coming back, wash all linen and clothing in hot water and dry your laundry in a dryer for 30 minutes before you use it again.

If you can't wash things like stuffed animals and toys, carefully vacuum them.

Soak all your combs and brushes in the lice shampoo diluted with water. A solution of 1 part bleach to 10 parts water will also work.

For body lice, all you may have to do is take off your clothing and shower carefully. Body lice live in clothing, not on the skin. Before you put your clothing back on, you should wash your clothes in hot water and dry them in a dryer for 30 minutes. Do not put your clothing back on or sleep in the same bed after you shower until everything is clean.

If you have lice, you should see a nurse or a doctor after about a week to make sure the lice are gone. Sometimes you have to get treated again.

How can you keep from getting lice?
The best way to keep from getting lice is not to share clothing, hats, combs, and other personal things. Tell people who complain about itching or rashes to see a doctor or nurse.

If you have been close to a person with lice, ask a doctor or nurse to evaluate you for lice.

Measles

What is measles?

Measles is a virus that is easy to get. Measles can make you or your child very sick.

What does measles look like?

Measles often begins like a cold. You can have a cough, high fever, runny nose, and red, watery eyes. Four days later, you get a rash that is red and blotchy. The rash starts on your face and then spreads to your body.

How do you get measles?

When someone who has measles coughs or sneezes, the virus can be spread through the air to other people.

You or your children can get measles if:
- you've never had measles or have never been vaccinated;
- you were vaccinated before 1968, because some early vaccines did not give lasting protection;
- your child has never had measles and has not been vaccinated.

If you're near someone who has measles, you should ask a doctor or nurse about the disease.

What should you do if you have measles?

When you see symptoms of measles on yourself or your child, you should go to a doctor immediately. The doctor can tell you if you or your child has measles. There is no medicine to get rid of the measles, but you can make sure that others don't get the disease.

If you have measles, don't go into public places like stores, buses, subways, and medical clinics. You could spread the disease to someone who had not yet had it. About 4 days after you get the rash, you can no longer give the disease to anyone else. It is then safe to go out in public.

How can you keep your children from getting measles?

You can prevent your children from getting measles by having them vaccinated. A vaccine to protect against measles is usually given to children at 12 to 15 months of age and again at 4 to 6 years of age. Children who have not been given a second dose of vaccine at 4 to 6 years of age are usually vaccinated when they go to middle school. The vaccine is combined with one for mumps and rubella (MMR) and will protect your child against all three diseases.

What is meningococcal disease?

Meningococcal disease is a serious infection caused by a bacteria. It can lead to meningitis, a swelling of the lining around the brain. It can also cause an infection of the blood.

What are the symptoms of meningococcal disease?

Meningococcal disease can begin as a cold, or it may start very quickly, with a fever, chills, and tiredness. Often, tiny red or purple splotches show up on your skin.

Older children and adults also get headaches with stiffness or pain in the neck. Very small children may be cranky and not want to feed. Their cry can sound much higher than normal.

How do you get meningococcal disease?

You can get infected when someone coughs or sneezes the bacteria that cause meningococcal disease into the air you breathe. Your children can get the bacteria when they put objects in their mouths which have been mouthed by other children carrying the germ.

The bacteria can live in the nose and throat of some people who do not get sick. They can still spread it to others.

How do you keep from getting meningococcal disease?

If you or your children spend a lot of time with someone who gets this illness, you can take an antibiotic called rifampin to reduce your changes of getting the disease. It only needs to be taken for two days. Talk to your health provider about this.

You should not take rifampin if you are pregnant, have severe liver disease, or have had previous problems with this medicine.

Rifampin can stain your urine, sweat, saliva, tears, and stool an orange-red color. This goes away once the medicine is finished.

Rifampin can stain soft contact lenses, so you should wear glasses until the medicine is finished.

If you take rifampin, your birth control pills may not work. You should use another method like a condom or a diaphragm until the end of the birth control pill cycle.

Rifampin can also interfere with methadone doses. If you are on methadone, have your health provider call your clinic to adjust the dosage.

See a doctor or nurse right away if you or your family has been around someone with meningococcal disease in the last two weeks and:
- you or anyone in your family develops a fever, headache, or becomes confused;
- your baby gets a fever, becomes cranky, feeds poorly, or has a funny cry.

Pertussis (Whooping Cough)

What is pertussis?
Most people know pertussis by its common name: whooping cough. It is a prolonged cough illness. This disease can be very serious, especially in infants who have not completed their immunizations. In children under a year old, pertussis can cause serious lung or brain problems.

How do you get pertussis?
You can get pertussis when someone with the disease coughs into the air you are breathing. Also, you can get pertussis by touching the saliva or mucous of someone with the disease.

What does pertussis look like?
Pertussis starts like a cold. You get a runny nose and runny eyes, and you begin to sneeze and cough. The cough goes on for about 2 weeks and gets worse and worse.

Sometimes, especially with children, the coughing fits can end up in a big "whoop" when they take in a breath. They can turn blue while coughing or vomit afterwards.

In children younger than 6 months, teenagers, and adults, pertussis may look just like a cough illness that lasts a long time.

If you or your child has a cough that lasts for more than 14 days, you may have pertussis. If you or your child has a cough that makes you turn blue or vomit, you may have pertussis. See a doctor or nurse.

What do you do if you have pertussis?
If you have pertussis, see a doctor, drink plenty of fluids, and get lots of rest.

Your doctor or nurse will probably give you some antibiotic medicine. The medicine may lessen the symptoms and also keep you from spreading the germs to other people.

How do you prevent pertussis?
Usually, children get pertussis vaccine 5 times during their routine checkups between 6 weeks and 7 years. The vaccine is the "aP" in the "DTaP" shot.

Keep your children's vaccinations up to date. This is the best way to make sure they don't get pertussis.

The pertussis vaccine can wear off. Sometimes, an older child or adult may get whooping cough even though they have had all their shots. These people can give it to small children who have not had all of their vaccinations.

If you have been near someone who is sick with pertussis, you may need to take antibiotics also. They may prevent you from getting sick.

What is ringworm?

Ringworm is a common infection that can grow on your skin, hair, or nails. It's a fungus, not a worm. Ringworm can appear as small red sores, red circles, or areas of scaling or crusting.

Many children get ringworm on their scalps. Sometimes the small rings get bigger and make hair fall out. The skin in these areas can get scaly and crusted.

Ringworm on your skin can look like many small circles. Or your skin can just be scaly and very crusted. It can itch a lot.

Ringworm on the feet is common for teenagers and adults. If you have ringworm, your feet will look red and scaly, especially between the toes. These places also itch a lot.

How do you get ringworm?

You or your children can get ringworm of the scalp if you touch another person's ringworm sores and then touch your head. You can also get ringworm on your head if you use an infected person's hat, comb, or anything else they had used in or on their hair.

You can get ringworm on your skin and feet by touching another person's sores. You can also get ringworm on your skin or feet by touching something they touched. Often this happens when you go into the bathroom and walk in your bare feet on a wet floor, take a bath in a tub that wasn't rinsed out, or sit on a changing bench that wasn't washed.

You can't get ringworm just by being in the same room with someone who has it.

If you have ringworm, you can give it to someone as long as you have sores. Once your sores heal, it can no longer be spread to others.

What do you do if you have ringworm?

If you have ringworm, your doctor or your nurse will give you some pills or a cream. The length of treatment depends on where the infection is and how severe it is.

If you're taking care of someone who has ringworm, wash your hands often. Wash your hands every time you touch infected skin or put lotion on the sores of someone who has ringworm.

Wash in hot water the clothes and linens of anyone with ringworm. Do not let anyone else use these items until they have been washed.

If you or your child has anything on your skin that looks like ringworm, tell someone in the shelter and see a doctor or a nurse. Also, look for the same signs in the rest of your family and in other children who play with your child.

What are scabies?

Scabies are tiny bugs called mites. Scabies burrow under the skin and make you itch and feel uncomfortable, especially at night. They can live anywhere on your body.

How do you get scabies?

Scabies are easy to get, especially in places where a lot of people live or play together. They spread when someone with scabies touches your skin. This can also happen when people sleep in the same bed or share clothing or bed linen. Scabies can spread from the infected person until he or she gets treated.

What do you do if you have scabies?

Scabies may be difficult to treat. A doctor or nurse practitioner or physician assistant can give you a lotion that kills scabies.

If you have scabies:

1) Trim your nails so the scratching doesn't hurt your skin.
2) Take a shower.
3) Wait a few minutes for your skin to cool down.
4) Spread the lotion on your skin as directed.
5) Do not put on any other cream, ointment, or body lotion.
6) Wait 8 to 12 hours. If you wash your hands during this time period, reapply the lotion to your hands.
7) Take another shower to rinse off the lotion.
8) Put on new or clean clothes that have been washed and dried according to the instructions below.
9) Wash your linen and bedclothes the morning after the treatment is finished. Everything should be washed in hot water and dried in a hot drier for 30 minutes.
10) You may need to repeat the treatment in 1 week – ask your doctor, nurse practitioner, or physician assistant.

For a child with scabies:

1) Trim the child's nails so the scratching doesn't hurt his or her skin.
2) Bathe or shower the child.
3) Wait a few minutes for the skin to cool down.
4) Spread the lotion on skin as directed.
5) Do not put on any other cream, ointment, or body lotion.
6) Wait 8 to 12 hours. If the child washes his or her hands during this time period, reapply the lotion to the hands.
7) Bathe or shower the child again to rinse off the lotion.
8) Put on the child new or clean clothes that have been washed and dried according to the instructions below.
9) Wash the linen and bedclothes the morning after the treatment is finished. Everything should be washed in hot water and dried in a hot drier for 30 minutes.
10) The child may need to repeat the treatment in 1 week – ask your doctor, nurse practitioner, or physician assistant.

Vacuum anything you or your child may have touched if it can't be washed (toys, rugs, pillows).

Even after treatment, you may continue to itch for a couple of weeks. This is normal. If itching is bad, ask your doctor or nurse for a medicine to control the itch.

How do you keep from getting scabies?

Try not to share your clothing or your children's clothing and bed linen with others.

If you know someone who complains about a rash or itching, urge them to see a doctor or nurse.

If you or your children have been around someone with scabies, see a doctor or nurse.

What is syphilis?
Syphilis is a sexually transmitted disease or STD, like gonorrhea and Chlamydia.

What does syphilis look like?
Syphilis can be hard to notice, especially for women. When you first get syphilis, you may see a sore on your penis, on or around your vagina, in your rectum, or in your mouth. Often, the sore is on a place you can't see, like your vagina or rectum, so you don't notice it. The sore is painless and goes away after a while. But the disease is NOT gone after the sore fades away.

The disease can go through many stages. The stages can take up to 40 years.

What happens when you get syphilis?
If you have syphilis and you don't treat it, the disease can spread almost anywhere in your body. The disease can cause very serious complications like stroke, heart attack, loss of hearing, insanity, and blindness.

Syphilis can be very bad for people with HIV infection. If you are infected with HIV, make sure you get a blood test for syphilis.

Babies can be born with syphilis if the mother is infected. If you are pregnant, make sure you get a test for syphilis on your first prenatal visit and again in the last 3 months of your pregnancy.

What do you do if you have syphilis?
If you have syphilis, tell your present and past sexual partners that you have the disease. They need to see their doctors even if they don't have any symptoms.

If you have syphilis, your doctor will usually give you penicillin. You will probably get a shot once a week for 2 to 3 weeks.

Penicillin cures syphilis. The earlier you and your partners begin treatment, the better your changes for cure.

If you are being treated for syphilis, your partner must be treated before you can safely have sex together.

If you have syphilis, you should talk to an HIV counselor about HIV testing. HIV is the virus that causes AIDS.

How can you keep from getting syphilis?
Condoms, diaphragms, and spermicides do not keep people from giving syphilis to one another.

People can get syphilis and not know it. If you are sexually active, get a blood test for syphilis every 2 to 3 years at your clinic or health center.

Streptococcal Pharyngitis (Strep Throat)

What is strep throat?
Strep throat is an infection caused by bacteria. It is called "strep" because the bacteria that causes the infection is called Streptococcus.

What are the signs of strep throat?
Adults with strep throat may have a sore throat, a fever, and swollen neck glands. They usually don't have a cough or a runny nose.

Children with strep throat have a sore throat and may have tummy pain or a red rash with small spots. The rash is worse under the arms and in skin creases.

How is strep throat treated?
Your doctor may give you or your child an antibiotic. Antibiotics kill bacteria, which helps strep throat go away a little faster. It can also prevent a few rare but serious conditions that people with strep throat might get. It is important to take all of the medicine your doctor gives you.

Should all sore throats be treated with antibiotics?
No. Not every sore throat is strep throat. Bacteria only cause about 5%-10% of sore throats. The rest are caused by viruses or other problems, and antibiotics will not help. Your doctor can do a test to make sure it is strep throat.

Can other people catch my strep throat?
Yes. You can give the infection to other people until you have been treated with an antibiotic for 1 to 3 days. Children with strep throat should not go back to school or day care until their fever has gone away and they have taken an antibiotic for at least 24 hours.

What can make my sore throat feel better?
Here are some things that might help you feel better:

- Taking ibuprofen (brand names: Advil™, Motrin™, Nuprin™) or acetaminophen (brand name: Tylenol™). Children should not take aspirin. Aspirin can cause Reye syndrome (a serious illness) and, in some cases, death when it is used in children under 18 years of age who have the flu.
- Gargling with warm salt water (1/4 teaspoon of salt in 1 cup (8 ounces) of warm water).
- For adults and older children, sucking on throat lozenges, hard candy, or pieces of ice.
- Eating soft foods, drinking cool drinks or warm liquids, or sucking on Popsicles.

Adapted from the American Academy of Family Physicians Fact Sheets.

What is tuberculosis?

Tuberculosis, or TB, is a germ that most often infects your lungs. It can also grow in other parts of your body. TB of the lungs can make a person sick with a cough that doesn't go away, fevers, sweats at night, and weight loss.

How do you get TB?

TB spreads when someone sick with TB in the lungs coughs or sneezes. This puts the germs into the air, and then other people breathe them. If you spend a lot of time near a person who is sick with TB, you can get infected. Most people who get infected with TB do not get sick; their immune system keeps the infection in check, and the person doesn't know that he or she is carrying the TB germ.

How do you know if you have TB?

To be sure you don't have TB infection, you can take a skin test called the "PPD." If you are at risk for TB, you can take the skin test every 6 months. This test shows if you have TB germs in your body. If you have TB germs, the test is "positive." To be sure that these germs are not making you sick, a physical exam and a chest x-ray usually are needed.

What do you do if you have TB?

If your test is positive, get a check-up and a chest x-ray to see if the germs are making you sick.

Your TB germs may not be making you sick right now. But they can make you sick at anytime in your life. The doctor can give you an antibiotic to kill the germs so they don't begin to grow and make you sick.

If you are infected with TB, but not yet sick, you cannot spread the germs to other people.

If you are sick with TB, it is possible that you can spread the disease to other people. Your friends may need to take a PPD skin test to make sure they are not infected.

If you are sick with TB, you will need to take TB medicine for many months before all of the germs are killed. You should take the medicine even if you feel better. TB germs can hide out until the medicine is not around. Then, the germs grow back and make you sick again.

It isn't easy to take medicine in shelters. Ask the shelter staff about a safe place to store the pills. Ask someone to help you to remember to take your pills. The Health Department should be able to help you with your medicines.

Sometimes the TB medicine can cause side effects. You may have a fever and a skin rash. You may not want to eat, or your stomach may get upset and you throw up. The right side of your stomach may be sore. Your skin and eyes may turn yellow and your urine may look dark, like tea. This means the medicine is hurting your liver.

If you see any of these signs, stop the pills immediately and see your doctor.

Upper Respiratory Infection (URI/Common Cold)

What is an upper respiratory infection?

Upper respiratory infection is a medial term for the common cold. People get colds all the time. Adult can get 2 to 4 colds every year. Children can get as many as 6 to 8 colds every year.

How do you get a cold?

Colds are most likely spread when people cough or sneeze germs into the air, and then other people breathe those germs. Also, people with colds may touch their noses and then put their hands on other people or things like toys.

What are the signs of a cold?

If you have a cold, you may cough, have a stuffed and runny nose. You sneeze and your throat is sore. You may feel pressure in your ears.

Adults can sometimes have fevers up to 101°F (38.3°C). Sometimes, children can get a fever up to 102°F (38.9°C).

What do you do if you have a cold?

You should get rest and drink plenty of water or any type of fluids. If you have a sore throat, mix some salt in warm water and then gargle. You can also use throat lozenges.

If you feel sore everywhere, you can take Tylenol™.

Decongestants may help a stuffed or runny nose.

If you have a high fever, what do you do?

- If you or your children have a high fever (over 102°F/38.9°C), see a doctor or nurse immediately.
- If you have a fever, swollen glands, and a sore throat see a doctor or nurse immediately.
- If you have a fever and cough up yellow or green phlegm, see a doctor or nurse immediately.

How do you keep from spreading a cold?

If you or your children have a cold you should wash your hands often, (especially after blowing noses or wiping secretions) and throw the tissue away.

People without colds should also wash their hands a lot with warm water and soap, particularly before preparing, serving or eating food.

What is a vaccination?

When you get a shot to protect you against a certain disease, you are getting a vaccination.

In the USA children routinely get shots to protect them against measles, mumps, rubella (German measles), diphtheria, tetanus, pertussis (whooping cough), *Haemophilus influenzae* type b (Hib), and polio.

Certain individuals may also be targeted for other vaccinations, especially the influenza vaccine. This depends on your health history and your risk for getting these diseases.

Vaccination is very important for you and your children. Children usually receive most vaccines before their seventh birthday. If you didn't get vaccinated in childhood for one of these diseases, you may still be able to receive the vaccine as an adult.

What are the diseases?

Measles is a serious virus that causes a high fever, cold-like symptoms, runny eyes, and a body rash. Rarely, measles can lead to pneumonia, inflammation of the brain, deafness, or mental retardation.

Mumps is a virus that causes painful swelling of the glands in the neck and behind the ears. It can lead to inflammation of the lining around the brain (meningitis) and swelling of the testicles in men. Rarely, it causes deafness or sterility.

Rubella is also called German measles. Normally, the symptoms of rubella are mild and include a rash with a low fever. However, pregnant women with rubella can have miscarriages, stillbirths, or babies born with serious birth defects.

Polio is a virus that can lead to swelling of the lining around the brain (meningitis) or paralysis. It is extremely rare in the USA due to good vaccination practices. You can get polio if you are not immunized and you are exposed to infected people from other countries where polio is more common.

Diphtheria is an infection that starts in the throat and nose. It causes a thick gray covering over the back of the throat that can make breathing very difficult. This germ can also release a poison that causes paralysis and severe heart problems.

Tetanus is an infection that gets into the body when you get a serious cut, puncture wound, burn, or bite. It leads to stiffness in the muscles, especially those of the jaw ("lockjaw") and the breathing muscles.

Pertussis, or whooping cough, is a serious infection of the upper airway. It begins very much like a cold with a runny nose and cough. The cough may get worse at night and occur in "fits" that may end in a loud whoop or vomiting. Infants are most at risk for problems including seizures, pneumonia, and brain damage from pertussis.

Hib (*Haemophilus influenzae* type b) is a bacteria that can infect the blood, the lining of the brain, and the lungs and airways. It rarely infects adults, but it can be a very serious illness in infants and young children.

Pneumococcus is a bacterial infection that can cause pneumonia, blood infections, or meningitis in small children. PCV, or pneumococcal conjugate vaccine, protects against pneumococcus infection.

Hepatitis B is a virus that infects the liver. Some people with hepatitis B do not feel sick at all, but they can pass the disease on to others. The virus can lead to an inflammation of the liver, causing fatigue, nausea, lack of appetite, and a yellowing of the skin called jaundice. The inflammation can cause the liver to stop working, which is fatal.

Continued next page.

Varicella (chickenpox) is a common viral illness in children, causing fever, cold symptoms, and a rash. Most children recover from varicella without any problems. Adults who get varicella often get serious complications from the disease, including pneumonia, encephalitis (an inflammation of the brain), or kidney failure.

What are the side effects of these vaccines?

The side effects of these vaccines are usually mild, with some redness and swelling where you get the shot and possibly a fever. Rarely, more serious side effects can occur with any vaccine. You should talk to your health provider about any concerns you have. Health clinics can also give you information sheets on each vaccine.

What if I don't get my child vaccinated?

If you don't get your child vaccinated, they can get very sick. Also, they may not be able to enroll in a school or day-care center. Massachusetts state law requires all children enrolled in daycare centers, schools, and colleges to be up-to-date with immunizations.

Keep your child's immunization records updated and in a safe place. You will need them as your child grows up.

What is varicella?

Varicella is a virus known as chickenpox. The same virus causes shingles. Chickenpox spreads easily from one person to another and is contagious until all the chickenpox blisters are crusted over. Once you've had chickenpox, you can never get it again.

What does chickenpox look like?

Chickenpox looks like an itchy rash or bunches of small, red bumps. The bumps grow into blisters, ooze, and then crust over. After about a week, the blisters stop oozing and scabs usually form. People with chickenpox also can have a mild fever.

You can only get chickenpox once. Rashes from other viruses can often look like the one from chickenpox. It is easy to get them confused.

Most people have chickenpox when they are young. Children don't usually get very sick from chickenpox, but some adults do. Some people can get very sick, especially pregnant women or people with bad health.

How do you get chickenpox?

If you've never had chickenpox, you can get it by breathing near someone who has the disease. Children get chickenpox by being in the same classroom and playing or eating with each other. Adults get it by being in the same shelter or by visiting someone who has it.

You can also get chickenpox by touching the fluid on the blisters that come with chickenpox or shingles. Sometimes the fluid gets on clothing and bed sheets, and you can get chickenpox when you touch them.

The rash and fever begin 10 days to three weeks after being near someone who had chickenpox.

If you see a rash on yourself or your children, tell someone on the shelter staff.

What do you do if you have chickenpox?

If you have chickenpox, see a doctor or nurse if you:

- are over 15;
- are pregnant;
- have other health problems.

If you have chickenpox, you need to rest and drink plenty of fluids.

Wash the lesions with soap and cool water to keep them clean. Put on calamine lotion to stop the itching.

Take Tylenol™ (acetominophen) if the fever causes discomfort. Do not take aspirin or medicine with aspirin in it. Aspirin can cause problems when used for the symptoms of chickenpox.

Viral Meningitis

What is viral meningitis?
Viral meningitis is an infection that causes the lining around your brain to swell. The most common symptoms are severe headaches, unusual behavior, fever, vomiting, and excessive tiredness.

What causes viral meningitis?
Viral meningitis can be caused by many different viruses. One of the most frequent causes is a very common virus that also can cause mild diarrhea and colds. Only a few people who get sick with this virus will go on to get meningitis.

How do you keep from getting viral meningitis?
The best way to avoid getting this disease is to wash your hands often with warm water and soap. This is very important before preparing, serving, or eating food or before feeding your child. Hand washing is also important after you or your child go to the bathroom or you change a diaper.

Wash your hands after blowing or wiping your own or your child's nose. Don't share objects with others that might have been mouthed or chewed.

What if you know someone who has viral meningitis?
Not every type of viral meningitis can spread from one person to another. If you recently spent time with someone who came down with viral meningitis and you get a fever or a severe headache, tell the shelter staff and see a doctor or a nurse.

¿Que es Clamidia?

Clamidia es una enfermedad que se transmite sexualmente. Aunque es muy comun, mucha gente nunca han escuchado de esta enfermedad.

Muchas mujeres y hombres que tienen Clamidia no lo saben porque no parece causarles ningun problema obvio. Pueda que usted no sepa que tiene la enfermedad, pero aun asi puede causar muchos problemas, especialmente en las mujeres. Esta puede causar un embarazo heptópico, dolor crónico en los órganos vaginales de la mujer, o prevenir que las mujeres queden embarazadas.

Muchas personas que tienen Clamidia también tienen gonorrea. Cuando las personas se enferman con Clamidia, los síntomas son a menudo los mismos que causan la gonorrea.

¿Qué sucede cuando se enferma con Clamidia?

Si tiene Clamidia, puede que sienta ardor al orinar. Su pene o vagina puede segregar un fluido o mucosa aguosa, y sus organos sexuales le pueden picar.

Si usted es una mujer y tiene Clamidia, podra sentir dolor debajo del estómago. Le puede ser doloroso al hacer el amor, y a veces puede sangrar entre sus periodos menstruales.

Si está embarazada y tiene Clamidia, usted le puede transmitir la enfermedad a su bebé al nacer. Puede que su bebé se le infecten los ojos y pulmones.

¿Que puede hacer en caso de que tenga Clamidia?

Usualmente, es fácil de tratar la Clamidia. Usted y su parejo/a tendran que tomar antibióticos por una o dos semanas.

¿Cómo puedo evitar seguir enfermandome con Clamidia?

Existen dos maneras de evitar enfermarse con Clamidia:
1. no tenga relaciones sexuales;
2. Si va a tener relaciones sexuales, use un condon durante cada ocasión.

Asegúrese de que usted y su pareja/o usen condones al comenzar y al terminar cada vez que tenga relaciones sexuales.

Usted no puede enfermarse con Clamidia por sentarse en los inodoros, por tocar cerraduras, toallas, o al alzar objetos pesados y lastimarse los músculos.

Conjuntivitis (Ojos Colorados)

¿Qué es Conjuntivitis?

Conjuntivitis algunas veces llamada "ojo colorado," es una condición del ojo muy común.

¿Cómo se manifiestan los síntomas?

Si usted tiene conjuntivitis, uno u ambos ojos están colorados. Sus ojos y pestañas le arden o le pican. Puede que sus ojos se agüen dejando una costra que puede hacer que sus pestañas se peguen, especialmente cuando se levanta en la mañana.

¿Cómo se puede enfermar con conjuntivitis?

Los gérmenes están constantemente visitando nuestros ojos. Algunos gérmenes pueden crecer debajo de las pestañas. Cuando usted se estruja o toca los ojos, los gérmenes pueden infectar sus ojos fácilmente.

La conjuntivitis no es siempre causada por gérmenes. Algunos químicos, alergias u otras enfermedades también pueden causar conjuntivitis.

¿Qué puede hacer si su conjuntivitis es causada por una infección?

Un doctor/a o enfermera/o probablemente le recetará antibióticos en forma de gotas, ungüento o pastillas.

Sus ojos mejorarán en dos o tres días luego de haberse tomado sus medicinas. Sin embargo los gérmenes todavía permanecerán vivos. Usted necesita tomarse todas las medicinas (usualmente tarda entre 7 a 10 días) para deshacerse completamente de los gérmenes. De lo contrario, su conjuntivitis puede reincidir.

Usted no necesita cubrirse los ojos si tiene conjuntivitis.

Si sus ojos se mantienen colorados luego del tratamiento, siente dolor o su visión está borrosa vea a su Dr. /a o enfermera/o nuevamente.

¿Cómo puedo evitar seguir enfermándome con infecciones de los ojos?

Usted no debe compartir sus gotas o ungüento de ojos, ni tan siquiera con su familia.

No comparta toallas, toallitas para lavarse o maquillaje con nadie y en particular con alguien que tenga conjuntivitis.

Si su niño/a o su parejo/a tiene un ojo infectado, lávese las manos con mucha agua tibia y jabón antes y después de aplicar la medicina en el ojo infectado

Si su pareja/o, un amigo/a o alguien en su familia tienen conjuntivitis, tal vez usted también necesita medicamentos para evitar enfermarse.

¿Que es Diarrea?

La diarrea es usualmente un cambio del patrón normal de los movimientos intestinales, con cantidades anormales o líquidas. Usted puede contraer diarrea a través de virus, bacterias, o parásitos. Usted también puede obtener diarrea por otros problemas médicos.

¿Qué sucede cuando usted tiene diarrea?

Si usted tiene diarrea, usted tiene que ir al servicio sanitario a menudo. Los movimientos intestinales son blandos y pueden contener líquido. Algunas veces, la diarrea viene acompañada con retortijónes, vómitos, o fiebre. Puede que sus feces contengan sangre o mucosa.

Cuando la diarrea dura más de tres días, o si es severa, vea a un doctor/a o enfermero/a. Ellos pueden tomarle una muestra de sus feces para saber que tipo de diarrea usted tiene.

¿Qué debe de hacer si niño/a tiene diarrea?

Siempre que tenga diarrea, beba mucho líquido claro para reponer los fluidos que ha perdido. Si su niño/a tiene movimientos intestinales blandos más de lo normal o la cantidad de feces aumenta más de lo común, llame a su doctor/a ya que los/as niños/as se pueden enfermar rápidamente cuando tienen diarrea.

Si su niño/a tiene diarrea, medicamentos especiales, como Pedialyte™ o Enfalyte™, los cuales se consiguen en una farmacia, pueden prevenir que su niño/a se deshidrate. Si la diarrea no es muy severa, y el/la niño/a no está vomitando, deberá comer una dieta en moderación. Tenga en mente que los alimentos que contienen almidón se absorben mejor.

Si la diarrea de su niño/a es severa o no se detiene, contacte a un/a doctor/a o enfermero/a.

Si usted ve alguna de las siguientes señales lleve a su niño/a al hospital:

- si su niño no puede hacer lágrimas;
- si la boca del/la niño/a está seca;
- si los ojos de su niño/a se ven hundidos o tiene las ojeras oscuras;
- si su niño/a tiene demasiado sueño;
- si su niño/a tiene menos de 12 meses de edad y está defecando un tamaño más grande de lo normal o más frecuent- emente;
- si su niño/a no moja el pañal dentro de 8 horas.

Si su niño/a tiene diarrea, vómitos o tiene fiebre de más de 38.4°C (101°F), vea un doctor/a o enfermero/a.

¿Cómo puede evitar enfermarse con diarrea?

Lávese las manos:

- antes de mezclar cualquier alimento o fórmula;
- antes de comer o darle de comer al/la niño/a;
- después de cambiar los pañales o de ir al baño.

Los/las niños/as que se están entrenando a ir al baño deberán lavarse las manos después de que vayan al baño. Usted u otro adulto deberán observarlos y recordarle que se laven las manos. Si los/las niños/as se traen los juguetes a la boca, trate de evitar que los compartan con otros/as niños/as. Esto es de suma importancia si uno/a de los/as niños/as están enfermos/as.

Si usted tiene diarrea, no le de comida para llevar o le sirva a nadie fuera de su familia. Usted puede servir o dar comida para llevar cuando sus síntomas desaparezcan o su doctor/a o enfermero/a le diga que está bien.

Faringitis

¿Qué es faringitis?

La faringitis es una infección causada por una bacteria.

¿Cuáles son los síntomas de faringitis?

Las personas adultas con faringitis pueden tener la garganta inflamada, fiebre y las glándulas del cuello inflamadas. Usualmente no tienen catarro u la nariz aguosa.

Los/as niños/as con faringitis tienen la garganta inflamada y pueden tener dolor de estomago o un salpullido colorado con pequeñas manchas. El salpullido ataca más debajo de los brazos y en las áreas donde la piel se arruga.

¿Cómo se trata la faringitis?

Su doctor/a le podría recetar a usted y a su niño/a un antibiótico. Los antibióticos matan las bacterias, lo cual ayuda que la faringitis desaparezca y se cure un poquito más ligero. También, podría prevenir unas pocas de condiciones serias y raras que las personas con laringitis pudiesen desarrollar. Es importante tomarse todas las medicinas que el doctor/a le mande.

¿Se deberían tratar todos los tipos de inflamación de garganta con antibióticos?

No, no todas las inflamaciones de la garganta son faringitis. Solo entre un 5 y 10% de las gargantas inflamadas es causado por bacteria. El resto es causado por viruses u otros problemas, así que los antibióticos no van a ayudar. Su doctor/a le puede hacer la prueba para asegurarse de que es faringitis.

¿Podrían otras personas contagiarse con mi faringitis?

Si, definitivamente usted puede transmitir la infección a otras personas a menos que se haya tratado con antibióticos de 1 a 3 días. Los/as niños/as con faringitis no deberán de ir a la escuela o guardería infantil hasta que su fiebre desaparezca y hayan tomado un antibiótico por lo menos por 24 horas.

¿Cómo puedo hacer para que mi garganta inflamada se mejore?

A continuación lea varias cosas que le podrían ayudar a sentirse mejor:

- Tome Ibuprofen (Advil™, Motrin™, Nuprin™) o acetaminofen (Tylenol™). Los/as niños/as no deben de tomar aspirinas. Las aspirinas le podrían causar un síndrome llamado Reyes (una enfermedad seria) y en algunos casos, muerte cuando se usa en niños/as menores de 18 años.
- Haga gárgaras de sal en agua tibia (1/4 de cucharada de sal por una tasa de 8 onzas de agua tibia).
- Para adultos y niños/as mayores, el chupar pastillas, bombones o un pedazo de hielo le podría ayudar.
- Comer alimentos suaves, tomar bebidas frías, líquidos tibios o chupar helado.

¿Qué es gonorrea?

La mayoría de las personas conocen la gonorrea como "the clap" o "the drip". La gonorrea puede infectar sus ojos, garganta, vagina, recto, coyunturas, piel, pene, o su uretra. La gonorrea es muy común.

¿Cómo se obtiene la gonorrea?

La gonorrea es una infección que puede obtener teniendo relaciones sexuales con una persona que tenga gonorrea. Si usted está embarazada y tiene gonorrea, los gérmenes pueden ser transmitidos al/la bebé al nacer.

Usted tiene más probabilidades de enfermarse con gonorrea si tiene más de un/a parejo/a sexual. Si usted tiene relaciones sexuales con alguien que tiene relaciones sexuales con personas diferentes, usted está en alto riesgo de enfermarse con gonorrea.

¿Cómo la gonorrea le afecta?

Si usted es un hombre y tiene gonorrea, puede que su pene le duela, le arda o le pique cuando orina. También, puede que un flujo amarillo le gotee del pene.

Si usted es una mujer y tiene gonorrea, las probabilidades de que se sienta enferma son pocas, aunque esté infectada. Pero cuando se enferma con gonorrea, puede que sienta dolor, ardor y picor. Puede que también tenga una descarga vaginal. Algunas veces la infección se puede mover a los tubos de falopio, los ovarios y la pelvis. Es muy importante buscar tratamiento lo antes posible para evitar problemas a largo plazo.

La mayoría de las mujeres y algunos hombres con gonorrea no tienen síntomas. Las personas que no tienen síntomas todavía pueden transmitir la enfermedad.

¿Qué debe de hacer si tiene gonorrea?

El tratamiento para gonorrea es usualmente sencillo. A menudo le darán una inyección de antibióticos seguida de una o dos semanas de pastillas. Algunas veces, una infección necesita antibióticos fuertes o una estadía de un día en el hospital.

¿Cómo se puede prevenir la gonorrea?

Si usted no tiene relaciones sexuales, no se enfermará con gonorrea.

El uso de condones es la próxima opción para prevenir la gonorrea.

USE CONDONES DESDE EL PRINCIPIO HASTA EL FINAL CADA VEZ QUE TENGA RELACIONES SEXUALES. Los condones es la mejor manera de prevenir gonorrea y otras enfermedades sexualmente transmitidas.

Gripe

¿Qué es gripe?

La gripe es el flu, un virus que da una vez al año, usualmente en los meses de otoño y de invierno.

Cuando usted tiene el flu, se enferma con fiebre, escalofríos, dolores de cabeza, tos seca y a menudo la nariz segrega liquido. Su cuerpo se siente bien cansado y se puede sentir adolorido/a por varios días.

Para la mayoría de las personas, el flu viene y se va ligero. Sin embargo, si usted tiene problemas con su corazón o sus pulmones, se puede enfermar por más tiempo. De igual manera las personas que viven con el VIH, el virus que causa SIDA tardan más tiempo en recuperarse.

Es más fácil enfermarse con el flu cuando viven muchas personas juntas. Usted se enferma con el flu cuando respira los gérmenes de alguien que tose o destornuda o quedándose en un albergue donde mucha gente está enferma.

¿Qué puede hacer si se enferma con el flu?

Si usted tiene el flu, deberá de descansar y tomar bastante líquidos. Se puede ayudar si tiene la garganta irritada haciendo gárgaras de sal en agua tibia.

Tome Tylenol™ (acetaminofen) para la fiebre y el dolor muscular.

En caso de que su salud empeore, no siente mejoría varios días después o si tiene problemas con el corazón o pulmones, vea un/a doctor/a.

¿Cómo puede evitar seguir enfermándose con el flu?

Puede ponerse la vacuna del flu cada año para evitar enfermarse y enfermar a otras personas. Usualmente, los albergues comienzan a poner la vacuna para el flu en Noviembre.

Usted no podrá enfermarse con el flu por tan solo ponerse la vacuna. La mayoría de las personas no tienen efectos secundarios al ponerse la vacuna del flu. Sin embargo, a veces la vacuna le puede hacer sentir adolorido/a y cansado/a, o pudiese tener fiebre baja y escalofríos. Esto no es común y tan solo duraría 2 días. Puede que su brazo se inflame por dos días luego de haberle puesto la vacuna.

Si usted es alérgico/a a los huevos, no debería de ponerse la vacuna del flu.

Usted debe de lavarse las manos con agua tibia y jabón, luego de haberse soplado su nariz o la de su niño/a para evitar enfermar a otras personas con gripe.

¿Qué es hepatitis A?

Hepatitis A es un virus que irrita su hígado.

Las personas con hepatitis A pueden sentir cansancio y tener fiebre, falta de apetito, náusea, la piel y los ojos amarillos, la orina oscura y sus feces son de color blanco. Algunas personas, especialmente los /as niños/as, su piel o sus ojos no se tornan amarillos. Usted se va a sentir enfermo/a con hepatitis A usualmente en un promedio de 2 semanas, aunque algunas personas se pueden enfermar por varios meses y otras no se enferman para nada.

¿Cómo se transmite la Hepatitis A?

La hepatitis A se transmite a través de las feces de personas infectadas. Esto puede suceder cuando una persona infectada va al baño, no se lava las manos y luego toca objetos que otras personas se pueden poner en la boca. La hepatitis A se puede transmitir al cambiar los pañales de los bebés o cuando los/as niños/as tocan con sus manos los pañales y luego tocan objetos que otras personan pueden echarse a la boca.

Usted no puede enfermarse con hepatitis A cuando le habla, toca o duerme en el mismo cuarto con una persona que esté enferma.

¿Cómo se combate la Hepatitis A?

No existe tratamiento para la hepatitis A. Si usted se enferma puede que descansa mucho y consume alimentos altos en calorías se pueda sentir mejor.

¿Cómo puedo evitar seguir enfermándome con Hepatitis A?

Si usted está en riesgo de contraer hepatitis A o se puede enfermar seriamente con hepatitis A, usted puede vacunarse. Esta vacuna es para hombres que están sexualmente activos y que tienen sexo con otros hombres, usuarios de drogas ilegales (que se pueden inyectar o no), personas con enfermedades crónicas del hígado, y niños que viven donde existe una alta taza de hepatitis A.

Es importante que usted se lave las manos antes de tocar alimentos, de comer, de darle de comer a su bebé, de cambiarle los pañales o de ir al baño, este o no este vacunado contra la hepatitis A. Recuerde siempre de poner los pañales sucios en un canasto de basura que los niños/as no puedan alcanzar.

Si sus niños/as contraen hepatitis A o la persona con quien usted vive tiene hepatitis A, usted puede vacunarse de globulina para asegurarse que no se va a enfermar demasiado. La inyección se necesita poner entre dos semanas antes de haber estado expuesto/a a la misma, por la misma razón es que debe de ver a su doctor/a lo antes posible.

¿Me puedo enfermar con hepatitis A más de una vez?

Después que usted se enferma con hepatitis A, no se enfermará otra vez. Pero recuerde, que puede contraer otros tipos de hepatitis.

Hepatitis B

¿Qué es Hepatitis B?

La hepatitis B es un virus que afecta su hígado. Los síntomas primarios son como el catarro o la influenza. Después de un mes, su piel se puede tornar amarilla y comienza a picar. Su orina se ve como Coca Cola, pero el color de sus feces es color claro. Puede que usted no vea ninguno de estos síntomas entre un mes y medio y seis meses luego de que se enferme.

Estos síntomas pueden durar hasta uno y dos meses. Usualmente, luego que los síntomas desaparecen usted se sentirá saludable otra vez. Algunas personas mueren de hepatitis B, y otras viven toda una vida con problemas del hígado.

¿Qué debo de hacer si me enfermo con hepatitis B?

Usted necesita descansar y comer alimentos altos en calorías ya que pueden ayudar a bajar su fiebre y el picor. Usualmente, los alimentos se pueden digerir mejor en la mañana.

Evite medicinas tales como Tylenol™ (acetaminofen) ya que es procesada por el hígado. El alcohol y las drogas ilegales también pueden dañar el hígado.

¿Cómo me puedo enfermar con hepatitis B?

El virus no se transmite al hablar, tocar o dormir en el mismo cuarto con una persona enferma con hepatitis B.

El tener sexo sin protegerse con un condón o el compartir agujas con una persona con hepatitis B puede transmitir el virus fácilmente.

Algunas personas pueden tener el virus y nunca se sienten o se ven enfermas, sin embargo, todavía pueden transmitir el virus.

¿Cómo puede evitar enfermarse con hepatitis B?

La vacunación podría prevenir que se enferme con hepatitis B. Es recomendable en estos momentos que todos los niños/as y adolescentes reciban la vacuna de hepatitis B. La vacuna también es recomendable para adultos que están en riesgo, incluyendo a los usuarios/as de drogas intravenosas.

Si usted se inyecta drogas, puede evitar enfermarse con hepatitis B si no comparte las agujas. Si usted usase drogas, use una solución de cloro diluido con agua para limpiar los aparatos antes y después de inyectarse para matar el virus de hepatitis B en la aguja.

Pregúntele al personal del albergue donde puede conseguir cloro.

Use un condón cada vez que tenga relaciones sexuales. El personal del albergue sabe donde puede conseguir condones.

No comparta los cepillos de dientes o razuradoras.

Cubra cualquier cortadura o llaga con vendajes.

Su usted toca cualquier fluido que salga del cuerpo de otra persona, especialmente sangre y orina, necesita lavarse las manos bien.

Tenga cuidado cuando deseche las razuradoras y otros objetos afilados. El personal del albergue le puede informar donde colocarlas.

Cuide a los/as niños/as para asegurarse que no se muerdan o se arañen el uno al otro.

Si usted queda expuesto/a al virus de hepatitis B, pregúntele a su doctor/a o enfermero/a acerca de las vacunas.

¿Qué es hepatitis C?

Es un virus que se transmite primariamente a través de la sangre. Las personas que están en mayor riesgo son aquellas que han tenido transfusiones de sangre o un transplante de órgano antes del 1992, o personas que han usado agujas contaminadas por sangre (por ejemplo, usuarios de drogas intravenosas). Los pobres y los/as desamparados/as están en mayor riesgo de infecciones. Desde Julio de 1992, se ha estado cotejando cuidadosamente para este virus y se considera que la reserva de sangre está segura.

El virus de hepatitis C se puede transmitir cuando la sangre (o fluidos que contengan sangre) entra en contacto con una cortadura en la piel u otro tejido. Esto puede suceder aunque estas cortaduras no se puedan ver. El virus de hepatitis C también puede ser transmitido por contacto sexual, pero esto no sucede tan fácil como lo es la transmisión de VIH, el virus que causa el SIDA. Los tatuajes y agujerarse el cuerpo también son factores de riesgo.

El virus de hepatitis C se transmite por contacto casual como abrazando, destornudando, tosiendo u compartiendo alimentos. Al igual que todas las infecciones causadas por sangre, los cepillos de dientes y las bebidas no deben de ser compartidas. No se puede enfermar con hepatitis C al donar sangre.

¿Cuán serio es la hepatitis C?

La infección de hepatitis C puede ser bien seria. La mayoría de las personas que se infectan cargan el virus por el resto de sus vidas. Algunas de estas personas desarrollaran daños al hígado y se sentirán bien enfermos. Otras personas puede que se sientan saludables antes por muchos años luego de ser diagnosticados con la infección de hepatitis C. Eventualmente el virus puede causar cirrosis del hígado u cáncer del hígado en algunas personas que están infectadas. Mientras la mayoría de las personas con hepatitis C no desarrollan fallos en el hígado u cáncer, un número significativo de personas si lo desarrollaran, no podemos decir quien o quien no desarrollara estos problemas. Lo que si sabemos es que las personas desamparadas y pobres están en mayor riesgo de tener infecciones y complicaciones.

¿Quién está a riesgo de contraer hepatitis C?

Las personas están a riesgo de contraer la infección de hepatitis C si ellos/as:

- han usado drogas o han compartido agujas, aunque haya sido una sola vez;
- han recibido una transfusión de sangre, productos derivados de sangre o un transplante de órgano antes de Julio de 1992;
- han tenido muchos/as parejos/as sexuales, especialmente si no usaron condones;
- son trabajadores de salud (como doctores/as o enfermeros/as) que hayan sido expuestos/as a sangre o agujas;
- son bebés nacidos/as de madres que tienen hepatitis C;
- están desamparados/as;
- son alcohólicos/as;
- son veteranos de la guerra de Vietnam;
- se han hecho tatuajes o agujeros en su cuerpo con agujas o tinta infectada;
- han estado en diálisis de los riñones.

¿Existe algún tratamiento para la hepatitis C?

Una medicina llamada interferón se puede usar a veces para tratar la infección de hepatitis C. Usualmente se usa en combinación con otras medicinas, como Ribavirin™. Las personas diagnosticadas con la infección de hepatitis C no deben de tomar nada de alcohol o ciertas medicinas que puedan causar daños al hígado. Se recomienda que las personas infectadas con hepatitis C sean vacunadas contra la hepatitis A y B, otros dos virus que causan daño a su hígado si es que están a riesgo de estas infecciones. Los antibióticos, medicinas que combaten las infecciones bacteriales, no son efectivas para contrarrestar el virus de hepatitis C. Pregúntele a su doctor/a acerca de opciones para tratamiento y pasos a seguir para proteger su hígado.

Continua en la proxima página.

Hepatitis C

¿Cómo se puede prevenir la hepatitis C?

No existe ninguna vacuna contra la hepatitis C. La mejor manera de no adquirir la enfermedad es evitar cualquier contacto con sangre. Esto incluye no compartir agujas, razuradoras o cepillos de dientes. Hoy día los bancos de sangre cotejan, la sangre donada, contra el virus de hepatitis C, para que su riesgo de contraer la infección a través de una transfusión de sangre sea extremadamente baja. Usted podrá también contraer hepatitis C a través de relaciones sexuales con un/a parejo/a que este infectado/a; al usar la protección de condones podrá reducir el riesgo de infectarse.

Para prevenir la transmisión de hepatitis C:

* Si se inyecta drogas, nunca comparta los aparatos con nadie. No comparta la cocaína o los solvetos de inhalarla, ya que estos pueden contener sangre también. Busque programas de tratamiento que le puedan ayudar a parar de usar drogas;
* Use un condón de látex cada vez que tenga relaciones sexuales;
* Hágase tatuajes o agujérese su cuerpo en lugares que usen equipo esterilizado;
* Los/as trabajadores/as de salud y personas que trabajan en mantenimiento en los hospitales o lugares en donde se usan agujas u objetos afilados deben de seguir las precauciones universales de salud para cada paciente;
* Si tiene hepatitis C, no comparta las rasuradotas o cepillos de dientes;
* Si tiene hepatitis C, no done sangre, esperma, u órganos.

¿Qué es herpes simplex?

Herpes simplex es un virus. Este virus no es peligroso para la mayoriá de las personas, pero puede ser bien doloroso.

Una vez usted se enferma con herpes, usted tiene el virus por la vida. La mayoriá del tiempo, usted no se da cuenta que tiene herpes. De vez en cuando, le dan ampollas que se abren y duelen. El estrés, la luz del sol y a veces el enfermarse con otras cosas podrían activar las ampollas nuevamente.

Si usted tiene herpes, usualmente tiene unos grupitos de ampollas pequeñas. Su piel formará un anillo de color rojo claro alrededor de las ampollas. Las ampollas se abrirán causando dolor, formándose luego cascaritas que se secarán.

Usted puede tener las ampollas en sus labios o en las esquinas de su boca. La gente le llama a estas, llagas o ampollas. Los/as doctores/as le llaman herpes oral. Las ampollas se pueden encontrar en su pene, en los labios interiores de su vagina o alrededor del ano. También, se pueden dispersar en su trasero, espalda y muslos. Esto se llama herpes genital.

Las ampollas del herpes genital y labial se abren y se secan. El herpes labial tarda alrededor de una semana en desaparecer. El herpes genital puede tardar dos semanas en desaparecer.

Si usted tiene un salpullido que se ve como herpes, vea a un/a doctor/a o enfermero/a. Estos le pueden mostrar como mejorarse del salpullido.

¿Cómo se transmite el herpes?

Usted se enferma con herpes al tocar las ampollas de otra persona que tenga herpes.

Usted se enferma con herpes labial besando o acariciando alguna persona que tenga las ampollas o alguna persona que está infectada pero no tiene ampollas.

Usted contrae herpes genital teniendo relaciones sexuales con alguien que tenga las ampollas o que esté infectado pero que todavía no tiene las ampollas.

La mayoría de las personas que se enferman con herpes es por medio de personas que están infectadas pero que no tienen ampollas todavía.

Los/as bebés recién nacidos/as pueden obtener el herpes de su mamá, si es que las mamás tienen las ampollas/llagas.

¿Qué hacer en caso de tener herpes?

Lavese las manos a menudo con agua tibia y jabón. Usted necesita lavarse las manos cada vez que se toque las ampollas.

Cubra las llagas con un paño u vendaje hasta que se sequen.

Mantenga el salpullido limpio y seco. Cuando está limpio, el salpullido no se puede infectar.

Ninguna medicina cura el virus completamente. Algunas medicinas pueden ayudar a sanar las ampollas. No existe ninguna vacuna para prevenir herpes.

Si usted tiene herpes genital, una enfermera o un/a doctor/a le podrían dar alguna medicina que le pueda ayudar.

Por favor vea a un/a doctor/a o enfermera/o si tiene herpes y:
- su salpullido se dispersa;
- se siente enfermo/a con dolor de cabeza, fiebre, o su comportamiento es extraño;
- el salpullido se dispersa a sus ojos;
- piensa que puede estar en estado de embarazo.

Continua en la proxima página .

¿Cómo puede evitar enfermarse con herpes?

Muchas personas ya están infectadas con herpes pero no lo saben porque nunca han tenido las ampollas o las llagas.

La mayoría de las personas se contagian con herpes estando con personas que están infectadas pero que las llagas no son visibles, todavía.

No toque las ampollas/llagas o la saliva de alguien que tenga herpes.

No tenga relaciones sexuales o bese a su pareja/o cuando tengan ampollas/llagas.

Use siempre un condón en cada ocasión que tenga relaciones sexuales con cualquiera porque aun las personas que no tienen las ampollas/llagas en el presente o en el pasado pueden estar infectados/as y le pueden transmitir la infección.

¿Qué es herpes zoster?

Herpes zoster es un sarpullido que se conoce como culebrilla. La culebrilla proviene del mismo germen que causa la varicela. Después de haber tenido varicela, el virus "duerme" por muchos anos y puede "levantarse" en cualquier momento causando dolorosas ampollas en su piel y atacando los terminales de los nervios.

¿Cuáles son los síntomas de la culebrilla?

El sarpullido se ve como varicela pero usualmente se ubica en un área. También, le salen unas pequeñas ronchas que pueden picar y supuran.

Usted puede enfermarse con culebrilla más de una vez sin embargo, la varicela no se vuelve a repetir.

¿Como se puede enfermar con culebrilla?

Las personas se enferman primero con varicela antes de enfermarse con culebrilla. Si su sistema inmunológico es saludable y toca las ampollas de alguien con culebrilla, usted no se va a enfermar con culebrilla. Sin embargo, usted se puede enfermar con varicela si no se ha enfermado anteriormente.

El drenaje de las ampollas de la culebrilla puede transmitir los gérmenes a personas que nunca se han enfermado con varicela. Usted debe cubrir las ampollas que estén abiertas o mojadas, con un vendaje o un paño limpio.

Si usted no se ha enfermado con varicela y tiene contacto con alguien con sarpullido de culebrilla, vea un doctor/a o enfermera/o.

¿Que puede hacer si se enferma con culebrilla?

Usted necesita mantener las lesiones limpias con agua y jabón para evitar que se infecten. Tal vez necesite tomar medicamento para el dolor.

Visite a un doctor/a o enfermero/a con frecuencia. Ellos/as le pueden ayudar con el dolor. También, estos se aseguraran que su sarpullido no se empeore.

Vea a un/a proveedor/a de la salud inmediatamente si alguna de estas señales o síntomas aparecen:
- si las ampollas se mueven a sus ojos u otras partes de su cuerpo;
- si las ampollas continúan apareciendo después de una semana;
- si duerme más de lo normal, se siente mal humorado/a, o se siente confundido/a.

Impétigo

¿Qué es impétigo?

Es una infección común de la piel que se puede transmitir fácilmente en lugares donde las personas están cerca como por ejemplo los centros de cuidado diurno y los albergues.

¿Cómo se manifiesta?

Esta infección se manifiesta en ampollas coloradas que luego se convierten en llagas, y pueden aparecer en cualquier parte de su cuerpo, pero comúnmente salen alrededor de la boca, la nariz o en sus brazos o en las piernas. También se puede ver como si las ampollas estuviesen llenas de pus.

¿Cómo se transmite?

Usted puede enfermarse con impétigo cuando tiene una herida abierta en su piel, o cuando se rasca una picada de insecto. La irritación se puede extender a otras partes de su cuerpo. Usted puede enfermarse con impétigo si toca la piel irritada de otra persona.

¿Qué debe de hacer si tiene impétigo?

Si tiene impétigo el doctor/a o el enfermero/a le recetará antibióticos en forma de ungüento o pastillas. Usted necesita completar el tratamiento recomendado para evitar que la infección se vuelva a repetir.

Si tiene impétigo, limpie la irritación con agua tibia y jabón todos los días, luego cúbralas con un vendaje. No comparta su toalla o ropa con otras personas hasta que las llagas desaparezcan.

Si tiene impétigo, lave sus manos a menudo con mucho jabón y agua limpia para evitar que la infección continué esparciéndose. Cada vez que toque las zonas irritadas con impétigo, cambie sus vendajes o el paño que cubre la irritación lávese las manos.

Asegurese de desechar los vendajes sucios y mantenga su ropa incluyendo la de cama que pueda contener drenaje lejos de otras personas. Toda la ropa que contenga drenaje puede ser desinfectada lavándola con agua caliente y cloro.

¿Cómo puedo evitar seguir contagiándome con impétigo?

Usted necesita evitar rascarse las picadas de insectos y arrancarse las cascaritas después que la llaga se seca.

Por favor mantenga las picadas de insectos y cortaduras limpias con agua y jabón. Si la picada o cortadura está supurando o se está formando una capa, vea a su doctor/a o a su enfermero/a.

Infección Respiratoria Alta (IRA/Catarro Común)

¿Qué es una infección respiratoria alta?
Es un término médico para denominar el catarro común. Las personas se enferman con catarro todo el tiempo. Las personas adultas se enferman con catarro entre 2 y 4 veces al año. Los/as niños/as se pueden enfermar tanto como de 6 a 8 veces al año.

¿Cómo nos enfermamos con catarro?
El catarro se dispersa cuando las personas tosen o destornudan gérmenes en el aire, y las personas a su alrededor respiran esos gérmenes. Las personas con catarro pueden tocarse la nariz y colocar las manos a otras personas o cosas como juguetes.

¿Cuales son las señales de un catarro?
Si usted tiene catarro, puede toser, tener la nariz congestionada y goteando liquido. Su nariz y garganta se irritan, puede que sienta presión en los oídos.

Las personas adultas podrían tener fiebre hasta de 38.3°C (101° F). Algunas veces, los/as niños/as pueden tener fiebre hasta de 38.8°C (102° F).

¿Qué debo de hacer si tengo catarro?
Usted necesita descansar y tomar bastante agua o cualquier tipo de fluidos. Si tiene la garganta irritada, mezcle sal en agua tibia y haga gárgaras o chupe pastillas.

Si se siente con dolor en todo el cuerpo, puede tomar acetaminofen (Tylenol™).

Los descongestionantes le pueden ayudar con la nariz tapada o aguosa.

¿Si tiene fiebre alta, qué debe de hacer?
- Si la fiebre es mayor de 38.8°C (102° F) necesita ver a un/a doctor/a o enfermera/o inmediatamente.
- Si tiene fiebre, las glándulas inflamadas, y la garganta le duele, necesita ver a un/a doctor/a inmediatamente.
- Si tiene fiebre y está tosiendo flema verde o amarilla, necesita ver a un/a doctor/a inmediatamente.

¿Cómo hago para evitar seguir dispersando el catarro?
Si usted o su niño tienen catarro lávese las manos a menudo, especialmente luego de haberse soplado las narices o limpiado las secreciones al toser.

Las personas deberían de todas maneras lavarse las manos con agua tibia a menudo, particularmente antes de preparar, servir o comer cualquier alimento.

Enfermedad Meningocócica

¿Qué es una enfermedad meningocócica?

La enfermedad meningocócal es una infección séria causada por una bacteria. La misma puede conducir a meningitis, una hinchazón en la corteza del cerebro. También, puede causar una infección en la sangre.

La meningitis mayormente afecta a niños/as menores de 5 años de edad, especialmente a bebés entre los 6 y 12 meses de edad.

¿Cuáles son los síntomas de meningitis?

La meningitis puede comenzar como un catarro o puede comenzar rápidamente, con fiebre, escalofríos y cansancio. A menudo, aparecen en su piel pequeñas manchas coloradas o violetas.

Los/as niños/as de mayor edad al igual que los adultos se enferman con dolores de cabeza y tortícolis o dolores de cuello. Los/as niños/as muy pequeños se manifiestan malhumorados y sin apetito. Su llanto puede ser más alto de lo normal.

¿Cómo se transmite la meningitis?

Usted se puede infectar cuando alguien con la bacteria que causa meningitis, tose o estornuda, al aire que usted respira. Sus niños/as pueden contraer la bacteria al echarse a la boca objetos/juguetes que otros/as niños/as contagiados/as con el germen se hayan echado a la boca.

La bacteria puede vivir en la nariz y la garganta de algunas personas y estas no se enferman. Sin embargo, pueden enfermar a otras personas.

¿Cómo puedo evitar enfermarme con meningitis?

Si usted o sus niños/as pasan mucho tiempo con alguien que tenga la enfermedad, usted puede tomar un antibiótico llamado rifampin que le ayudará a reducir las oportunidades de enfermarse. Este medicamento solo se necesita tomar por dos días, consulte con su proveedor/a de salud acerca del mismo.

Usted no debe de tomar rifampin si está en estado de embarazo, tiene alguna enfermedad severa del hígado o ha tenido problemas anteriores con este medicamento.

El medicamento rifampin puede manchar su orina, sudor, saliva, y sus feces de color naranja-rojo. Este color desaparecerá una vez el medicamento se termine.

Este medicamento puede manchar sus lentes de contacto así que deberá de usar espejuelos hasta que la medicina se termine.

Si usted tiene que tomar rifampin, puede que sus anticonceptivos no le funcionen. Usted debe de usar otro método como un condón o diafragma hasta que se termine el ciclo de las pastillas anticonceptivas.

Este antibiótico también puede interferir con las dosis de metadona. Si usted está en tratamiento de metadona, dígale a su proveedor/a de salud que llame a la clínica para ajustar su dosis.

Si usted o su familia han estado alrededor de alguien con meningitis en las últimas dos semanas, vea un/a doctor/a o enfermero/a inmediatamente y además:

- si alguien en su familia tiene fiebre, dolor de cabeza, o se nota confundido/a;
- si su bebé se muestra de malhumor, no tiene apetito u muestra un llanto peculiar.

¿Qué es meningitis viral?

Meningitis viral es una infección que causa que el forro del cerebro se hinche. Los síntomas más comunes son dolores de cabeza severos, cambios de comportamiento, fiebre, vómitos y cansancio excesivo.

¿Que causa la meningitis viral?

La meningitis viral puede ser causada por muchos virus diferentes. Uno de las causas más frecuentes es un virus muy común que también puede causar diarrea y catarros. Solo unas pocas personas que se enferman con éste virus desarrollaran meningitis.

¿Como puede evitar seguir enfermándose con meningitis viral?

La mejor manera de evitar enfermarse con esta enfermedad es lavarse las manos a menudo con agua tibia y jabón. Esto es muy importante antes de preparar, servir o comer alimentos al igual que antes de darle de comer a su/s niños/as. El lavarse las manos es importante luego que usted o su niño/a vayan al baño, o de que se cambien pañales.

Lavese las manos luego de soplar o limpiar su nariz o la de su niño/a. No comparta objetos con otras personas que puedan haberlos mascado o echado a la boca.

¿Qué me sucedería si yo conozco alguna persona que tenga meningitis viral?

No todos los tipos de meningitis viral se transmiten de una persona a otra. Si usted recientemente compartió con alguien que fue diagnosticado/a con meningitis viral y a usted le da fiebre o dolores de cabeza fuertes, dígale al personal del albergue y vea a un/a doctor/a o enfermero/a.

Pertusis (Tos Seca)

¿Qué es la tos seca?

La tos seca es una enfermedad donde la tos se prolonga. Esta enfermedad puede ser séria especialmente en los/as infantes que todavía no han completado sus inmunizaciónes. En niños/as menores de un año, la tos seca puede causar problemas sérios en los pulmones y en el cerebro.

¿Cómo se transmite la tos seca?

Usted puede enfermarse con tos seca cuando alguien con la enfermedad tose al aire que usted está respirando. También, se puede enfermar tocando la saliva o mucosa de alguien que tenga la enfermedad.

¿Cuáles son los síntomas de la tos seca?

La tos seca comienza como un catarro. Su nariz y ojos se ponen aguosos, y se comienza a toser y a destornudar. La tos se extiende hasta dos semanas y se empeora.

Algunas veces, especialmente con los/as niños/as los ataques de tos pueden terminar en un chillido al inhalar aire. Se pueden poner azules mientras están tosiendo o pueden vomitar después de toser.

En los/as niños/as menores de 6 meses, adolescentes y adultos, la tos seca puede verse como una enfermedad de la tos que dura un largo tiempo.

Si usted o su niño/a tienen una tos que dure más de 14 días, pueda que usted tenga tos seca. Si usted o su niño/a tiene tos que lo hace ponerse azul o vomitar, puede que usted tenga tos seca. Por favor, vea a un/a doctor/a o un/a enfermero/a.

¿Qué hacer en caso de tener tos seca?

Si tiene tos seca, vea a un/a doctor/a, beba suficientes fluidos y descanse mucho.

Su doctor/a o enfermero/a probablemente le recetarán antibióticos. Esta medicina puede que aminore los síntomas y también evitará que disperse los gérmenes a otras personas.

¿Cómo se puede prevenir la tos seca?

Usualmente los/as niños/as toman la vacuna de la tos seca 5 veces durante sus chequeos rutinarios que cubren entre un mes y medio de nacimiento y los siete años. La vacuna es la "aP" la cual se añade a la vacuna de "DTaP".

Mantenga las vacunas de sus hijos/as al día. Esta es la mejor manera de asegurarse que no se enfermen con la tos seca.

La vacuna para la tos seca puede perder el efecto. Algunas veces, un/a muchacho/a o un adulto puede contraer la tos seca aun luego de haberse puesto todas las vacunas. Estas personas pueden transmitir la enfermedad a niños/as pequeños/as que todavía no tienen todas sus vacunas puestas.

Si usted ha estado cerca de alguien que esté enfermo/a con la tos seca, puede que también necesite tomar antibióticos. Los antibióticos pueden evitar que se enferme con la tos seca.

¿Qué son piojos?

Los piojos son pequeños insectos que viven en el cuerpo humano.

Existen tres tipos de piojos:
Los piojos de cabeza viven en el pelo de las personas y hacen que el cuero cabelludo pique. Los huevos a menudo parecen caspa, pero no se pueden sacar del pelo fácilmente.

Los piojos de cabeza se pasan cuando una persona con piojos entra en contacto con el pelo de otra persona. Se pueden pasar también cuando las personas comparten sombreros, peinillas, y otros objetos que toquen el pelo o la cabeza. Los piojos de la cabeza son común entre los/as niños/as.

Los piojos del cuerpo viven en la ropa de las personas, especialmente en las costuras. Usualmente no viven en la piel. Las personas se dan cuenta de que tienen piojos en el cuerpo cuando le dan ronchas al rascarse tanto.

Los piojos de cuerpo se pasan cuando usted toca o entra en contacto con una persona que tenga piojos. Se pueden transmitir también, al compartir la ropa o la ropa de cama que tenga piojos.

Los piojos púbicos se transmiten comúnmente por contacto corporal cercano o por contacto sexual. Si usted tiene piojos púbicos, debería de preguntarle a su doctor/a o enfermero/a que le examine para otras enfermedades sexualmente transmitidas.

¿Cómo se deshace de los piojos?

Para los piojos en la cabeza o en el área púbica, pregúntele a su doctor/a o enfermero/a por champú o acondicionadores que maten los piojos de su pelo. Usualmente tiene que dejarse el champú en su pelo hasta 10 minutos. Luego enjuague su pelo bien y séquelo con una toalla. Una vez su pelo está seco, usted tendrá que peinar cualquier huevo que quedo en su pelo con una peinilla de diente fino. Este proceso toma bastante tiempo. Algunas personas prefieren recortarse o afeitarse el pelo en vez de peinarse.

Para evitar que los piojos regresen, lave toda la ropa de cama y de vestir en agua caliente y seque su ropa por 30 minutos antes que la use otra vez.

Si usted no puede lavar cosas tales como peluches y juguetes, pásele un paño cuidadosamente.

Remoje todas sus peinillas y cepillos en el champú de piojos diluido con agua. Haga una solución de 1 tasa de cloro por 10 tasas de agua, esto trabajará también.

Para los piojos del cuerpo, todo lo que tendrá que hacer es quitarse la ropa y bañarse cuidadosamente. Los piojos del cuerpo viven en la ropa, no en la piel. Antes de ponerse su ropa, deberá lavarla en agua caliente y colocarla en la secadora por 30 minutos. No se ponga su ropa o duerma en la misma cama luego de haberse bañado hasta que todo esté limpio.

Si usted tiene piojos, usted debe de ver a un/a doctor/a o enfermero/a 1 semana después para asegurarse que los piojos se han ido. Algunas veces tendrá que ser tratado otra vez.

¿Cómo puedo evitar los piojos?

La mejor manera de evitar los piojos es no compartiendo ropa, sombreros, peinillas y otras cosas personales. Dígale a la gente que se queja de picor o salpullidos que vea a un/a doctor/a o enfermero/a.

Si usted ha estado cerca de una persona con piojos, pídale a su doctor/a que le evalué para saber si tiene piojos.

Sarampión

¿Qué es el sarampión?

El sarampión es un virus que se transmite fácilmente. El sarampión puede enfermar a usted y a sus niños/as severamente.

¿Cuáles son los síntomas del sarampión?

El sarampión comienza la mayor parte del tiempo como un resfriado. Usted puede tener tos, fiebre alta, los ojos colorados y aguados. A los cuatro días aparece un salpullido rojo y lleno de manchas. El salpullido comienza en la cara y luego se expande a todo su cuerpo.

¿Cómo se transmite el sarampión?

Si la persona con sarampión destornuda o tose, el virus puede transmitirse a través del aire a otras personas.

Usted y sus niños/as pueden contagiarse con sarampión si:

- nunca se ha enfermado con sarampión o ha sido vacunado/a;
- fue vacunado/a antes del 1968 porque las vacunas en ese entonces no tenían protección duradera;
- su niño/a nunca se ha enfermado con sarampión o no se ha vacunado.

Si usted está cerca de alguien enferma/o con sarampión, deberá preguntarle a su doctor/a o enfermero/a acerca de esta enfermedad.

¿Qué debe de hacer si tiene sarampión?

Cuando usted vea los síntomas en su cuerpo o el de su niño/a, usted debe de ver a un/a doctor/a inmediatamente. El/la doctor/a podrá informarle si usted o su niño/a tienen sarampión. No existen medicinas para curar el sarampión, pero usted puede asegurarse de que otras personas no contraigan la enfermedad.

Si usted tiene sarampión no salga a lugares públicos como tiendas, autobuses, trenes subterráneos o clínicas médicas. Si sale fuera de la casa estaría transmitiendo la enfermedad a otras personas que están sanas todavía. Luego de haber tenido el salpullido por cuatro días, ya no es contagioso y entonces podrá salir fuera de su casa.

¿Cómo usted puede mantener a sus niños/as sin enfermarse con sarampión?

Usted puede ayudar a prevenir que sus niños/as contraigan sarampión llevándolos/as a vacunar. Las vacunas que protegen del sarampión usualmente se inyectan a los/as niños/as de 12 a 15 meses de nacidos/as y por segunda vez entre los 4 y 6 años de edad. Los/as niños que no se han sido vacunados/as con la segunda dosis (entre los 4 y 6 años de edad) usualmente son vacunados en la escuela cuando están entre los 12 y 14 anos de edad. Esta vacuna es una combinación con una para paperas y rubéola que protegerán a sus niños/as contra estas tres enfermedades.

¿Qué es sarna?

La sarna son chinches diminutos llamados ácaros. Los chinches escarban debajo de la piel causando picor y se siente bastante incómodo, especialmente de noche. Estos ácaros pueden vivir en cualquier parte de su cuerpo.

¿Cómo se transmite la sarna?

La sarna es fácil de transmitirse, especialmente en lugares donde mucha gente vive o juega juntos/as. La sarna se propaga cuando alguien con la enfermedad toca su piel. Esto también puede suceder cuando las personas duermen en la misma cama o comparten ropa o ropa de cama. La sarna puede transmitirse de la persona hasta que el/ella se empiece a tratar.

¿Qué puede hacer si tiene sarna?

La sarna puede ser difícil de tratar. Un/a doctor/a o enfermero/a práctico/a o un asistente al médico le pueden recetar una loción que mata la sarna.

Si usted tiene sarna:

1) Corte sus uñas para cuando se rasque no irrite su piel.
2) Deze un baño.
3) Espere varios minutos en lo que su piel se refresca.
4) Esparza la loción en su piel según las instrucciones.
5) No se ponga otra crema, ungüento o loción de cuerpo.
6) Espere entre 8 a 12 horas. Si se lava las manos durante este periodo de tiempo, reaplique la loción en las manos.
7) Tome otro baño para sacarse la loción.
8) Pongase ropa nueva o limpia que haya sido lavada y secada de acuerdo con las instrucciones a continuación.
9) Lave su ropa de cama en la mañana luego que termine el tratamiento. Todo debe de ser lavado en agua caliente y secado en caliente por 30 minutos.
10) Puede que usted necesite repetir el tratamiento dentro de una semana – pregúntele a su doctor/a, enfermero/a práctico/a o al asistente del doctor.

Para un/a niño/a con sarna:

1) Corte las unas de su niño/a para que al rascarse no se haga daño en la piel.
2) Bañe o déle una ducha a su niño/a.
3) Espere vários minutos en lo que la piel se refresca.
4) Esparza la loción en su piel según se le indique.
5) No le ponga ninguna otra crema, ungüento o loción de cuerpo.
6) Espere de 8 a 12 horas. Si el/la niño/a se lava las manos durante este periodo de tiempo, reaplique la loción en las manos.
7) Bañe nuevamente al/la niño/a para sacarle la loción.
8) Vista al/la niño/a con ropa nueva o limpia que haya sido lavada y secada de acuerdo con estas instrucciones a continuación.
9) Lave la ropa de cama la mañana después que se termine el tratamiento. Toda la ropa deberá ser lavada en agua caliente y secada en caliente por 30 minutos.
10) Puede que el/la niño/a necesite repetir el tratamiento en una semana – consulte con su doctor/a, su asistente o enfermero/a práctico/a.

Limpie cualquier cosa que usted o su niño/a puedan haber tocado si es que se puede lavar (juguetes, alfombras, almohadas).

Puede que aun después del tratamiento, la picazón continué por dos semanas. Esto es normal. Si el picor es muy severo, consulte con su doctor/a o enfermero/a acerca de medicinas para controlar la picazón.

¿Cómo puedo evitar enfermarme con sarna?

Trate de no compartir su ropa, la de su niño/a y la ropa de cama con otras personas.

Si usted conoce a alguna persona que se queja de salpullido o picazón, dígale que es urgente que vea a un/a doctor/a o enfermero/a.

Si usted o su niño/a han estado alrededor de alguien con sarna, vea a un/a doctor/a o enfermero/a.

Sífilis

¿Qué es sífilis?

Sífilis es una enfermedad sexualmente transmitida, al igual que gonorrea y clamidia.

La sífilis puede ser difícil de detectar, especialmente en las mujeres. Cuando contrae sífilis los hombres podrán notar una llaga en su pene, las mujeres podrán notar una llaga en o alrededor de la vagina, en su recto, o en su boca. A menudo, la llaga está ubicada en un lugar que usted no puede ver, como en su vagina o recto, por lo tanto no se puede notar. La llaga no duele y desaparece al cabo de un tiempo. Sin embargo, la enfermedad no se cura hasta que la llaga desaparece.

La sífilis puede pasar por diferentes etapas. Las etapas pueden tomar hasta 40 años.

¿Qué sucede cuando se enferma con sífilis?

Si usted tiene sífilis y no se trata, la enfermedad puede esparcirse casi a cualquier parte del cuerpo. La enfermedad puede causar complicaciones sérias como un infarto, un ataque del corazón, sordera, insanidad y pérdida de la visión.

La sífilis puede ser peligrosa para las personas que viven con el virus de VIH. Si usted vive con el virus, asegurese de hacerse una prueba de sangre para sífilis.

Los/as bebés pueden nacer con sífilis, si la mamá está infectada. Si usted está embarazada, tome una prueba para sífilis en su primera visita prenatal y por segunda vez durante los últimos tres meses de su embarazo.

¿Qué puede hacer en caso de enfermarse con sífilis?

Si usted tiene sífilis, comuníquele a su parejo/a sexual del presente y del pasado que usted tiene la enfermedad. Ellos/as tienen que ver a su doctor/a aunque no tengan los síntomas.

Si usted tiene sífilis, usualmente su doctor le recetará penicilina. Tal vez, tendrá que ponerse una inyección una vez a la semana durante dos o tres semanas.

La penicilina cura la sífilis. Usted tendrá mejor oportunidad de curarse, dependiendo de cuanto ligero usted y su parejo/a empiecen el tratamiento.

Si usted está recibiendo tratamiento médico para sífilis, su parejo/a necesita ser tratado/a antes de que puedan tener relaciones sexuales seguras juntos/as.

Si usted tiene sífilis, usted debe de hablar con un/a consejero/a acerca de la prueba del VIH. El VIH es el virus que causa el SIDA.

¿Cómo puedo evitar seguir enfermándome con sífilis?

Los condones, diafragmas, y espermicidas no evitan que las/os parejas/os se transmitan sífilis el/la uno/a al/la otro/a.

Las personas pueden tener sífilis y no saberlo. Si usted está sexualmente activo/a, hágase una prueba de sangre para sífilis de cada dos a 3 años en su clínica o centro de salud.

¿Qué es tiña?

La tiña es una infección común que puede crecer en su piel, cabello u en sus uñas. Es un hongo, no un gusano. La tiña puede aparecer en forma de llagas coloradas pequeñas o en pequeños círculos.

A muchos/as niños/as se le manifiesta la tiña en su cuero cabelludo. Algunas veces los anillos pequeños se agrandan y hacen que el pelo se caiga. La piel en estas áreas se puede tornar escamosa y costrosa.

La tiña puede verse en su piel como círculos pequeños o puede que su piel se torne escamosa, áspera y le pique mucho.

El hongo de la tiña en los pies es común entre los adolescentes y personas adultas. Si usted tiene tiña sus pies se ven rojos y escamosos especialmente entre los dedos de los pies. En esta área también pica mucho.

La tiña es contagiosa y durante el primer y segundo día se cura con crema o medicina por la boca.

¿Cómo se transmite la tiña?

Usted y sus niños/as se pueden contagiar con tiña del cuero cabelludo si usted toca las llagas, que contiene el hongo de la tiña, de otra persona y luego se toca la cabeza. Usted también puede contraer la tiña en su cabeza si usted usa el sombrero, peine o cualquier otra cosa que hayan usado en el pelo.

Usted también puede contraer tiña en su piel y pies, al tocar las llagas de otra persona o al tocar algo que la persona haya tocado. Esto sucede a menudo cuando se va al baño y se camina descalzo en el piso mojado, si toma un baño en una bañera que no se haya enjuagado o se sienta en una banqueta para cambiarse de ropa que no se haya lavado.

Usted no podrá contraer tiña por tan solo estar en el mismo cuarto con alguien que la tenga.

Si usted tiene tiña, la podrá transmitir si todavía tiene llagas. Una vez sus llagas se sanen, no es contagioso.

¿Qué debe de hacer si contrae la tiña?

Si usted contrae tiña, su doctor/a o enfermero/a le recetarán pastillas o una crema medicinal. La duración del tratamiento depende de donde se ubica la infección y de su severidad.

Si usted está cuidando a alguien enfermo/a con tiña, lávese las manos a menudo. Cada vez que toque la piel infectada o le ponga loción en las llagas del/la enfermo/a lávese las manos.

Si alguien tiene tiña usted necesita lavar toda la ropa incluyendo la de cama en agua caliente. No deje que nadie use esta ropa hasta que se lave.

Si usted o su niño/a tiene algo en la piel parecido a la tiña, comuníquele a alguien en el albergue y vea a un/a doctor/a o a un/a enfermera/o. También, busque las mismas señales en el resto de su familia y en otros/as niños/as que juegan con los suyos.

Tuberculosis (TB)

¿Que es tuberculosis?
Tuberculosis o TB es un germen que a menudo infecta sus pulmones. Puede también crecer en otras partes de su cuerpo. La TB de los pulmones tiene varios síntomas, entre ellos tos crónica, fiebre, sudores nocturnos y perdida de peso.

¿Como se adquiere la tuberculosis?
La TB se dispersa cuando alguien enfermo/a con TB en los pulmones tose o destornuda. Cuando los gérmenes pasan al aire la gente los respira. Si usted pasa mucho tiempo cerca de una persona con TB, se podría infectar. La mayoría de las personas que se infectan con TB no se enferman; su sistema inmunológico mantiene la infección en control, y la persona desconoce que está cargando el germen de TB.

¿Cómo puede saber si tiene TB?
Este seguro/a de que no está *infectado/a* con TB, usted puede hacerse una prueba de piel llamada "PPD". Si está a riesgo de TB, puede hacerse la prueba de piel cada 6 meses. Esta prueba determina si tiene gérmenes de TB en su cuerpo. Si tiene gérmenes de TB, la prueba es "positiva". Para asegurarse que estos gérmenes no le están enfermando, necesita hacerse un examen físico y placas de pecho.

¿Qué debe de hacer si tiene TB?
Si su prueba es positiva, hágase un chequeo y una placa de pecho para saber si los gérmenes le están enfermando.

Puede que sus gérmenes de TB no lo/a estén enfermando en el momento. Sin embargo, lo/a pueden enfermar en cualquier momento de su vida. El/la doctor/a le puede dar un antibiótico para matar los gérmenes, evitando así que no crezcan y le enfermen.

Si está infectado/a con TB, pero no está enfermo/a todavía, no podrá transmitir los gérmenes a otras personas.

Si está enfermo/a con TB, es posible que pueda transmitirle la enfermedad a otras personas. Puede que sus amistades necesiten hacerse la prueba de piel, PPD, para asegurarse que no están infectados/as.

Si está enfermo/a con TB, necesitará tomar medicinas por muchos meses antes que todos los gérmenes mueran. Necesita tomarse la medicina aunque se sienta mejor. Los gérmenes de TB se pueden esconder si para de tomar la medicina. Entonces, los gérmenes crecen otra vez enfermándole nuevamente.

No es fácil tomar medicinas en los albergues. Pregúntele al personal del albergue si existe un lugar seguro donde pueda guardar las pastillas. El Departamento de Salud debería de ayudarle con sus medicinas.

Algunas veces los medicamentos para TB causan efectos secundarios. Usted podría enfermarse con fiebre y salpullido en la piel. Puede que pierda el apetito, o que su estomago se descomponga y vomite. El lado derecho de su estomago podría estar inflamado. Su piel y sus ojos se podrían tornar amarillos y su orina se podría ver obscura, como el té. Si le dan estos síntomas quiere decir que la medicina no está ayudando a su hígado.

Si ve alguno de estas señales, pare las pastillas inmediatamente y vea a su doctor/a.

¿Qué es una vacuna?

Cuando a usted le inyectan para protegerle contra cierta enfermedad, a usted le están vacunando.

En los EE.UU., los/as niños/as son vacunados/as rutinariamente para protegerles contra la varicela, paperas, difteria, tétano, tos seca, hemofilia, gripe y polio.

Ciertas personas podrían ser el blanco para otras vacunaciones, especialmente la vacuna para el flu. Esto depende de su historial de salud y del grado de riesgo que está usted para contraer estas enfermedades.

La vacunación es importante para usted y sus niños/as. Los/as niños/as usualmente reciben la mayoría de sus vacunas antes de cumplir sus 7 años. Si en su niñez, no le vacunaron contra algunas de estas enfermedades, tal vez pueda recibir la vacuna como adulto.

¿Cuales son las enfermedades?

Sarampión es un virus serio que causa fiebres altas, síntomas de gripe, ojos llorosos y un salpullido en su cuerpo. Muy raras veces el sarampión conlleva a pulmonía, inflamación del cerebro, sordera o a retardación mental.

Las paperas es un virus que causa una hinchazón dolorosa en las glándulas del cuello y detrás de las orejas.

Rubéola se llama también Sarampión Alemán. Los síntomas de la rubéola son normalmente leves e incluyen un salpullido con fiebre baja. Sin embargo, las mujeres embarazadas con rubéola pueden perder su bebé, la criatura puede nacer muerta o con defectos serios.

Polio es un virus que puede resultar en la hinchazón del revestimiento alrededor del cerebro (meningitis) o en parálisis. El polio es raro en los EE.UU. debido a las buenas prácticas de vacunación. Usted puede enfermarse con polio si no está inmunizado/a y está expuesto/a a personas infectadas que llegan de otros países donde el polio es más común.

Difteria es una infección que empieza en la garganta y en la nariz. La difteria causa una cubierta espesa y de color gris por encima de la garganta que puede dificultar la respiración. Este germen también puede soltar un veneno que causa parálisis y problemas severos del corazón.

Tétano es una infección que entra al cuerpo cuando usted tiene una cortadura seria, una herida que haya sido perforada, una quemada, o una mordida. Esto conlleva a rigidez en los músculos, especialmente los de la quijada y los de respirar.

Tos ferina es una infección seria en las vías respiratorias superiores. Empieza casi como un catarro con la nariz goteando y tos. La tos puede empeorar en la noche, y ocurre en "repeticiones" que pueden terminar en una tos ruidosa o vómitos. Los infantes son los que están más a riesgo con problemas que incluyen ataques, neumonía y daños en el cerebro debido a la tos ferina.

Hib (Hemofilia influenza tipo b) es una bacteria que puede infectar la sangre, el revestimiento del cerebro, y los pulmones y vías respiratorias. Es raro que afecte a la población adulta, pero puede ser una enfermedad muy seria en los/as infantes y niños/as pequeños/as.

Neumococus es una infección bacterial que puede causar neumonía, infecciones en la sangre o meningitis en niños/as pequeños/as. La vacuna neumococal, sirve de protección contra la infección neumococal.

Hepatitis B es un virus que infecta el hígado. Algunas personas con hepatitis B no se sienten enfermos en lo absoluto, pero pueden transmitir la enfermedad a otras personas. El virus puede causar inflamación del hígado, causando fatiga, nausea, falta de apetito, y una condición donde la piel se pone amarilla llamada ictericia. La inflamación puede causar que el hígado para de funcionar, lo cual es fatal.

Varicela es una enfermedad viral común en los/as niños/as, que causa fiebre, síntomas de catarro y salpullido. La mayoría de los/as niños/as se

Continua en la proxima página.

recuperan de varicela sin ningún problema. Las personas adultas que se enferman con varicela tienen a menudo complicaciones serias, que incluyen neumonía, encefalitis (inflamación del cerebro) o paro riñonal.

¿Cuáles son los efectos secundarios de estas vacunas?

Los efectos secundarios de estas vacunas son usualmente leves, incluyen una hinchazón, la piel colorada y tal vez fiebre en el lugar donde se inyecto. Raramente, podrían ocurrir otros efectos secundarios más serios que con cualquier vacuna. Usted debe de hablar con su proveedor/a de salud acerca de cualquier preocupación que tenga. Las clínicas también le pueden dar volantes informativos de cada vacuna.

¿Qué sucede si no vacuno a mi niño/a?

Si usted no vacuno a sus niños/as, ellos/as se pueden enfermar. Al igual que no podrían matricularse en la escuela o en un centro de cuidado infantil. Las leyes estatales de Massachussetts, requieren que todos/as los/as niños/as matriculados en centros infantiles, escuelas, y colegios estén al día con sus inmunizaciones.

Mantenga los registros de inmunizaciones al día y colóquelos en un lugar seguro. Los va a necesitar según sus muchachos/as vayan creciendo.

Varicela

¿Qué es varicela?

La varicela es un virus. Este virus también causa culebrilla/herpes zoster. La varicela se transmite fácilmente de persona a persona y es contagiosa hasta que las ampollas se sequen. Una vez usted haya tenido varicela, nunca más se enfermará de nuevo con varicela.

¿Cuáles son los síntomas de la varicela?

Los síntomas son: sarpullido con picazón o un mazo de pequeñas ronchas. Las ronchas crecen hasta convertirse en ampollas, luego supuran hasta convertirse en una llaga. Luego de una semana, las ampollas pasan de ser llagas a unas cascaritas. Las personas podrían contraer fiebre.

Usted podrá enfermarse de varicela solamente una vez. El sarpullido de otros virus es parecido al de la varicela y a veces se confunden con facilidad.

La mayoría de las personas se enferman con varicela cuando son jóvenes. Usualmente los/as niños/as no se enferman severamente con varicela, sin embargo algunos adultos sí. Algunas personas se pueden enfermar severamente, especialmente las mujeres embarazadas o las personas que están poco saludables.

¿Cómo se transmite la varicela?

Si usted nunca ha tenido varicela, se puede enfermar si respira cerca de una persona que tenga la enfermedad. Los niños/as se enferman con varicela al estar en el mismo salón de clases, jugando u comiendo todos juntos. Los adultos se enferman al estar en el mismo albergue o visitando a alguien que esté enfermo/a con varicela.

Usted se puede enfermar también con varicela al tocar el fluido dentro de la ampolla que contiene varicela o culebrilla. Algunas veces éste fluido mancha su ropa o la ropa de cama, y si las tocamos nos podemos enfermar con varicela.

Luego de haber estado cerca de una persona con varicela, el sarpullido y la fiebre tardan entre 10 días a tres semanas para manifestarse.

Si usted o su niño/a tienen sarpullido, hable con el personal del albergue.

¿Que puede hacer si tiene varicela?

Vea un/a doctor/a o enfermera/o si usted:
- tiene más de 15 anos;
- está embarazada;
- tiene otros problemas de salud.

Si usted tiene varicela, necesita descansar y tomar mucho líquido. Las lesiones necesitan lavarse con jabón y agua fría para mantenerlas limpias. Para que no le pique póngase loción de calamina.

Si la fiebre le causa malestar tome acetaminofen (Tylenol™). No tome aspirina o medicina que contenga aspirina. La aspirina puede causar problemas cuando se usa para los síntomas de varicela.

VIH y SIDA

¿Qué es el (VIH) virus de inmunodeficiencia humana?

El VIH es un virus que se transmite a través de contacto sexual y contacto de sangre. El virus también puede ser transmitido de una mujer embarazada a su bebé o a su bebé a través de la leche materna.

¿Qué es SIDA?

El SIDA significa "síndrome de inmunodeficiencia adquirida". El SIDA es el resultado de cuando el sistema inmunológico del cuerpo no funciona debido al virus de inmunodeficiencia humana (VIH). Esto puede resultar en infecciones y ciertos tipos de cáncer. *¡El SIDA puede ser prevenido!*

¿Cómo se transmite el virus de VIH?

El VIH es un virus que se transmite por medio del contacto corporal entre dos personas, a través de fluidos corporales, tales como, sangre, semen, fluidos vaginales o de la leche materna.

El virus es mayormente transmitido a través del contacto sexual, de compartir jeringas y otra parafernalia de drogas. También, puede ser transmitida a un/a recién nacido/a durante el estado de embarazo o durante el nacimiento de la criatura.

El contacto sexual puede ser a través de un hombre a una mujer o entre parejas del mismo sexo.

¿Cómo otras enfermedades sexualmente transmitidas afectan el VIH?

Cuando una persona tiene otra enfermedad sexualmente transmitida como gonorrea, clamidia, o herpes, el/ella está en mayor riesgo de contraer VIH.

¿Cómo puedo saber si mi parejo/a tiene el virus de VIH?

No hay manera de saber si una persona está infectada con el VIH. El/ella puede verse y sentirse saludable.

¿Cómo yo puedo saber si he sido infectado/a con VIH?

Cuando una persona se infecta inicialmente con VIH, el/ella podría tener fiebre, escalofríos, inflamación en los nódulos linfáticos y erupción de la piel. Usualmente, estos síntomas desaparecen en varios días. Puede que las personas con VIH no lo sepan. Ellos/as se pueden ver y sentir saludables. Sin embargo, pueden transmitir el virus. La única manera de saberlo es haciéndose la prueba del VIH mediante una muestra de saliva o de sangre.

¿Una prueba positiva de VIH significa que tengo SIDA?

No, significa que ha sido infectado/a con el virus de VIH. Un tratamiento con un buen régimen de medicamentos puede prevenir el desarrollo de SIDA. Si su prueba de VIH es positiva, usted puede transmitir el virus a parejas sexuales, parejas que son usuarios de agujas o su bebé dentro del vientre.

¿Qué puedo hacer si estoy embarazada y tal vez pueda estar infectada con VIH?

Si usted está embarazada o está planeando embarazarse, consulte con su doctor/a acerca de hacerse la prueba de VIH. Si usted es VIH positivo/a, su doctor/a puede ayudarle a usted y a su bebé si usted comienza tratamiento lo antes posible.

¿Qué puedo hacer si soy VIH positivo/a?

Es importante recordar que el VIH en estos momentos es una enfermedad que se puede tratar. Usted necesita buscar cuidado medico lo antes posible. Si no necesita medicación, es importante mantenerse saludable y asistir a sus chequeos médicos regulares.

Continua en la proxima página.

¿Qué puedo hacer si algún conocido es VIH positivo/a?

Las personas con VIH necesitan apoyo y comprensión, como también el respeto a su confidencialidad. Si alguien le comunicase que tiene VIH, ofrézcale su amistad y respete su privacidad.

¿Cómo puedo cuidarme para no contagiarme con el VIH?

Usted puede infectarse si no practica sexo seguro. Los hombres siempre deben de usar condones (profilácticos). Siempre lubrique el condón con substancias a base de agua tales como el lubricante K-Y Jelly™, For-Play™, PrePair™ o Probe™. No le ponga al condón ningún aceite o vaselina porque se puede romper. Evite el espermicida nonoxynol 9. Nunca use un condón más de una vez. No se ponga en riesgo, usted vale mucho. Use un condón desde que comience hasta que termine cada vez que tenga relaciones sexuales.

Si tiene sexo oral con un hombre también, debe de hacerlo protegiendose con un condón. Para tener sexo oral con una mujer, use un dental dam. No deje que la sangre o fluidos sexuales toquen su boca o la de su parejo/a.

El besarse en seco, masturbarse, tocarse y juguetear son actividades seguras. No se han visto casos donde se transmita el virus a través del beso (Francés) cuando se efectúa profundamente pero puede ser arriesgado, especialmente si hay llagas o sangre en la boca de alguien.

¡NO SE INYECTE DROGAS! La mejor protección contra el VIH es buscar ayuda a través de un programa para el abuso de substancias controladas. Cuando use drogas, NUNCA COMPARTA LAS AGUJAS, sorbetos o los aparatos. Siempre limpie sus aparatos con cloro antes y después de usarlos.

Ya que el VIH se transmite a través de la sangre, no comparta objetos afilados como razuradoras y cepillos de dientes que puedan tener sangre.

Usted no se infectará con el virus por el mero hecho de ser picado/a por un insecto, por sentarse en la tapa del inodoro, lavar platos o al estar alrededor de alguien con SIDA. El virus no se transmite al compartir baños, trastes o ropa. Una persona infectada con VIH no puede transmitirlo abrazando, tocando o estornudando cerca de usted.

¿Dónde puedo buscar información acerca de VIH/SIDA?

Hoy día existe mucha información disponible acerca del VIH/SIDA. Los albergues tienen información y algunas veces videos. Hoy en día existen revistas con información acerca del VIH/SIDA. Si tiene acceso al Internet, las siguientes redes le podrán dar información fácil de comprender:
www.projectinform.com
www.thebody.com
www.aegis.com